CRF	Chronic renal failure
CSF	Cerebrospinal fluid
CSF	Colony stimulating factors
CT	Computed tomography
CVA	Cerebrovascular accident
CVP	Central venous pressure
D&C	Dilatation and curettage
DDT	Dichlorodiphenyltrichloroethane
DI	Diabetes insipidus
DIC	Disseminated intravascular coagulation
DM	Diabetes mellitus
DMD	Duchenne's muscular dystrophy
DNA	Deoxyribonucleic acid
DST	Dexamethasone suppression test
DUB	Dysfunctional uterine bleeding
EBV	Epstein-Barr virus
ECG	Electrocardiogram
ECMO	Extracorporeal membrane oxygenation
EEG	Electroencephalogram
ELISA	Enzyme-linked immunosorbent assay
EMG	Electromyogram
ESWL	Extracorporeal shock wave lithotripsy
FDA	Food and Drug Administration
FRC	Functional residual capacity
FU	Flourouracil
FVC	Forced vital capacity
G6PD	Glucose-6-phosphate dehydrogenase
GBS	Guillain-Barré syndrome
GER	Gastroesophageal reflux
GFR	Glomerular filtration rate
GI	Gastrointestinal
HAM	Hypoparathyroidism, Addison's disease, and moniliasis
HAV	Hepatitis A virus
Hb	Hemoglobin
HbsAG	Hepatitis B surface antigen
HBV	Hepatitis B virus
Hct	Hematocrit
HCV	Hepatitis C virus
HDV	Hepatitis D virus
HELLP	Hemolysis, elevated liver enzymes, low platelet count

Continued on inside back cover

Mo

HANI
OF DI

Mosby's
HANDBOOK
OF DISEASES

Rae W. Langford, EdD, RN

Private Practice
Rehabilitation Nurse Consultant
Legal Nurse Consultant
Research and Statistics Consultant
Houston, Texas

June D. Thompson, DrPh, RN

Former Director of Nursing Research,
Education, and Standards
University Hospital
University of New Mexico Health Sciences Center
Albuquerque, New Mexico

Second Edition

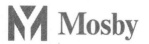

A Harcourt Health Sciences Company

St. Louis   Philadelphia   London   Sydney   Toronto

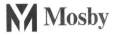
Mosby

A Harcourt Health Sciences Company

Editor-in-Chief: Sally Schrefer
Executive Editor: Barbara Nelson Cullen
Senior Developmental Editor: Sandra Clark Brown
Project Manager: Deborah L. Vogel
Designer: Bill Drone

Mosby, Inc.
A Harcourt Health Sciences Company
11830 Westline Industrial Drive
St. Louis, Missouri 63146

Printed in the United States of America

International Standard Book Number 0-323-00895-X

00 01 02 03 04 GW/FF 9 8 7 6 5 4 3 2 1

Linda Foley, RN, PhD
Associate Professor
Associate Chairperson of Curriculum
Nebraska Methodist College
Omaha, Nebraska

Patricia J. Giordano, MS, RT (R) (T)
Assistant Professor/Program Director
Radiation Therapy
Gwynedd-Mercy College
Sumneytown Pike
Gwynedd Valley, Pennsylvania

Kathy Russell, RNC, MSN
Nursing Professor
Front Range Community College
Westminster, Colorado

Wanda E. Wesolowski, RT, MA
Professor/Chairperson
Radiologic Technology Program
Community College of Philadelphia
Philadelphia, Pennsylvania

Imagine this . . .

Finally, the kids are grown and you decide to return to work.
  You normally work on the pediatric unit, but because of
  the flu epidemic, you are asked to work on the adult medical-
  surgical unit.
You receive a telephone call from Mr. Sansone asking you to
  interpret his diagnostic study findings to him.
Your best friend calls you telling you that her brother was just
  diagnosed with Gastroesophageal Reflux Disease, but she
  doesn't know much about it and wants you to tell her more.

You are in charge; you need to be in the know. However, so
much is evolving in health care, that it is impossible to know it
all. Wouldn't it be great to have a little supplemental brain in
your pocket or on your shelf? A "little brain" that is easy to
access, organized for quick and ready reference, and chuck full of
vital information about the pathogenesis, etiology, diagnosis,
and treatment of diseases and conditions. Well, look no more,
the second edition of *Mosby's Handbook of Diseases* is the crown
jewel that fits the bill.

This edition of *Mosby's Handbook of Diseases* provides an
up-to-date profile of more than 230 diseases and conditions,
including 39 new entries. Many of the new diseases or conditions
include emerging health care problems such as *Latex Allergies*
and *Ebola Virus*. Also realizing that many health care problems
may be avoided by maintaining a healthy lifestyle and avoiding
risks, we have added *risk factor* and *prevention strategy* information where applicable.

The *Handbook* is designed for you, the reader. All diseases
and conditions are listed in alphabetical order starting with
Abruptio Placentae and ending with Zollinger-Ellison Syndrome. A cross reference is indicated where applicable so that
whether you know the disease or condition by its scientific
name, *Herpes Zoster,* or by its common name, *Shingles,* you can
still look it up quickly.

Each disease and condition is organized in a consistent format
so that you can immediately find essential information: (1) a
definition of the disease or condition; (2) the etiology and
incidence of the problem; (3) the pathophysiology; (4) risk
factors; (5) clinical manifestations; (6) frequently ordered diag-

nostic studies; (7) therapeutic management, including indications for surgery, common medications, and general interventions; and (8) prevention.

So whenever you need just a little more information to "get smart fast" or if you just want to learn a little more about a disease or condition, you will find this handy little "supplemental brain" to be a crown jewel in your pocket or on your bookshelf.

Rae Langford, EdD, RN

June M. Thompson, DrPH, RN

contents

abruptio placentae

A premature separation of a normally implanted placenta from the uterine wall, usually occurring in the third trimester of pregnancy

Etiology and incidence: The etiology is unknown but is believed to be related to hypertensive and cardiovascular disease processes or use of cocaine. Abruptio placentae occurs in 0.5% to 3.5% of all deliveries. It accounts for 15% of all perinatal deaths. About one third of all infants born to women with abruptio placentae die either from prematurity or intrauterine hypoxia.

Pathophysiology: The placenta releases from the wall of the uterus, and retroplacental bleeding occurs. The degree of release may vary from a few millimeters to complete detachment. Blood can accumulate under the placenta (concealed hemorrhage) or can be passed behind the membranes and out the cervix (external hemorrhage).

Risk Factors

History of a prior reproductive loss (abortion, stillbirth, neonatal death)
Hypertension
Multiparity (three times more likely after five pregnancies)
Previous separation of placenta (risk of recurrence is 30 to 40 times general population)
Use of tobacco, alcohol, cocaine, and caffeine during pregnancy

Clinical Manifestations

The signs and symptoms vary with the degree of separation and the resultant amount of hemorrhage. Severe cases involve slight-to-profuse vaginal bleeding; maternal shock (hypotension, dizziness, rapid pulse, dyspnea, pallor); sudden, severe pain; tender, tightly contracted uterus; and fetal distress or fetal death.

Complications

Hypofibrinogenemia with disseminated intravascular coagulation, uteroplacental apoplexy (Couvelaire uterus), and renal failure are possible, particularly if the woman has preexisting toxemia.

Diagnostic Tests

History and physical examination
Abdominal ultrasound to rule out placenta previa

Therapeutic Management

Surgery	Cesarean section (unless vaginal delivery is imminent) when bleeding cannot be controlled
Drugs	None
General	Bed rest until bleeding stops; monitor fetal heart rate; fluid and volume replacement by intravenous administration; blood replacement if necessary to prevent shock; rupture of membranes if delivery is imminent to reduce the possibility of DIC

abuse, domestic

Abuse or violence commonly describing spouse or partner abuse; includes physical abuse, sexual violence, and psychological and/or emotional abuse

Etiology and incidence: Domestic abuse is a form of family violence. This cause of violence has been reported as the leading cause of injury and death to American women. Accurate data about the incidence of spouse/partner abuse are difficult to calculate. Estimates report that annually, husbands and partners batter 3 to 4 million women in the United States. It is a crime committed every 15 seconds. Domestic violence is also the most common unreported crime in America. Victims of domestic violence are primarily in heterosexual relationships, but new data show that domestic violence is now also being reported in both male and female homosexual relationships.

Pathophysiology: *Physical abuse* is the deliberate infliction of injury to a spouse or partner. Common behaviors of the spouse or partner include kicking, biting, hitting, pushing, choking, and assaulting with weapons. Pregnant women often sustain injuries to the abdomen and potentially to the unborn child.

Sexual violence may also be referred to as *marital* or *partner rape*. This is a form of violence whereby sex is used to hurt, degrade, dominate, humiliate, and gain power over the victim. It is an act of aggression.

Emotional or *psychological abuse* is a form of violence that has the power to destroy the victim's self-esteem over time. This form of abuse is almost always present in families where physical and/or sexual domestic violence occurs.

Risk Factors

The victim
Has feelings of worthlessness and being degraded
Feels isolated, which keeps her cut off from family and friends
Feels that leaving spouse or partner is not an alternative
Feels that it is her job to keep the family together at any cost
Lacks positive self-esteem, which may prevent sharing of what is
    happening
Often completely dependent on the abuser and may face severe
    economic hardship if she were to leave

The batterer

Denies the existence of violent behavior

Exhibits extreme possessiveness and jealousy

Has history of violence in the family

Refuses to accept responsibility for the abuse, blaming behavior on stress, alcohol, drugs, or victim

Uses alcohol and/or drugs

Society and the environment

A lack of understanding exists that verbal and physical violence are behaviors that are often learned from parents, relatives, or friends.

A lack of understanding exists that violence is often used as a way to reduce emotional stress.

After hundreds of years, some segments of American society still believe "women are property" and that the spouse or partner has the "right" to use physical force in relating to her.

Continued exposure to violent behavior is seen in entertainment, sports, and the media.

A lack of public awareness exists regarding the severity of the problem.

Society reinforces sexual roles that condone aggressive and violent behavior in men.

Clinical Manifestations

Physical abuse	Physical signs include bruising (face, neck, arms, legs, abdomen, or back), cuts, broken bones, black eyes, burns, marks of strangulation, wounds or bruises at different stages of healing, and swelling or puffiness in the face or around the eyes. Other signs include a history that does not match the presenting injuries and reports of being hit or injured.
Sexual violence	Physical signs include bruising around the breasts or genitalia; genitalia, vaginal, or rectal swelling or lacerations; torn, stained, or bloody underclothing; and reports of being assaulted or raped.

Emotional and/or psychological abuse	Reports of being intimidated are evident, as are given looks or gestures, being yelled at, or being in an environment where things are being thrown or smashed. Threats to harm a child or children or to keep them from the victim are made. Victim is isolated from family and friends, and there is economic domination.

Diagnosis

Diagnosis is typically made by social service, health care, and legal experts after history, investigation, and physical examination.

Therapeutic Management

Surgery	None
Drugs	None
General	If serious signs are obvious, report the situation to the local authorities for immediate investigation and victim protection.
	If the signs are vague or inconsistent, document observations and report to appropriate local authorities for investigation.
	If the individual is perceived to be in an immediately dangerous situation, seek protection through the local Adult Protective Services or the county Department of Social Services.
Prevention	Raise awareness by conducting education about the incidence and causes of abuse. Provide education to teens and young adults. Observe for early signs of abuse and offer assistance if necessary.

abuse and neglect, child

An act or failure to act that results in serious harm, risk of serious harm, or death of a child (under the age of 18) by a parent or caretaker who is responsible for the child's welfare

Sexual abuse, a subset of abuse, is the use of a child to engage in, or assist any other person to engage in, sexually explicit conduct or simulation of such conduct (e.g., rape, molestation, prostitution, sexual exploitation, or incest). Each state provides specific legal definitions of child abuse and neglect.

Etiology and incidence: Precise causal mechanisms are unknown but history of abuse to the abuser is strongly linked, as are poverty, stress, lack of parenting skills, and emotional instability. An estimated 2 million reports on child maltreatment are filed with the Child Protection Service (CPS) annually. Nearly 1 million of these cases are substantiated, with 15 children per 1000 victims of abuse and neglect in the United States each year. Estimates indicate that child abuse and neglect are underreported and that each year, as many as 42 per 1000 children are at risk. The incidence has increased 18% from 1990 to 1996. Of these, 50% were less than 7 years of age. Younger children were more likely to be targets of neglect, whereas older children were more likely to be abused. The perpetrators were most likely to be parents (77%), relatives of the child (11%), and other caretakers (2%).

Pathophysiology: Child abuse is the deliberate infliction of injury on a child and may be characterized as physical, sexual, or emotional. *Physical abuse* is the infliction of physical injury as a result of punching, beating, kicking, biting, burning, shaking, or otherwise harming the child. The parent or caretaker may not have intended to hurt the child; rather the injury may have resulted from overdiscipline or physical punishment. *Sexual abuse* includes fondling a child's genitals, intercourse, incest, rape, sodomy, exhibitionism, and commercial exploitation through prostitution or the production of pornographic materials. Many experts believe that sexual abuse is the most under-reported form of child maltreatment because of the secrecy or "conspiracy of silence" that so often characterizes these cases. *Emotional abuse* (psychological or verbal abuse and/or mental injury) includes acts or omissions by the parents or other caregivers that have caused or can cause serious behavioral, cognitive, emotional, or mental disorders. In some cases of emotional abuse, the acts of parents or other caregivers alone, without any harm evident in the child's behavior or condition, are sufficient to warrant child protective services intervention.

Child neglect is characterized by failure to provide for the child's basic needs. Neglect can be physical, educational, or emotional. *Physical neglect* includes refusal of or delay in seeking health care, abandonment, expulsion from the home, refusal to allow a runaway to return home, and inadequate supervision. *Educational neglect* includes the allowance of chronic truancy, failure to enroll a child of mandatory school age in school, and failure to attend to a special educational need. *Emotional neglect* includes such actions as marked inattention to the child's needs for affection, refusal of or failure to provide needed psychological care, spouse abuse in the child's presence, and permission of drug or alcohol use by the child. The assessment of child neglect requires consideration of cultural values and standards of care, as well as recognition that the failure to provide the necessities of life may be related to poverty.

Risk Factors

Child
Unwanted child
Child who appears unkempt or unclean, or who has torn, dirty
    clothes
Child who is different in any way from his/her siblings
"Difficult" child or unruly child
Parent or caregiver
Caucasian (more than 50%)
Inappropriate or negative parental comments or indifference to
    the child's welfare
Lack of parenting skills
Parent or caregiver history of being abused as a child
Parents who express little tolerance for irritation, the child, or
    child care; have poor impulse control; and/or seem angry
    and depressed
Environmental and socioeconomic issues
Family discord resulting in living in a stressful household,
    divorce, unemployment, or poor housing
Poverty and/or lack of financial resources

Clinical Manifestations

Physical abuse	Physical signs include unexplained bruising on soft tissue areas such as the face, back, neck, buttocks, upper arms, thighs, ankles, and back of legs; multiple bruises at different stages of healing; burns; bites; cuts; unexplained head or abdominal injuries; multiple fractures; or x-ray evidence of multiple old fractures. Child's comments or behavior exhibit fear of being hit or hurt. Child is wearing long-sleeve shirts or similar clothing to hide injuries.
Sexual abuse	Patterns are evident, such as torn, stained, or bloody underclothing; bruising, redness, swelling, or bleeding of the genitalia, vagina, or rectum; statements that it hurts to walk or sit; and complaints of pain or itching in the genital area. The child may play out their abuse with dolls or playmates.
Emotional abuse (psychological, verbal, or mental)	Child exhibits inappropriate behavior or developmental delays with speech or social interactions, facial tics, rocking motions, and odd reactions to persons in authority. Emotional abuse may often be seen in combination with other forms of abuse and neglect.
Child neglect (physical, medical, educational, or emotional)	Patterns are evident for a lack of care and attention. The child may be having to provide care for self, which is inappropriate for his/her age or developmental level. The child may be unresponsive or withdrawn or may not respond to the caregivers' coaxing. Nonorganic failure to thrive or malnutrition should be considered when a healthy baby at birth appears to have lost weight or physical tone, especially when the infant has declined 25% from the growth curve.

Diagnosis

Diagnosis is typically made by social service, health care, and legal experts after history, investigation, and physical examination.

Therapeutic Management

Surgery	None
Drugs	None
General	If serious signs are obvious, report the situation to the local source for immediate investigation.
	If the signs are vague or inconsistent, document observations and report to appropriate local source for investigation.
	If the child is perceived to be in immediate danger, seek child protection through the local child protection agency.
Prevention	Mechanisms of prevention include risk factor identification, parenting classes, home visits, early intervention, support groups for parents, and counseling.

abuse and neglect, elder

An act or failure to act that results in risk of harm, harm, neglect, or exploitation of the elders. Elder abuse may occur in many forms such as physical, emotional, psychological, or sexual abuse; neglect; abandonment; financial or material exploitation; and self-neglect. *Domestic elder abuse* refers to several forms of maltreatment of an older person by someone who has a special relationship with the elder (i.e., spouse, sibling, child, friend, or caregiver). *Institutional abuse* refers to any of the previously mentioned forms of abuse occurring in residential facilities (e.g., nursing, foster, or group homes, or board and care facilities).

Etiology and incidence: Precise causal mechanisms of elder abuse and neglect are unknown, but three basic categories of elder abuse are observed: domestic, institutional, and self-neglect. In 1996 the National Center on Elder Abuse (NCEA) reported 500,000 cases of elder abuse. This is a 150% increase over the previous 10 years. Despite these data, it is speculated that only one in five cases actually get reported.

Pathophysiology: *Physical* abuse is the deliberate infliction of injury on an elder that results in bodily injury, physical pain, or impairment. Physical abuse may include but is not limited to such acts of violence as striking, hitting, beating, pushing, shoving, shaking, slapping, kicking, pinching, and burning. In addition, the inappropriate use of drugs and physical restraints, force-feeding, and physical punishment of any kind are also examples of physical abuse. *Sexual* abuse is nonconsensual sexual contact of any kind with an elderly person. Sexual contact with any person incapable of giving consent is also sexual abuse. This includes but is not limited to unwanted touching, sexual assault or battery such as rape, sodomy, coerced nudity, and sexually explicit photographing. *Emotional* or psychological abuse is the infliction of anguish, pain, or distress through verbal or nonverbal acts such as insults, threats, intimidation, humiliation, and harassment. *Neglect* is the refusal or failure to fulfill any part of a person's obligations or duties to an elder. Refusal or failure to provide life necessities such as food, water, clothing, shelter, personal hygiene, medicine, comfort, and personal safety may be evidence of this. *Abandonment* is the desertion of an elderly person by an individual who has assumed responsibility for providing care. Financial or material exploitation occurs when illegal or improper use of an elder's funds, property, or assets is being conducted. Examples include cashing an elder's personal check without authority, forging the person's signature, misusing or stealing the individual's possessions or money, and coercing or deceiving the elder into signing documents. *Self-neglect* is characterized if the elderly person acts to threaten his or her own health or safety. The individual's refusal or failure to provide self with adequate food, water, clothing, shelter, personal hygiene, medication, and personal safety may be evidence of this.

Risk Factors

Elders

Elders 80 years and older are abused and neglected two to three times more often than younger elders.

Elders often have poor personal health.

Female elders are abused at a higher rate than males.

Ninety percent of abused and neglected elders are abused by a family member, and of those, two thirds are adult children or the spouse.

Victims of self-neglect are usually depressed, confused, or extremely frail.

Family or caregiver

Caregiver experiences stress such as mental or emotional disorders, alcoholism, and drug addiction.

Caregiver is in poor personal health or incapable of providing adequate care.

Environmental and socioeconomic factors

A history of violence is transmitted from one generation to another.

Family is in poverty and having financial difficulty.

Clinical Manifestations

Physical abuse	Cuts, lacerations or other wounds; bruises; welts; black eyes; broken bones, sprains, or dislocations; any injury that is incompatible with the history; broken eyeglasses/frames; physical signs of being subjected to punishment or being restrained; laboratory findings of medication overdose or underuse of prescription drugs; elder

	report of being hit, slapped, kicked, or maltreated; caregiver's refusal to allow visitors to see elder alone
Sexual abuse	Bruises around the breasts or genitalia; unexplained venereal disease or genital infections; unexplained vaginal or rectal bleeding; torn, stained, or bloody underclothing; elder report of being assaulted or raped
Psychological/ emotional abuse	Appearance of being emotionally upset or agitated; hesitation to talk openly; extremely withdrawn and noncommunicative; unusual behavior usually attributed to dementia, implausible stories, and/or report of being verbally or emotionally abused
Neglect	Dirt, feces/urine, or other health and safety hazards in the elder's living environment; dehydration; malnutrition; untreated bed sores; poor personal hygiene; untreated health care problems; elder report of being mistreated
Abandonment	Desertion of an elder at a hospital, nursing facility, or similar institution; desertion at a shopping center or other public location; elder's own report of being abandoned
Financial or material exploitation	Unusual, sudden, or inappropriate activity in bank accounts; signatures on checks that do not resemble the older person's signature; unusual concern by caregiver that an excessive amount of money is being spent on care of the older person; numerous unpaid bills; overdue rent; abrupt changes in a will or other financial documents; unexplained disappearance of funds or valuable possessions; unexplained or sudden transfer of assets to a family member or someone outside the family

| Self-neglect | Dehydration; malnutrition, untreated or improperly attended medical conditions, poor personal hygiene, hazardous or unsafe living conditions, inappropriate or inadequate clothing, overall lack of self-care |

Diagnosis

Diagnosis is typically made by social service, health care, and legal experts after history, investigation, and physical examination.

Diagnostic Tests

Laboratory tests and drug screening may be done to determine the extent of malnutrition, dehydration, and medication drug levels.

Therapeutic Management

Surgery	None
Drugs	None
General	If serious signs are obvious, report the situation to the local authorities for immediate investigation and elder protection.
	If the signs are vague or inconsistent, document observations and report to appropriate local authorities for investigation.
	If the elder is perceived to be in an immediately dangerous situation, seek elder protection through the local Adult Protective Services or the county Department of Social Services.
Prevention	Skill-building workshops for family members, coordinated care of elderly needs, public education about the problem, and coordination among state agencies and service providers are all mechanisms for prevention.

acne vulgaris

An inflammatory disease of the sebaceous glands and hair follicles that is characterized by comedones, papules, pustules, nodules, and pus-filled cysts on or under the skin on the face, neck, chest, or upper back

Etiology and incidence: The etiology is unknown, although genetics, hormonal dysfunction, and oversecretion of sebum are strongly implicated. Predisposing factors include cosmetics, stress, steroids and other drugs, oral contraceptives, mechanical skin irritants, and climate. Acne usually begins in puberty and affects about 80% of adolescents in some form. Males are affected more often, but females have more severe and more prolonged cases.

Pathophysiology: Androgenic activity increases oil production and the size of the sebaceous glands. Intrafollicular hyperkeratosis occurs, and the hair follicles in the sebaceous gland are blocked, as comedones (blackheads and whiteheads), consisting of sebum, keratin, and microorganisms, are formed. As these comedones enlarge, they become visible and palpable on the skin's surface, often forming cysts. The enlarged follicle eventually ruptures and the contents are released into the dermis, setting up an inflammatory reaction and forming abscesses. Chronic and recurring lesions form distinctive acne scars.

Clinical Manifestations

Typical presenting symptoms of superficial acne include comedones and pustules. Deep acne is characterized by inflamed nodules, pus-filled cysts, abscesses, and sometimes scarring.

Complications

Permanent scarring is the most common complication.

Diagnostic Tests

Diagnosis is by physical examination.

Treatment varies, depending on the severity of the acne. Mild cases are often self-treated with over-the-counter preparations.

Surgery	Excision of large cysts and abscesses, cryosurgery to freeze cysts and nodules, dermabrasion for scarring
Drugs	Topical antimicrobial and antiinfective drugs, as well as comedolytics, for pustules; oral antiinfective drugs to reduce and prevent pustules; isotretinoin if antibiotics are unsuccessful; oral estrogen-progesterone for unresponsive, menses-related acne
General	Extraction of comedones, instruction not to pick or squeeze comedones or pustules, emotional support to boost self-esteem

acquired immune deficiency syndrome (AIDS)

A terminal, secondary immunodeficiency syndrome characterized by dysfunction of cell-mediated immunity and manifested by opportunistic infections and malignancies. The CDC uses a case surveillance definition for AIDS that lists diseases indicative of a definitive diagnosis of AIDS with or without laboratory evidence and diseases that are presumptive for AIDS with laboratory evidence. (See also Kaposi's sarcoma and *Pneumocystis carinii* pneumonia.)

Etiology and incidence: The cause is the human immunodeficiency retrovirus (HIV-1 or HIV-2) that converts viral ribonucleic acid into a proviral deoxyribonucleic acid (DNA) copy, which is incorporated into the DNA of the host cell. The proviral copy then is duplicated with normal cellular genes during each cellular division. The cell primarily infected is the CD4 lymphocyte. HIV is a blood-borne virus and commonly is transmitted through exchange of body fluids during sexual contact, through parenteral exposure or fetal exposure to blood, and through select body fluids from an individual with HIV. Individuals with HIV who are asymptomatic are in a carrier state and may transmit the disease without displaying any of the characteristic signs of AIDS.

AIDS is a global pandemic, and it is estimated that more than 1 million people in the United States and more than 10 million people worldwide have HIV. In the United States, the incidence of HIV has steadily increased from 3.46 per 100,000 population in 1985 to 12 per 100,000 population in 1996. It is the leading cause of death in males age 25 to 44 and the second leading cause of death in females age 25 to 44. All races and ethnic groups are affected. Currently men far outnumber women as victims of the disease. However, the fastest rise in cases is occurring among minority women. The median age range for all individuals with AIDS is 30 to 39 years.

Pathophysiology: The current theory holds that as HIV is reproduced, it affects the immune system by infecting the helper T-cell lymphocytes, which usually coexist in a 2:1 ratio with suppressor T-cells. As the viruses replicate, masquerading as helper cells, the number of real helper cells declines, and the suppressor T-cells eventually dominate, leading to immunosuppression and a lowering of the body's prime defense mechanism against intracellular pathogens and the formation of malignant tumors.

Risk Factors

An individual is placed at risk when exposed to bodily fluids from an individual with the HIV virus. High-risk behavior for HIV exposure includes unprotected sexual activity (oral, anal, or vaginal) and IV drug use with shared needles. Unprotected sex with multiple partners or multiple modes of exposure increases the risk. Infants are at risk of acquiring HIV during fetal development, delivery, or breastfeeding from a mother with HIV. Occupational transmission to health care workers is possible through needle sticks or other exposure to HIV-infected blood. Transfusion from contaminated blood products is a risk factor that has been mediated by testing of donated blood.

Clinical Manifestations

The CDC states that HIV infection is a chronic, progressive, terminal illness that can be divided into four stages:

Stage I	An acute, flulike syndrome that develops at the time of initial infection and lasts from days to weeks
Stage II	An asymptomatic, HIV-positive carrier state that may persist for years; may have generalized persistent lymphadenopathy
Stage III	Persistent fever, involuntary weight loss, chronic diarrheas, fatigue, night sweats, thrush
Stage IV	The development of AIDS as manifested by (1) neurological disease (peripheral neuropathies, paresthesia, myelopathy, dementia); (2) opportunistic infections (bacterial, viral, fungal, or protozoal) and their accompanying clinical features; (3) secondary neoplasms; and (4) other conditions (e.g., endocarditis, interstitial pneumonitis, immune thrombocytopenic purpura)

Complications

The complications are numerous and are associated with the various opportunistic infections or neoplasms, as well as the repetitive nature of the infections. These infections eventually overwhelm the body's compromised immune system, leading to massive infectious invasions in every body system and eventually death.

Diagnostic Tests

Clinical evaluation	Any of the above manifestations, history of high-risk behavior
Enzyme-linked immunosorbent assay (ELISA)	Screening test for HIV antibody (may be positive from 0 to 12 months after exposure); if results are positive, then it should be repeated twice on same sample
Western blot/immunofluorescent assay test	To confirm reactive seropositive results obtained by ELISA
p24 antigen test	Detects HIV p24 antigen in serum plasma or cerebrospinal fluid; can be detected before seroconversion
Reverse transcription polymerase chain reaction (RT-PCR), branched chain deoxyribonucleic acid (bDNA), and nucleic acid sequence-based amplification (NASBA)	Detects HIV and measures viral load and disease progression
WBCs/lymphocytes	Depressed
T-cell studies	Reduced reactivity and function of T-cells; reduced number of helper T-cells, increased number of suppressor T-cells

B-cell studies	Numbers and function of cells normal or increased
Natural killer (NK) cells	Reduced activity
Complement	Normal or increased

Therapeutic Management

Surgery	Tumor excision of some related neoplasms
Drugs	Treatment with combinations of various retroviral drugs such as zidovudine (Retrovir), didanosine (Videx), alcitabine (Hivid), stavudine (Zerit), lamivudine (Epivir), Siquinavir (Invirase), ritonavir (Norvir), indinavir (Crixivan), and evirapine (Viramune), using CD4 lymphocyte counts as a treatment guide; prophylaxis with trimethoprim-sulfamethoxazole tablets to prevent *Pneumocystis carnii* pneumonia; rifabutin prophylaxis for *Mycobacterium avium* infection; drugs specific for various opportunistic infections; and chemotherapy for carcinomas
	Prophylactic use of zidovudine after exposure through penetrating injuries is controversial.
General	Measures to improve overall health (e.g., smoking cessation; balanced nutrition; drug rehabilitation; and influenza, pneumococcal, and hepatitis B vaccines); supportive measures for coping with and adapting to the effects of the disease (e.g., counseling, support groups)
Prevention	Instruction in how the disease is spread to promote prevention, particularly among high-risk groups; emphasis on elimination of high-risk behaviors such as unprotected sexual activity and sharing needles when engaging in IV drug use; promotion of safe-sex practices such as use of latex condoms and/or barriers treated with viracidal spermicides; use of universal precautions by health care workers and family members to prevent transmission

adenovirus

A family of viruses that causes conjunctivitis and/or upper respiratory infections

Etiology and incidence: Adenoviruses are a cluster name for more than 40 specific viruses that cause common illnesses. For example, adenovirus is the causative agent for 4% to 5% of all respiratory illnesses. The most common respiratory diseases are acute febrile respiratory disease in children, acute respiratory diseases in adults, and viral pneumonia in both children and adults. Occular diseases caused by adenovirus include acute follicular conjunctivitis and epidemic keratoconjunctivitis (mostly seen in Japan).

Pathophysiology: Acute febrile respiratory disease is the most common of the adenoviruses. Infection is spread by air, water, or direct contact. Viral pneumonia in infants causes pneumonia in a lobe of the lung, and depending on severity, it may be considered lobular pneumonia. Acute pharyngoconjunctival fever commonly has a water-borne transmission and a 5-to-8-day incubation, and lasts 1 to 2 weeks. Conjunctivitis is a common manifestation of infections with several different adenovirus serotypes. It occurs most often in young adults and typically parents of children with acute pharyngoconjunctival fever.

Clinical Manifestations

Manifestations vary depending on the type of adenovirus and the body system affected.

Acute febrile respiratory disease (seen in children)	The most common outbreak occurs in the home or day-care center. Some children have fever only, some have fever and pharyngitis, and others have fever, pharyngitis, bronchitis, and nonproductive cough. Regional lymph nodes may be swollen and tender.
Acute respiratory disease (seen in adults)	Symptoms include malaise or tiredness, fever (lasting 2 to 4 days), chills, and headache.

Respiratory signs include nasopharyngitis, hoarseness, and dry cough. Cervical lymph nodes may be swollen and tender. A fine, red macular rash may appear on the body.

Viral pneumonia (seen in infants)

It is rare, but when seen, it is sudden and affects infants from a few days to 1 month old.

Acute pharyngocon-junctival fever

A triad of symptoms result, including fever, pharyngitis, and conjunctivitis.

Conjunctivitis

This is the sensation of a foreign body in the eye. Watering and local redness of the palpebral and bulbar conjunctiva are symptoms. Discharge from the eye is not purulent. A mild sore throat may also develop.

Complications

Secondary bacterial infections

Diagnostic Tests

Clinical evaluation

Identification that an infection is caused by an adenovirus is usually presumptive and is made on clinical examination.

Virus isolation

Although rarely done, except in military situations, it is possible to isolate the virus in 7 to 10 days using respiratory or occular secretions.

Therapeutic Management

Surgery   None
Drugs   Acetaminophen may be necessary for febrile episode. Aspirin should be avoided in children because of concerns of developing Reye's syndrome.

General   *Mild symptoms:* Supportive rest is recommended,
             including bed rest if needed.
             Severe symptoms: Children may become quite ill.
             Severe pneumonia in children may require hospi-
             talization and supportive care.

Careful handwashing and cleanliness is required when around
or caring for infected individuals. Air, water, or direct contact
may spread the virus. When possible, separate ill child or adult
from others in the household or classroom.

adrenal insufficiency, primary (Addison's disease)

A progressive, chronic disease process resulting from a decline in the production of adrenocortical steroids as the adrenal cortex is destroyed

Etiology and incidence: Most cases are the result of idiopathic atrophy of the adrenal cortex; the rest result from destruction of the entire gland. Clinical signs often are manifested during periods of metabolic stress. About four in 100,000 individuals across all age groups are affected.

Pathophysiology: A decline in cortisol and corticosterone production by the adrenal cortex results in multiple disturbances in fat, protein, and carbohydrate metabolism, which in turn give rise to diminished production of liver glycogen and increased production of insulin. This leads to hypoglycemia and muscle weakness. Electrolyte imbalances and dehydration are caused by an increase in sodium (Na) secretion and a decrease in potassium (K) secretion, leading to low serum concentrations of sodium and chloride (NaCl) and high serum concentrations of K. The decrease in cortisol also leads to an increase in adrenocorticotropic hormone (ACTH) and beta-lipotropin, which stimulates melanin production and causes hyperpigmentation. Over time, resistance to infection and stress diminishes. Dehydration may lead to reduced cardiac output and ultimately circulatory collapse.

Clinical Manifestations

Early	Weakness, fatigue, orthostatic hypotension, tanning, freckles, vitiligo, darkened mucosal areas
Midcourse	Nausea, vomiting, diarrhea, abdominal pain, headaches, dizziness, fainting, intolerance to cold
Late	Weight loss, dehydration, hypotension, confusion, restlessness, emotional lability, small heart size

Complications

Acute stress or trauma, in which the body's store of glucocorticoids is exhausted, may trigger an adrenal crisis, which is characterized by generalized muscular debility; severe abdominal, back, and leg cramps; peripheral vascular collapse; and acute renal failure.

Diagnostic Tests

ACTH stimulation test	No increase in cortisol
	Blood chemistry
	Elevated K and blood urea nitrogen; decreased Na, bicarbonate, and fasting glucose; Na:K ratio less than 30:1; elevated hematocrit, eosinophils, and lymphocytes
CBC	Decreased WBCs
Radiology	Small heart, adrenal size and calcifications; renal or pulmonary tuberculosis

Therapeutic Management

Surgery	None
Drugs	IV hydrocortisone, NaCl replacement; vasopressors to elevate blood pressure; hydrocortisone/fludrocortisone PO maintenance for life; antibiotics with evidence of infection; antitubercular drugs with evidence of tuberculosis
General	Fluid replacement IV and PO; high-calorie diet; cardiac monitoring for peaked T waves; rest; monitoring for signs of infection; monitoring of urine output; instruction about the disease and maintenance medications

adult respiratory distress syndrome (ARDS)   A

Acute respiratory failure associated with pulmonary injury and characterized by noncardiogenic pulmonary edema, hypoxemia, and severe respiratory distress

Etiology and incidence: ARDS is precipitated by a variety of acute processes that injure the lung. Trauma is the most common cause; other causes include anaphylaxis, aspiration of gastric reflux, pneumonia, inhalation burns from fire or chemicals, drug reactions, drug overdose, near-drowning, and oxygen toxicity. The condition may also develop as the result of an underlying disease process (e.g., leukemia, tuberculosis, pancreatitis, uremia, or thrombocytopenic purpura) or as a byproduct of a medical procedure (e.g., coronary artery bypass, multiple blood transfusions, mechanical ventilation, or hemodialysis).

Because ARDS is often misdiagnosed, the incidence and mortality are elusive. ARDS is also called *shock lung, wet lung, stiff lung, white lung, Da Nang lung,* or *adult hyaline membrane disease.* Recent studies place the survival rate at about 50% with treatment.

Pathophysiology: The initial injury to the lung is poorly understood. It is hypothesized that activated WBCs and platelets accumulate in the capillaries, interstitium, and air spaces and release prostaglandins, oxygen radicals, proteolytic enzymes, and other products. These injure the cells, increase fibrosis, and reduce bronchomotor tone, leading to capillary leakage of blood and plasma into the interstitial and alveolar spaces. This results in alveolar flooding and reduced surfactant activity, producing atelectasis. Bronchial inflammation and proliferation of epithelial and interstitial cells follow. Collagen accumulates, resulting in severe interstitial fibrosis (stiff lung) with low lung compliance, reduced FRC, pulmonary hypertension, perfusion maldistribution, and hypoxemia.

Clinical Manifestations

Early	Dyspnea, particularly on exertion, followed by rapid, shallow respirations, inspirational chest retractions, and wheezing

Late   Bloody, sticky sputum; racing heart rate; clammy, mottled, cyanotic skin; severe difficulty breathing; confusion; coma

Complications

Complications include secondary bacterial superinfections, tension pneumothorax, multiple-system organ failure, metabolic and respiratory acidosis, and cardiac arrest.

Diagnostic Tests

Pulmonary function	Decreased FRC and compliance, low/normal pulmonary capillary web pressure, increased shunt fraction
Arterial blood gases	Decreased Pao_2, low/normal $Paco_2$, elevated pH
Lactic acid	Elevated
Radiology	Blurred margins and alveolar infiltrates on early chest x-rays, normal cardiac silhouette

Therapeutic Management

Mechanical ventilation with positive end-expiratory pressure and continuous positive airway pressure is generally required until the underlying problem has been identified and treated.

Surgery	None
Drugs	No specific drugs; morphine and pancuronium bromide (Pavulon) are used in the management of mechanical ventilation; antiinfective drugs may be used for underlying infections
General	Correction of underlying cause of injury; hyperalimentation to prevent nutritional depletion; blood gas monitoring to prevent oxygen toxicity; careful aseptic technique and monitoring of secretions to prevent superinfection; intubation and ventilation; tracheobronchial suctioning to clear secretions; cardiac monitoring; bed rest; fluid volume replacement; regulation of activity to reduce hypoxia; instruction in communicating with intubated patient; communication tools (e.g., alphabet or picture boards, response switches)

aldosteronism, primary (Conn's syndrome)

A hypertensive disorder resulting from excess production of aldosterone by the adrenal gland

Etiology and incidence: Most cases are caused by an adenoma of the adrenal gland. Other causes are adrenal nodular hyperplasia and adrenal carcinoma. Only 0.5% to 2% of those with hypertension are affected. The condition is three times more likely to affect women, and the typical age ranges from 30 to 50 years.

Pathophysiology: Excess production of aldosterone leads to hypernatremia, hypervolemia, and hypokalemic alkalosis. Mild to severe arterial hypertension occurs because of the increased volume and arteriolar sodium levels. Hypokalemia results from increased renal excretion of potassium, and metabolic alkalosis occurs because of an increase in hydrogen ion secretion. Over time, this leads to transient paralysis and tetany.

Clinical Manifestations

In many cases the only manifestation is a mild to moderate hypertension. Other signs and symptoms include episodic weakness, fatigue, paresthesia, polyuria, polydipsia, and nocturia. Glycosuria, hyperglycemia, and personality disturbances are occasionally manifested.

Complications

Marked alkalosis with transient paralysis, tetany, and positive Chvostek's and Trousseau's signs.

Diagnostic Tests

Plasma renin activity	Decreased (measured after restricted sodium/diuretic therapy)
Aldosterone levels	Increased (measured after sodium loading)
Blood chemistry	Normal/increased sodium, decreased potassium
CT scan	To detect presence of adenoma
Blood pressure	Elevated
Edema	Absent

Therapeutic Management

Surgery	Adrenalectomy
Drugs	Spironolactone (Aldactone)
General	Low-sodium diet; instruction about medication, diet, and surgery

Alzheimer's disease   A

A chronic, progressive, neurological disorder characterized by degeneration of the neurons in the cerebral cortex and subcortical structures, resulting in irreversible impairment of intellect and memory

Etiology and incidence: The cause is not fully known; however, three genes have been linked to the disorder and are in some way responsible for removing toxic protein fragments from the brain. Theories involving aluminum poisoning, autoimmune disease, and viruses have also been advanced. Alzheimer's disease is the ninth leading cause of death among those age 65 and older in the United States claiming over 21,150 lives a year. Approximately 5% of individuals over age 65 show signs of the disease; the proportion climbs to 20% in those over age 80. The incidence is higher in women.

Pathophysiology: Selective neuronal cells, primarily those involved in the transmission and reception of acetylcholine, degenerate in the cerebral cortex and basal forebrain, resulting in cerebral atrophy of the frontal and temporal lobes, with wide sulci and dilated ventricles. Senile plaques and neurofibrillary tangles are present. The basic pathophysiological processes accompanying the brain damage are unknown.

Clinical Manifestations

Early	Short-term memory loss, impaired insight/judgment, momentary disorientation, emotional lability, anxiety, depression, decline in ability to perform activities of daily living
Midcourse	Apraxia, ataxia, alexia, astereognosis, auditory agnosia, agraphia, prolonged disorientation, progressive memory loss (long and short term), aphasia, lack of comprehension, decline in care abilities, insomnia, loss of appetite, repetitive behavior, socially unacceptable behavior, hallucinations, delusions, paranoia
Late	Total dependence in ADLs, bowel and bladder incontinence, loss of speech, loss of individua-

tion, myoclonic jerking, seizure activity, loss of consciousness

Complications

The end stage of Alzheimer's disease invites complications commonly associated with comatose conditions (e.g., skin breakdown, joint contractures, fractures, emaciation, aspiration pneumonia, infections).

Diagnostic Tests

Definitive diagnosis can be made only through autopsy.

Clinical evaluation	Any of the above manifestations after depression, delirium, and other dementia disorders (e.g., head injury, brain tumor, alcoholism, drug toxicity, arteriosclerosis) have been ruled out; family history
Mental status examination	Decreased orientation, impaired memory, impaired insight/judgment, loss of abstraction/calculation abilities, altered mood
CT scan/MRI	Brain atrophy; symmetrical, bilateral ventricular enlargement
EEG	Slowed brain wave activity, reduced voltage

Therapeutic Management

Surgery	None at present but experimental trials with fetal neuronal transplants are being conducted.
Drugs	Tacrine (Cognex) and donepezil (Aricept) used to improve memory and other cognitive deficits in individuals with mild to moderate dementia. These drugs do not alter the underlying dementia. Medications are used for treating specific symptoms or behavioral manifestations (i.e., antidepressants, stimulants, antipsychotics, sedatives); experimental drugs include cholinergic, dopamine, and serotonin precursors; neu-

ropeptides; and transcerebral dilators. Gene
therapy is on the horizon.

General   Structured, supportive, familiar environment; ori-
entation and cueing program for daily tasks; safety
program; family support and counseling; respite
care; institutionalization when home care is
no longer possible

amyotrophic lateral sclerosis (ALS) (Lou Gehrig's disease)

A rapidly progressive, degenerative disease of the upper and lower motor neurons characterized by atrophy of the hands, arms, legs, and eventually the entire body. Seventy percent of individuals die within 5 years of diagnosis.

Etiology and incidence: The etiology of ALS is unknown, but proposed explanations include genetics, metabolic disturbances, and external agents. Although the incidence worldwide is 60 to 70 people per 100,000, with large clusters of cases in the western Pacific, the incidence in the United States is only about 5 in 100,000. The disease usually occurs in men between 40 and 70 years of age.

Pathophysiology: Patterns of degeneration occur in the brain and spinal cord. The anterior horn cells deteriorate, resulting in denervation of muscle fibers. Atrophy of the precentral gyrus and loss of Betz's cells occur in the cortex. Motor neurons are lost in the brainstem, although neurons that control the sensory and urinary sphincters are spared. The corticospinal tract and large motor neurons in the spinal cord also atrophy.

Clinical Manifestations

Early	Weakness, cramps in the hands and forearms
Midcourse	Fatigue, dyspnea, slurred speech, dysphagia, asymmetric spread of muscle weakness to the rest of the body, spasticity, fasciculations, hyperactive deep tendon and extensor plantar reflexes
Late	Paralysis of vocal cords; paralysis of chest muscles, necessitating ventilatory support

Complications

The end stage of ALS can be complicated by disuse syndrome, contractures, skin breakdown, and aspiration pneumonia.

Diagnostic Tests

Clinical evaluation	Any of the above manifestations, motor involvement unaccompanied by sensory abnormalities
Electromyography (EMG)	Fibrillation, positive waves, fasciculations, giant motor units
Blood	Possible elevation in creatinine phosphokinase
Spinal tap	Elevated total protein, normal cell and IgG concentrations
CT scan	Normal until cerebral atrophy late in disease
Myelogram	Normal; spinal cord atrophy late in disease

Therapeutic Management

Surgery	Cricopharyngeal myotomy to alleviate dysphagia, tracheostomy, esophagostomy/gastrostomy
Drugs	Muscle relaxants (e.g., baclofen) to control spasticity; tricyclic antidepressants to control saliva; phenytoin to reduce cramping
General	Physical therapy to maintain muscle strength; occupational therapy for ADL support; speech therapy to aid communication; splints for neutral joint alignment; leg braces, canes, or walkers to aid ambulation; nutritional support/tube feedings; cardiac monitoring; mechanical ventilation; counseling for individual and family; respite care or placement if family is unable to provide care

anal fissure

A small ulceration, tear, or slitlike crack in the lining of the anus

Etiology and incidence: Anal fissures are most common in young and middle-aged adults. The exact cause of anal fissures is unknown. Commonly these may be associated with passing large and hard stools, laxative abuse, scarring from anal surgery, and chronic diarrheal diseases such as ulcerative colitis and Crohn's disease.

Pathophysiology: The fissures may be acute or chronic. The fissure rests on the internal sphincter and causes it to go into spasm, which is believed to perpetuate the fissure. An external skin tag may be present at the lower end of the fissure. Defecation stimulates spasms of the internal anal sphincter that causes the sphincter to contract and trap drainage. Any problem that causes local trauma or a loss of elasticity of the anal canal may predispose the individual to anal fissures.

Risk Factors

Chronic diarrheal diseases
Frequent passing of large, hard stools
Frequent and/or abusive use of laxatives
Frequent anal intercourse or other anal dilators

Clinical Manifestations

Pain	Complaints of pain, tearing, or burning sensation during bowel evacuation
Bowel habits	Change in bowel habits with evacuation spasms that result in prolonged gnawing discomfort
Rectal examination	Slight bleeding may be present with bowel evacuation, rectal discharge, skin tags

Complications

Constipation secondary to painful bowel evacuation or secondary infection of fissure area

Diagnostic Tests

Digital rectal examination	To assess sphincter tone, anal papillae, tenderness, and presence of blood and stool
Proctoscopy	To visualize the anorectal area and locate the anal fissure

Therapeutic Management

Surgery	This is used only when conservative measures fail. The internal anal sphincter is divided, hypertrophied papillae and anal tags are removed, and the fissure is left to heal.
Drugs	Bulk stool agents, emollient suppositories, analgesic ointments
General	Treat the underlying cause
	Topical application of silver nitrate, sitz baths, warm topical compresses, medicated pads (e.g., Tucks) or witch hazel pads to cleanse

anaphylaxis

An immediate, acute, systemic reaction resulting from an IgE-mediated antigen-antibody response that can range from mild to life threatening

Etiology and incidence: The most common causes are insect stings, drugs, blood products, and parenteral enzymes. Anaphylaxis occurs in both genders and across all age groups and races. Individuals with known allergies or previous sensitivity reactions are at greater risk.

Pathophysiology: Histamine, leukotrienes, and other mediators are released when the antigen agent reacts with the IgE (antibody) on the basophils and mast cells. This causes smooth muscle contraction and vascular dilation. Vasodilation and escape of plasma into tissues causes urticaria and angioedema, as well as a decrease in plasma volume, leading to shock. The escape of fluid from the alveoli causes pulmonary edema and angioedema. A prolonged reaction can produce cardiac arrhythmias and cardiogenic shock.

Clinical Manifestations

Mild	Queasiness, anxiety, hives, itching, flushing, sneezing, nasal congestion, runny nose, cough, conjunctivitis, abdominal cramps, tachycardia
Moderate	Malaise, urticaria, periorbital edema; pulmonary congestion; hoarseness; edema of the tongue, larynx, and pharynx; dysphagia; bronchospasm; dyspnea; wheezing; nausea; vomiting; diarrhea; hypotension; syncope; confusion
Severe	Cyanosis, pallor, stridor, occluded airway, hypoxia, respiratory arrest, cardiac arrhythmia, circulatory collapse, seizures, incontinence, coma, death

Complications

Lack of timely and appropriate treatment results in shock, cardiac and respiratory collapse, coma, and death.

Diagnostic Tests

Clinical evaluation	Rapid development of above signs and symptoms after exposure to a likely offending agent
CBC	Normal or elevated Hct
Blood chemistry	Normal until circulatory collapse
Radiology	Normal or hyperinflation, edema
ECG	Normal until hypoxemia develops

Therapeutic Management

Treatment centers around immediate and aggressive management of emerging symptoms. Maintaining the airway and blood pressure is critical.

Surgery	Tracheostomy
Drugs	Epinephrine and other drugs to counteract effects of mediator release and to block further mediator release, vasopressors to maintain blood pressure
General	Maintenance of airway; suctioning; monitoring of vital signs; monitoring of blood gases for acidosis; IV volume replacement; ECG monitoring for dysrhythmias
Prevention	Instruction in prophylaxis for those at risk (i.e., avoid known allergens, wear a medical-alert identification bracelet or necklace that identifies allergies, and ensure that all medical records have allergies highlighted in a prominent place)
	If allergic reaction is severe, investigate the possibility of carrying an anaphylaxis kit with preloaded epinephrine syringes.

anemia (aplastic, hemolytic, iron deficiency, pernicious, posthemorrhagic)

An inadequate number of circulating RBCs and an insufficient amount of Hgb to deliver oxygen to tissues, resulting in pallor, fatigue, shortness of breath, and predisposition to cardiac complications. The type and cause dictate manifestations and treatment; various types are addressed below.

aplastic anemia

A reduction in the number of circulating RBCs resulting from bone marrow failure and generally accompanied by agranulocytosis and/or thrombocytopenia

Etiology and incidence: The etiology is unknown in half of diagnosed cases; the other half is induced by chemicals, drugs, viruses, or radiation. The incidence is low.

Pathophysiology: Exposure to a known or unknown toxin depresses production of erythrocytes, platelets, and granulocytes in the bone marrow. Common toxins include ionizing radiation, chemical agents (e.g., benzene, DDT, carbon tetrachloride), and drugs (e.g., antitumor or antimicrobial agents).

Clinical Manifestations

The onset is usually insidious, occurring weeks or months after exposure to the toxin. Fatigue, weakness, dyspnea, and waxy pallor of the skin and mucous membranes are characteristic. Thrombocytopenia causes hemorrhage into mucous membranes, skin, and optic fundi. Agranulocytosis leads to severe infection.

Complications

Chronic anemia leads to increasing hemorrhage and repeated infections, which result in death in about half of those diagnosed.

Diagnostic Tests

CBC	Decreased RBCs (normochromic, normocytic), WBCs, and Hgb
Platelet count	Decreased

Serum iron	Increased
Bone marrow biopsy	Hypocellular/hypoplastic; fatty, fibrous tissue
Reticulocyte count	Markedly decreased

Therapeutic Management

Surgery	None
Drugs	Corticosteroids to stimulate granulocyte production; antibiotics for infection; androgens to stimulate bone marrow
General	Removal of causative agent; bone marrow transplant from an HLA-matched donor (sibling); blood transfusions; hemorrhage precautions

hemolytic anemia

Abnormal or premature destruction of RBCs and the inability of the bone marrow to produce sufficient RBCs to compensate

Etiology and incidence: The etiology is typically related to an extracorpuscular factor (e.g., trauma, burns, surgery, chemical agents, drugs, infectious organisms, systemic diseases). Less common are intracorpuscular causes such as a G6PD deficiency.

Pathophysiology: The precipitating factor results in a shortened life span for erythrocytes and an increase in erythrocyte destruction by the reticuloendothelial system. The bone marrow is unable to produce sufficient replacement cells to keep pace with the destruction, and anemia ensues.

Clinical Manifestations

Hemolysis can be acute or chronic. The symptoms of chronic hemolysis resemble those of other anemias: fatigue, weakness, dyspnea, and pallor. Individuals with chronic symptoms may suffer from a physiological or emotional stressor that triggers a hemolytic crisis. Acute hemolytic crisis, which is rare, is characterized by chills; fever; headache; pain in the back, abdomen, and joints; splenomegaly; hepatomegaly; lymphadenopathy; and reduced urinary output.

Complications

Chronic symptoms can lead to jaundice, arthritis, renal failure, and other organ failure. Crisis can lead to paresthesia, paralysis, chills, vomiting, shock, and organ failure.

Diagnostic Tests

Sickle cell test	To rule out sickle cell anemia
CBC	Decreased Hgb and Hct
Serum tests	Elevated lactate dehydrogenase and bilirubin
Bone marrow aspiration	Hyperplasia
Reticulocyte count	Elevated
Urine/fecal urobilinogen	Elevated

Therapeutic Management

Surgery	Splenectomy
Drugs	Corticosteroids to depress extracorpuscular factors and diminish inflammatory response; diuretics to prevent tubular necrosis; folic acid to increase RBC production
General	Elimination of causative agent; erythrocytopheresis (RBC exchange); transfusion; oxygen therapy for hypoxemia; fluid and electrolyte management

iron deficiency anemia

A chronic anemia characterized by depleted iron stores and small, pale RBCs lacking in Hgb

Etiology and incidence: Iron deficiency anemia is usually caused by chronic blood loss or by an increased need for or decreased intake of iron. It is the most common of the anemias, with a high worldwide incidence. It occurs most often in women, children, and the elderly in underdeveloped countries.

Pathophysiology: Some factor (e.g., chronic blood loss, a decrease in iron intake) leads to iron deficiency. This occurs in orderly steps. Initially, iron loss exceeds intake, and the iron stores in the bone marrow are used and depleted. A compensatory mechanism increases absorption of dietary iron but depletion continues, and insufficient iron is available for RBC formation. This leads to a decrease in Hgb production, microcytosis, and a decrease in oxygenation of the tissues.

Risk Factors

Acute/chronic blood loss
Iron-deficient diet

Clinical Manifestations

Usual signs and symptoms associated with anemia (pallor, fatigue, weakness) plus symptoms specific to the iron deficiency, such as glossitis, cheilosis, koilonychia (spoon-shaped fingernails), and pica.

Complications

Exhaustion, infection, and respiratory and cardiac complications are possible if the condition goes untreated.

Diagnostic Tests

CBC	Decreased RBCs, Hgb, and Hct
Peripheral blood smear	Decreased mean corpuscular volume and mean corpuscular Hgb concentration, microcytosis, hypochromia
Iron capacities	Decreased serum iron, serum ferritin, and iron ferritin; increased iron-binding capacity
Bone marrow aspiration	Erythrocyte:granulocyte ratio of 1:1 (normal, 1:3 to 1:5); lack of marrow iron; ringed sideroblasts

Therapeutic Management

Surgery	None
Drugs	Iron replacement PO or parenterally
General	Correction of underlying cause (e.g., treatment of bleeding, increased dietary intake of iron); nutritional education

pernicious anemia

A chronic, progressive anemia characterized by the production of megaloblasts, which are enlarged RBCs with immature nuclei

Etiology and incidence: Pernicious anemia usually is caused by a deficiency in or underuse of vitamin B_{12}. It is a fairly common anemia in adults over age 50 who are of Scandinavian origin.

Pathophysiology: Most commonly, the gastric mucosa develops a defect caused by an unknown factor and atrophies. This inhibits the secretion of intrinsic factor (IF), which binds and transports dietary vitamin B_{12} to the ileum for absorption. The lack of IF prevents vitamin B_{12} from entering the body, and existing stores of the vitamin are depleted, leading to the production of enlarged, immature RBCs.

Clinical Manifestations

Usual signs and symptoms associated with anemia (pallor, fatigue, weakness, dyspnea) plus symptoms that stem from the physiological changes in the gastrointestinal tract (e.g., glossitis, gingivitis, indigestion, epigastric pain, loss of appetite, diarrhea, constipation, weight loss); peripheral neurological changes occur, with paresthesia in the hands and feet.

Complications

If the condition goes untreated, the neurological changes become more profound, with involvement of the spinal cord and loss of vibratory sense, ataxia, spasticity, and disturbances in bowel and bladder function. Depression, paranoia, and delirium may follow. Splenomegaly and hepatomegaly occur, as well as organ failure, neurological degeneration, or infection, eventually causing death.

Diagnostic Tests

Peripheral blood smear	Oval macrocytes, hypersegmented neutrophils, enlarged platelets
Schilling test	Radioactive-tagged vitamin B_{12} is not excreted in urine
CBC	Decreased Hgb, leukocytes, erythrocytes, and thrombocytes

| Bone marrow aspiration | Hyperplasia; increased large-cell megaloblasts |
| Gastric analysis | Lack of free hydrochloric acid |

Therapeutic Management

Surgery	None
Drugs	Lifelong parenteral vitamin B_{12} replacement (dietary vitamin B_{12} replacement is not effective); oral iron if Hgb does not rise
General	Treatment of underlying cause of gastric atrophy, if possible; oxygen to increase arterial levels; oral hygiene; orientation if confused; safety precautions for neurological effects; instruction about vitamin B_{12} replacement as a life change

posthemorrhagic anemia

An anemia characterized by a decrease in Hgb in the blood and related to rapid, massive hemorrhage

Etiology and incidence: Rapid blood loss may be caused by traumatic rupture, incision, or erosion of a large blood vessel (ulcer, tumor). The prognosis depends on the rate and site of bleeding and the total blood loss.

Pathophysiology: With blood loss, blood volume diminishes, hemodilution occurs, and oxygenation of the tissues declines.

Clinical Manifestations

The rate of blood loss determines the signs and symptoms, which may include dizziness; faintness; weakness; pallor; thirst; sweating; rapid, weak pulse; rapid respiration; and orthostatic hypotension.

Complications

Lack of prompt treatment or failure to control the bleeding results in shock, coma, and death.

Diagnostic Tests

| CBC | RBCs, Hgb, and Hct are deceptively high |

	during initial period of hemorrhage because of vasoconstriction; values begin to decline within hours of the onset of bleeding if hemorrhage is not controlled
Peripheral smear	Normocytic cells, agranulocytosis
Coagulation time	Reduced

Therapeutic Management

Surgery	If indicated to control hemorrhage
Drugs	Iron replacement
General	Control of bleeding; blood transfusions; IV fluids, oral fluids as tolerated; oxygen; absolute bed rest; diet high in protein and iron

angina pectoris

Transient chest pain resulting from myocardial ischemia. (See also Coronary Artery Disease and Myocardial Infarction).

Etiology and incidence: Angina is caused by an imbalance in the demand for oxygen and the myocardial oxygen supply. Coronary atherosclerosis is often an underlying factor. Aortic stenosis, hypertension, and cardiomyopathy can also play a role.

Pathophysiology: In the usual pathogenic process, atherosclerosis eventually causes an obstruction, which leads to diminution of the coronary blood flow, which in turn reduces the myocardial oxygen supply and delivery. An increase in oxygen demand through exertion, exercise, or an underlying pathological condition causes oxygen demand to outstrip supply, and pain results.

Clinical Manifestations

The chief symptom is a highly variable, transient, substernal pain that typically arises with exertion (e.g., exercise, heavy meal, emotional excitement, sexual intercourse) and subsides with rest. It may be a vague ache or an intense crushing sensation that may or may not radiate to the left shoulder, arm, or jaw or through to the back. Attacks are exacerbated by cold. Because characteristics tend to be constant for a given individual, a change in symptom patterns (e.g., an increase in the frequency or intensity of attacks) should be viewed as serious. When these changes occur, the condition is called *unstable angina*.

Complications

Angina, particularly unstable angina, is often a precursor to myocardial infarction (MI).

Diagnostic Tests

The chief diagnostic parameters are (1) clinical evaluation of the nature of the pain; (2) the type of electrocardiographic changes seen during an attack; and (3) whether the pain is relieved promptly by a test dose of nitroglycerin.

Therapeutic Management

Surgery	Coronary artery bypass for selected cases with severe angina, localized coronary artery disease (CAD), no history of MI, and good ventricular function; angioplasty to remove obstructive atherosclerotic lesion
Drugs	Nitrates, beta-blockers, and calcium antagonists to prevent myocardial insufficiency and relieve pain; prophylactic aspirin in daily doses for individuals with known CAD; heparin to treat intracoronary clotting in cases of unstable angina
General	Reduction of risk behaviors (e.g., smoking); diet to reduce cholesterol levels and/or weight if necessary; consistent exercise program

ankylosing spondylitis

A systemic inflammatory disorder affecting primarily the spinal column and the large peripheral joints and eventually resulting in hardening and deformity of the affected skeleton

Etiology and incidence: Studies support a genetic basis with environmental links, but the exact cause is unknown. A higher than expected level of HLA-B27 tissue antigen is seen in 90% of individuals with the disease. It is three to four times more common in men than in women, and onset typically occurs between ages 20 and 40.

Pathophysiology: The disease most commonly begins in the sacroiliac area of the spine. The intervertebral discs become inflamed and cartilage and bone deteriorate, leading to the formation of fibrous tissue, which infiltrates the disc space and then ossifies. This inflammation and ossification process gradually progresses up the lumbar, thoracic, and cervical spine, leaving behind bamboo-like vertebral calcifications.

Clinical Manifestations

Early	Recurrent pain in the lower back or large peripheral joints; morning stiffness that is relieved by activity; stooped posture; limited motion of lumbar spine or limited ROM in affected joints; fatigue; fever; anorexia; weight loss; diminished chest expansion; red, painful eyes
Late	Kyphosis, fixed flexion of hips, vertebral fractures, impotence, incontinence, diminished bladder and rectal sensation, angina, pericarditis, pulmonary fibrosis (rare)

Complications

Occasionally the disease is severe and rapidly progressive, resulting in severe, pronounced skeletal deformities that greatly inhibit performance of activities of daily living (ADLs). In rare cases atlantoaxial subluxation occurs, resulting in compression of the spinal cord. Development of secondary amyloidosis, a rare event, can cause death.

Diagnostic Tests

Clinical evaluation	Spine/joint pain or limitation, any manifestations described above, family history
Radiology	Narrowing in sacroiliac joints, vertebral squaring, calcification, demineralization
HLA-B27 antigen	Positive in 90% of cases
Erythrocyte sedimentation rate	Mildly elevated
Immunoglobulin M rheumatoid factor	Negative

Therapeutic Management

Surgery	Rare, done to correct kyphosis or hip flexion or for cervical fusion to keep neck upright
Drugs	Analgesics; NSAIDs to reduce pain, spasm, and swelling and to facilitate exercise
General	Physical therapy, regular stretching, ROM and strength-building exercises, straight posture, proper alignment of joints, use of firm mattress in prone position with no pillows, avoidance of prolonged time in any one position, traction/back brace in special cases

anorectal abscess

A local abscess (cavity containing pus, surrounded by inflamed tissue) in the area of the rectum and anus

Etiology and incidence: An anorectal abscess is an infection that can occur anytime there is trauma and a break in the anal/rectal wall tissue. Anorectal abscesses are more common in men. Causes include traumatic anal intercourse, chronic diarrheal conditions such Crohn's disease, and hematological and immune-deficient conditions.

Pathophysiology: The abscess commonly develops from an infection beginning in an anal crypt and moving along anal ducts through the internal sphincter. The infection may also develop in an anal fissure, prolapsed internal hemorrhoid, traumatic injury, and superficial skin lesions. If not treated, the abscess may progress to an anorectal fistula.

Risk Factors

Chronic diarrheal or inflammatory bowel diseases
Traumatic anal intercourse or use of anal dilators
Passing large and/or hard stools

Clinical Manifestations

Early signs include a change in bowel habits with purulent discharge and increased odor. As the abscess becomes worse, increased throbbing, constant pain exacerbated by sitting or walking, anorectal swelling, and redness are present. Fever and malaise may also be present.

Complications

Secondary and/or systemic infection

Diagnostic Tests

Proctoscopy	To visualize the lesion and determine the extent of the abscess

Therapeutic Management

Surgery	Prompt surgical drainage of the abscess is required.
Drugs	Stool softeners or antibiotics may be used depending on the causative organism and the extent of infection.
General	Perianal area should be kept clean, packing and irrigation of abscess after surgery if required, Sitz bath, rubber ring or pillow for sitting

anorectal fistula

A tubelike tract with one opening in the anal canal or rectum and the other in a secondary, or external, opening such as the perianal skin

Etiology and Incidence: Anorectal fistulas usually arise spontaneously and occur secondary to drainage of a perirectal abscess. Predisposing causes include traumatic injury, Crohn's disease, chlamydial infections, tuberculosis, cancer, and radiation therapy.

Pathophysiology: The primary, or internal, opening is usually at a crypt near the pectinate line. The exit of the fistula may be to the outside via the skin, vagina, buttocks, or bladder. Feces may enter the fistula and cause an infection.

Risk Factors

Cancer and/or radiation therapy
Chlamydial infection
Crohn's disease
Traumatic injury
Tuberculosis

Clinical Manifestations

Pain and/or discomfort or history of recurrent abscess, followed by intermittent or constant discharge are present. If the fistula drains to the outside, persistent, blood-stained, and purulent and/or stool drainage may occur.

Complications

Secondary and/or systemic infections

Diagnostic Tests

Rectal examination	Inspection of the skin may reveal one or more secondary openings. A cordlike track may be palpated. A probe may be inserted into the tract to determine depth and direction.

| Proctoscopy or sigmoidoscopy | Required to determine internal point of origin and to rule out other fistula formation sources |

Therapeutic Management

Surgery	Surgery is considered the primary treatment and may include one of two techniques: fistulotomy (involves opening and cleaning the fistula so healthy tissue can granulate in) or fistulectomy (excision of the entire fistulous tract).
Drugs	Analgesics Organism-specific antibiotics Stool softeners
General	Treat underlying cause Sitz baths and wound irrigation Packing and wound care as required Pillow or rubber ring for sitting comfort

anorexia nervosa

An eating disorder characterized by drastically reduced food intake and intense exercise, leading to marked weight loss and eventual emaciation. Anorectic individuals have a disturbed sense of body image and attempt to achieve control, autonomy, and competence in their lives by manipulating their food intake and body weight.

Etiology and incidence: Etiology is unknown, but various psychological theories suggest societal factors, dysfunctional family systems, or disturbed mother/child relationships. Onset usually occurs in adolescence in young white women of middle or upper socioeconomic status. Men account for only 5% of cases, and the disorder is not seen in areas where food is in short supply. Estimates of the incidence of anorexia in the United States range from 1 in 800 to 1 in 100 among adolescent girls. Reports of anorexia in young black women with professionally educated and employed parents are increasing. The incidence among men and adults is also rising. The mortality rate averages about 15% of reported cases.

Pathophysiology: The pathological processes are those seen in malnutrition and starvation. Eventually all body systems become involved as they are deprived of vital nutrients.

Risk Factors

Adolescence
Characteristics such as perfectionism, overachievement, and
   meticulousness
Female gender
Preoccupation with weight, food, or diets

Clinical Manifestations

Early signs and symptoms include meticulousness; perfectionism; preoccupation with weight; increase in physical activity; restriction of intake; preoccupation with food, recipes, and meal planning; hoarding and hiding food; and meal preparation for others. This is followed by marked weight loss, amenorrhea, social isolation, increasingly secretive behavior, and denial of any problem.

Complications

As malnourishment continues, all body systems are affected. Cachexia ensues, and endocrine disorders, electrolyte imbalances, metabolic acidosis, and cardiac dysfunction appear. Sudden death from ventricular dysrhythmia is possible, as is eventual death from total system failure.

Diagnostic Tests

Diagnosis is made through a constellation of symptoms and patterns described above, in concert with loss of at least 15% of body weight, particularly in individuals in high-risk groups.

Therapeutic Management

Surgery	None
Drugs	Doxepin to reduce anxiety and depression
General	*Short term:* Hospitalization to stabilize fluid and electrolytes and stop weight loss
	Long term: Psychotherapy, family therapy, dietary supplements to induce weight gain

anxiety disorders

A group of disturbances in which anxiety is the predominant experienced symptom

Etiology and incidence: Anxiety is a subjective experience that is a normal part of everyday living. Normal anxiety is proportionate to a given threat or situation and is used constructively to alter a situation or object. Approximately 3% of the general population experience pathological anxiety, which is disproportionate to a threat and can actually paralyze a person's problem-solving, daily functioning, and overall productivity. Anxiety disorders include generalized anxiety disorder (the incidence for men and women is equal); panic disorder with agoraphobia (the incidence for women is three times that of men); and obsessive-compulsive disorder (equally common in men and women).

Pathophysiology: Anxiety ranges from a healthy state of alertness and attention to a pathological state. The biology of anxiety disorders is obscure, although it appears that some biochemical heredity traits are apparent. Psychological and interpersonal factors may predispose a person to anxiety disorders. These include early psychic trauma, pathogenic parent-child relationships, pathogenic family patterns, and loss of social supports. Generalized chronic anxiety is a continuous hyperalert and hyperanxiety state that produces apprehension and dread that are disproportionate to the situation. Panic states are acute, sudden anxiety attacks that may last for a few minutes to 1 hour or more. The frequency of these attacks may range from several times a day to less than one per month. During the attack, the person has fears of imminent death or physical catastrophe. Other fears include humiliation or appearing foolish or stupid. Obsessive-compulsive behavior is not necessarily pathological. It becomes pathological when the individual feels compelled to carry out an activity over and over. Obsessions are persistent, intrusive, and inappropriate ideas, thoughts, and/or actions.

Risk Factors

Chronic stressful situations
Isolation

Family members with anxiety disorders
Feelings of being overwhelmed
Low self-esteem or threats to self-esteem

Clinical Manifestations

Behavioral	Expressed feelings of apprehension disproportionate to the external risk; dread; irritability; anger; frustration; terror; blocking; panic; incapacitation, immobilization; impaired memory, attention, and concentration; irrational fear with avoidance of a dreaded activity, event, or object; scattered thoughts or lack of focus to details; lack of confidence; low self-esteem; sense of worthlessness and rejection; stuttering; blocking; rapid, pressured speech; repetitive questioning about same thing; being petty or complaining
Physical	Heart palpitations; tachycardia; dizziness; light-headedness; dyspnea; gasping for air; heartburn; tremors; generalized weakness; nausea; vomiting; change in appetite; insomnia; difficulty falling asleep; restlessness; elevated blood pressure and pulse; urinary frequency; diarrhea or occasional constipation

Complications

Individuals with undiagnosed and/or untreated anxiety disorders may have difficulty coping with average activities of daily living. Over time, they may exhibit signs of other psychological or physiological conditions. To prevent possible complications, early and significant intervention is required.

Diagnostic Tests

Laboratory	Screen for other medical disorders or conditions such as thyroid dysfunction
ECG	Screen for cardiopathology

Therapeutic Management

Surgery	None

Drugs	Antianxiety medications such as alprazolam; other psychotropic medication as indicated.
General	Provide quiet, nonstressful, nondemanding environment; speak calmly and directly.
	Assist to calm individual and reduce physiological stressors.
	Encourage individual to evaluate own actions and causes of actions; help individual learn coping strategies.
	Acknowledge individual's strengths and abilities.
	Teach behavior modification, problem-solving and assertiveness skills, and other coping strategies to enhance self-esteem and block anxiety episodes.

aortic aneurysm

A localized dilation or ballooning of the aorta

Etiology and incidence: Most cases are caused by arteriosclerosis. Smoking and hypertension contribute to the formation of aneurysms. Trauma, syphilis, infection, connective tissue disorders, and arteritis are also causes. Aneurysms can develop anywhere along the aorta, but 75% occur in the abdominal aorta. About 25% develop in the thoracic aorta, and the remainder occur in peripheral aortic branches. White men over age 40 have the highest incidence of aortic aneurysms in the United States.

Pathophysiology: With arteriosclerosis, fibrosis and intimal thickening develop as a result of long-term hypertrophy and atrophy of the smooth muscle coat, generally as a result of aging. The vessel becomes less elastic, and the vessel wall thins in spots. Pressure on these spots causes ballooning, which increases over time. Aneurysms caused by infection occur when the infection infiltrates and damages the aortic wall. Aneurysms caused by blunt chest trauma arise from damage to the aorta and subsequent leakage and hematoma formation.

Clinical Manifestations

Many people are asymptomatic, even with huge aneurysms. Signs and symptoms, when present, are dictated by location and compression or erosion of adjacent tissues.

Abdominal	Deep, boring, steady visceral pain in lumbosacral area, often relieved by positioning; feeling of abdominal pulsation or pain; tenderness on palpation; wide aortic pulsation on palpation
Thoracic	Pain in spine or rib cage, cough, wheezing, hemoptysis, dysphagia, hoarseness, tracheal deviation, abnormal chest wall pulsations

Complications

The most serious threat posed by an aneurysm is rupture. Depending on the severity of bleeding, hypovolemic shock and death usually follow quickly. The success rate for surgery for a ruptured abdominal aortic aneurysm is only 50%.

Diagnostic Tests

Abdominal/chest x-ray	Calcification of aneurysm wall
Ultrasound/CT scan/ MRI	To determine extent and size of aneurysm
Contrast aortography	To determine origin of major vessels arising from aortic site; useful for resection

Therapeutic Management

Surgery	Resection and replacement with a synthetic conduit is recommended for all aneurysms >6 cm and for most 4 to 6 cm.
Drugs	Intensive antibiotic therapy for mycotic aneurysms before resection, antihypertensives to decrease blood pressure and myocardial contractility
General	Monitoring if surgery is not done

appendicitis

An acute inflammation of the appendix

Etiology and incidence: The etiology is not clear but appears to be related to obstruction of the appendiceal lumen by a fecal mass, stricture, or infection. Acute appendicitis is one of the most common reasons for abdominal surgery. The incidence is about 1:1000 persons in the United States, and the condition is most common in adolescents and young adults and is slightly more prevalent in men.

Pathophysiology: The lumen is obstructed, blood flow is diminished, hypoxia develops, the mucosa ulcerates, and bacteria invade the wall, causing an infection and producing edema, which further impedes blood flow, causing tissue necrosis, gangrene, and perforation.

Clinical Manifestations

The typical symptom is progressively severe abdominal pain, which begins in the midabdomen and shifts to the lower right quadrant after 6 to 10 hours. The pain may be accompanied by a low-grade fever, malaise, nausea, and vomiting.

Complications

Perforation causes peritonitis.

Diagnostic Tests

Clinical examination	Localized rebound tenderness at McBurney's point
WBCs	Moderately elevated with left shift
Laparoscopy	For visualization when diagnosis is in doubt

Therapeutic Management

Surgery	Appendectomy, which may be done by laparoscope, decreasing recovery time
Drugs	Antibiotics for prophylaxis after surgery
General	None

arthritis (osteoarthritis, rheumatoid)

osteoarthritis (degenerative joint disease)

A chronic, degenerative disease process occurring primarily in the hips and knees and characterized by deterioration of the joint cartilage, formation of new bone in subchondral areas and joint margins, and joint hypertrophy

Etiology and incidence: The etiology is unknown in primary osteoarthritis but is believed to be related in some way to aging and genetics. Secondary osteoarthritis usually follows a predisposing event such as trauma, disease, developmental processes, or obesity. Osteoarthritis is the most common of all articular disorders, affecting more than 33 million Americans. Men and women are equally affected, but the onset in men occurs earlier. In women, the incidence increases after menopause.

Pathophysiology: The water content of the hyaline cartilage increases, and the protein-carbohydrate molecules decrease. The cartilage becomes softer and sheds flakes into the joint. The shedding rubs away the cartilage and increases the friction coefficient in the joint, setting up an erosive cycle. As the cartilage erodes, underlying bone is exposed. Fibrous tissue forms in the joint capsule, causing inelasticity and limiting joint movement. New bone, formed in the subchondral area and at joint margins, is stiff and subject to microfractures and callus formation. Deterioration of the weight-bearing surface combined with the bony overgrowth leads to joint hypertrophy and deformity.

Clinical Manifestations

Early	Deep, aching joint pain that is aggravated by exercise and that worsens as the day progresses; stiffness after inactivity
Midcourse	Reduced joint motion, tenderness, crepitus, grating sensation, flexion contractures, joint enlargement

| Late | Tenderness on palpation, pain with passive ROM, increase in degree and duration of pain, joint deformity, and subluxation |

Complications

Osteoarthritis of the spine can cause compression of the spinal cord, leading to weakness in the extremities, incontinence of bowel and bladder, and impotence.

Diagnostic Tests

Clinical evaluation	Any of above manifestations, Heberden's or Bouchard's nodules of finger joints
Gait analysis	Altered motion patterns
Radiology	Narrowed joint space, increased density of subchondral bone, pseudocysts in subchondral marrow, osteophytes at joint periphery
Erythrocyte sedimentation rate	Normal/moderate increase
Synovial analysis	High viscosity; yellow, transparent color; negative culture; WBC 200-2,000/µl; <25 polymorphonuclear leukocytes

Therapeutic Management

Surgery	Osteotomy, laminectomy, fusion, total joint replacement if conservative therapy fails
Drugs	Aspirin, muscle relaxants, and intraarticular steroid injections provide some transient relief. Cytokinine is being evaluated in clinical trials.
General	*Exercise:* Isometric, isotonic, isokinetic, strengthening, stretching, ROM, and balance exercises; rest; massage, moist heat for pain; elastic bandages for support; canes and walkers to aid mobility *Teaching:* Avoid soft chairs, recliners, and pillows under knees; use firm bed and hard chairs; wear sturdy, low-heeled shoes

rheumatoid arthritis

A chronic, systemic, degenerative disease characterized by inflammation of the connective tissues and manifested primarily in and around peripheral joints

Etiology and incidence: The etiology is unknown, although the disease often is characterized as an autoimmune disorder, and a familial link is suspected. Approximately 6.5 million people in the United States are affected, with women three times more likely to be affected than men. Onset usually occurs between ages 35 and 50, although the disease has been diagnosed in children between ages 8 and 15.

Pathophysiology: Joint inflammation begins with congestion and edema of the synovial membrane and joint capsule, which develops into synovitis. Thickened layers of granulation tissue invade and destroy the cartilage and joint capsule. The fibrous granulation tissue deforms, ossifies, occludes, and immobilizes the joint. Eventually the disease spreads to major organ systems, including the heart, lungs, kidneys, and eyes.

Clinical Manifestations

Early	Nonspecific symptoms of fatigue, malaise, low-grade fever, anorexia, and weight loss
Midcourse	Tenderness, pain, and stiffness in affected joints (most often the fingers) that occurs in a bilateral, symmetric pattern and spreads to the wrists, elbows, knees, and ankles; diminished joint function; paresthesia; joint contractures and deformities
Late	Subcutaneous rheumatoid nodules, leg ulcers, lymphadenopathy, inflammation and dryness of mucous membranes, episcleritis, pericarditis, valvular lesions, splenomegaly, pneumonitis

Complications

Acute rheumatoid arthritis is characterized by abrupt onset and progressive, relentless deterioration of joints and then other major body systems without remission and with poor or no response to medical treatment. The prognosis in these cases is poor.

Diagnostic Tests

Clinical evaluation	The American Rheumatoid Association (ARA) looks for a presence of four or more of the following: (1) morning stiffness lasting more than an hour; (2) inflammation in at least three joints with swelling observed in fingers, wrist, elbow, knee ankle, and/or toe joints; (3) the swelling in at least one joint should be the wrist, fingers, or toes; (4) symmetric joint swelling; (5) subcutaneous nodules; (6) positive rheumatoid factor; (7) bone erosion; or (8) decalcification seen on x-ray.
Rheumatoid factor	Positive in 95% of cases
Synovial analysis	Opaque color; increased volume and turbidity; decreased viscosity and complement; 3000 to 50000 WBCs/µl; polymorphonuclear cells predominant
Erythrocyte sedimentation rate	Elevated in 90% of cases
CBC	Hypochromic anemia, elevated WBCs
Radiology	Soft tissue swelling, narrowed joint space, marginal erosions

Therapeutic Management

Surgery	Synovectomy for pain relief, repair of ruptured tendon sheaths to prevent deformity and subluxation, osteotomy to change weight-bearing surfaces, total joint replacement to increase mobility
Drugs	Aspirin, NSAIDs, and gold compounds/penicillamine to reduce pain and inflammation; oral or intraarticular injections of corticosteroids to reduce inflammation; immunosuppressive/antineoplastic agents

General   Whirlpool, moist compresses, paraffin gloves to reduce pain and edema; therapy and exercise to increase ROM, strength, and endurance; balance of activity and rest; splints, canes, or walkers to aid mobility; emotional support to adapt to disability

asbestosis

A diffuse, interstitial pulmonary fibrosis resulting from inhalation of asbestos

Etiology and incidence: The cause is prolonged exposure to airborne asbestos particles. Susceptibility increases with increasing length and intensity of exposure. The incidence is greatly increased by chronic occupational exposure. Families of workers are also at risk from fibers carried home on clothing. The general public is at risk from long-term exposure to asbestos dust in old buildings in which asbestos was used as insulation or from asbestos in shingling or building material.

Pathophysiology: Asbestos particles are deposited on bronchiole or alveolar walls and are ingested by cells, leading to an edematous process in the wall that results in non-nodular alveolar and interstitial fibrosis, reduced lung volume and compliance, and impaired gas transfer.

Risk Factors

Exposure to asbestos fibers in an occupational setting that
    involves the mining, milling, or use of asbestos, where
    the suppression of asbestos dust is poorly controlled and
    exposure is not adequately limited
Smoking

Clinical Manifestations

Symptoms begin with exertional dyspnea and decreased exercise tolerance. As the disease progresses, dyspnea is chronic even at rest and a dry cough may develop.

Complications

Asbestos is a cocarcinogen with tobacco, and asbestos workers who smoke are 90 times more likely to develop lung cancer than smokers who are not exposed to asbestos.

Diagnostic Tests

Clinical examination   History of long-term exposure to
                                 asbestos

Radiology	Interstitial markings in lower lung, thickening, plaques, calcification
Pulmonary function	*Early:* Normal
	Later: Reduced lung capacity and compliance
Arterial blood gases	*Early:* Normal
	Later: Decreased Po_2, increased Pco_2

Therapeutic Management

Surgery	None
Drugs	None
General	Exposure elimination; chest physiotherapy, increased fluids, and steam inhalation to loosen secretions; oxygen therapy
Prevention	Enforce industrial safety regulations to control exposure such as adequate dust suppression measures, respirators.
	Remove asbestos from public buildings when it poses a health threat.
	Smoking cessation

asthma

A chronic obstructive disorder of the airways characterized by airway hypersensitivity to a variety of stimuli, resulting in transient bronchospasm and constriction of the airways

Etiology and incidence: Asthma is triggered by either extrinsic or intrinsic agents. Extrinsic agents include allergens such as dust, smoke, pet dander, mold spores, chemicals, and foods. Intrinsic agents include underlying respiratory infections, emotional stress, and fatigue. Many attacks are triggered by a combination of agents. Asthma affects more than 14.5 million people in the U.S. population and 5500 people a year die as a result of the disease. It is the most common chronic disease of children and adults, beginning in childhood about half the time and in adolescence or adulthood half the time. In children, boys are affected twice as often as girls, but this ratio evens out by adolescence. The prevalence and mortality rate are increasing rapidly worldwide. The last two decades have seen close to a 50% increase in incidence of this disease. It is theorized that this increase is related to the shift to urban living centers and the increase in pollution.

Pathophysiology: Various agents trigger a reaction in the tracheal and bronchial linings, which causes bronchospasm of the smooth muscle and constricts the airways. The airways become inflamed and edematous and produce excess thickened secretions, which aggravate the blockage. Eosinophils infiltrate the airway walls, injuring and desquamating the epithelial lining. Expiratory capacity is reduced, causing trapping of gas in the airways, hyperinflation, and labored breathing. Because the obstruction is not uniform, blood flow continues in some areas of hypoventilation, producing a ventilation-perfusion imbalance and resulting in arterial hypoxemia.

Clinical Manifestations

Symptoms vary from mild to pronounced, depending on the acuteness and severity of the attack

Mild   Diffuse wheezing, slight dyspnea, chest tightness

| Moderate | Marked wheezing; dyspnea at rest; hyperpnea; chest tightness; nostril flaring; dry cough; upright, forward-leaning posture; prolonged expiration |
| Severe | Decreased wheezing; severe dyspnea; chest retractions; nasal flaring; shallow, rapid respirations; anxiety; fatigue; inability to speak more than a few words before stopping for breath; upright posture; cyanosis |

Complications

Atelectasis, pneumothorax, and status asthmaticus with respiratory failure are common complications.

Diagnostic Tests

The following tests are done for acute attacks. The individual is also assessed for severity of disease based on frequency and severity of attacks, response to bronchodilators, degree of lung damage seen on x-ray, and exercise tolerance.

Clinical evaluation	Above-mentioned manifestations plus pulsus paradoxus; decrease in airway exchange, rhonchi, wheezes; increased pulse and respirations
Arterial blood gases	*Mild:* pH, Pao_2, $Paco_2$ normal; forced vital capacity (FVC) 80% of normal
	Moderate: pH increased; Pao_2, $Paco_2$ decreased; FVC 50% of normal
	Severe: pH, Pao_2 decreased; $Paco_2$ increased; FVC 25% of normal
Sputum	Increased viscosity, plugs
Complete blood count	Increased Hct, eosinophilia
Radiology	Chest x-ray normal to hyperinflation, increase in lung markings, possible atelectasis
Pulmonary function	Total lung capacity, functional reserve capacity, and respiratory volume increased; vital capacity normal or decreased

| Peak expiratory flow rate (PEFR) | Decreased; also used to monitor treatment effectiveness |

Therapeutic Management

Surgery	None
Drugs	*Acute attack:* Bronchodilators (aerosol, parenteral); corticosteroids (oral, parenteral)
	Maintenance: Long-acting bronchodilators (oral, aerosol); corticosteroids (aerosol); cromolyn sodium(nasal spray); allergy injections
General	*Acute attack:* Oxygen, fluid and electrolyte replacement, maintenance of patency of airway
	Maintenance: Avoid triggering agents, obtain influenza shots, avoid or obtain early treatment of respiratory infections, obtain education about disease and long-term drug therapy, attend support groups

Bell's palsy

Unilateral facial paralysis with sudden loss of the ability to use the muscles that control expression on one side of the face

Etiology and incidence: The cause is unknown but is thought to be related to a virus or immune disorder. Most individuals are 20 to 60 years of age, and men and women are affected equally.

Pathophysiology: Cranial nerve VII (facial nerve) is compressed at the temporal bone pathway by edema produced by an unknown cause. As a result, the muscles controlling expression on one side of the face are paralyzed.

Clinical Manifestations

Facial weakness, numbness, and heaviness, as well as pain behind the ear, followed by inability to work facial muscles on one side, are apparent. The extent of the symptoms depends on the severity of compression; symptoms can include inability to wrinkle the forehead, upward rolling of the eyeball, inability to close the eyelid, and unilateral lack of smile or frown expression. Taste, lacrimation, and salivation may also be affected.

Complications

Facial contractures, corneal ulceration, and synkinesia are possible complications. Paralysis may be transient or permanent. Any return of function usually occurs in 1 to 6 months.

Diagnostic Tests

Diagnosis is based on clinical examination and history of onset.

Therapeutic Management

Surgery	Hypoglossal-facial nerve anastomosis to restore partial facial function if none has returned by 6 to 12 months
Drugs	Methylcellulose drops for affected eye, analgesics as required for pain, steroids to reduce edema of facial nerve
General	Patching of affected eye; stimulation of facial nerve, and physical therapy to prevent facial contracture

black lung disease (coal worker's pneumoconiosis)

Chronic, progressive nodular pulmonary disease involving diffuse deposition of coal dust in the lungs

Etiology and incidence: The cause is inhalation and prolonged retention of bituminous or anthracite coal dust. Susceptibility increases with length and intensity of exposure, smallness of inhaled particles, and silica content of the coal. Anthracite coal miners in the eastern United States have the highest incidence.

Pathophysiology: The deposition of coal dust triggers a phagocytic reaction and increases the production of macrophages. As the dust overwhelms the pulmonary clearing mechanism, fibroblasts appear and lay down a network of reticulin fibers that enmesh the dust. The collections of macrophages and reticulin fibers around the bronchioles, known as coal macules, lead to dilation of the alveoli; this is known as the simple disease phase. If allowed to progress, the macules enlarge and coalesce, and a massive fibrosis occurs, which destroys pulmonary structures as the vascular bed, alveoli, and airways are invaded; this is the complicated phase.

Risk Factors

Prolonged exposure to coal dust

Clinical Manifestations

Simple phase	Asymptomatic
Complicated phase	Exertional dyspnea, hypoxia, black sputum

Complications

Pulmonary hypertension and cor pulmonale may develop in severe cases. Smoking, bronchitis, emphysema, and other respiratory diseases aggravate the disease process.

Diagnostic Tests

Clinical examination	History of exposure to coal dust, usually at least 10 years underground

Radiology	*Simple phase:* Small, rounded opacities in both lung fields
	Complicated phase: Large opacities >1 cm mixed with numerous small opacities
Pulmonary function	*Simple phase:* Normal vital capacity
	Complicated phase: Decreased
Arterial blood gases	*Simple phase:* Normal, decreased Po_2
	Complicated phase: Increased Pco_2

Therapeutic Management

Surgery	None
Drugs	None
General	*Simple phase:* Eliminate further exposure, prevent secondary infections
	Complicated phase: Chest physiotherapy and steam inhalation to loosen and remove secretions; increased fluid intake to thin secretions; oxygen (advanced stage)

bladder cancer

Transitional cell carcinomas account for 90% of all bladder cancers, while squamous cell tumors and adenocarcinomas account for the remaining 10%. It is also classified as invasive or noninvasive (superficial). Invasive tumors grow in the bladder wall, spreading quickly to the underlying musculature, whereas noninvasive tumors occur on the superficial surface of the bladder wall.

Etiology and incidence: Known carcinogens include tobacco tars and industrial chemical agents found in rubber and dye, as well as in paint shops and chemical manufacturing, petrochemical, and printing plants. Chronic irritants (e.g., schistosomiasis, bladder calculi) are predisposing factors. Bladder cancer is the fourth most common cancer in men and the eighth most common in women. More than 50,000 new cases are diagnosed each year in the United States and 10,000 people die annually. The morbidity and mortality is three times higher for men and the median age for diagnosis is 65.

Pathophysiology: Transitional cell tumors are characterized by multicentric and papillary growth into the bladder lumen, with potential invasion into the bladder muscle, pelvis, pelvic structures, and surrounding lymph nodes. The lungs, bones, and liver are common sites of metastasis.

Risk Factors

Chemical exposure (Benzidine, 2-naphthylamine, *p*-aminodiphenyl, 4-nitrobiphenyl)
Chronic bladder irritation (bladder calculi, schistosomiasis)
Diet high in fried, fatty meats and other fats and low in vitamin A
History of multiple urinary tract infections
History of treatment with cyclophosphamide (Cytoxan) or pelvic radiation
Occupational exposure (e.g., aluminum worker, dry cleaner, worker in a plant producing preservatives or polychlorinated biphenyls, chimney sweep, miner, exterminator)
Overuse of drugs such as acetaminophen or phenacetin
Tobacco use (increases two-to-four-fold)

Clinical Manifestations

Frequency of and burning on urination, hematuria, dysuria, and pyuria are the most common presenting signs and symptoms. Pain in the legs, pelvis, and lower back may develop with invasion and metastasis.

Complications

Fistulas of the ureter or small bowel (or both) and obstruction of the small bowel are possible.

Diagnostic Tests

Filling defects on a cystogram and positive results on urine cytologic tests suggest a neoplasm. The definitive diagnosis is made by cystoscopy and transurethral resectional biopsy. CT scan or MRI with bimanual examination is used for staging.

Therapeutic Management

Surgery	*Noninvasive tumors:* Endoscopy and fulguration; laser therapy for noninvasive tumors
	Invasive tumors: Radical cystectomy with urinary diversion usually an ileal conduit with external pouch
Drugs	**Chemotherapy**
	Noninvasive tumors: Intravesical instillations with bacille Calmette-Guérin (BCG), doxorubicin, thiotepa, or mitomycin-C for noninvasive tumors
	Invasive tumors: Systemic chemotherapy with multidrug combinations such as cisplatin, methotrexate, doxorubicin, and vinblastine (CMDV) and methotrexate, vinblastine, and cisplatin (MVC)
General	Radiation as a preoperative regimen or as adjunct to chemotherapy; care of and instruction about ileal appliance

blepharitis

An inflammation of the eyelid margins

Etiology and incidence: A common chronic condition associated with seborrheic dermatitis of the scalp, eyebrows, and external ears. Severe cases may be bacterial in origin (commonly staphylococcal). Allergies may aggravate the condition. It is often impossible to isolate the exact causative agent. Other common conditions associated with chronic blepharitis are diabetes, gout, anemia, and rosacea. Infections of the nose and mouth may also be transferred to the eyes and lids by frequent eye rubbing.

Pathophysiology: Blepharitis may be seborrheic or ulcerative. Seborrheic (nonulcerative) blepharitis is commonly associated with seborrhea of the face, eyebrows, external ears, and scalp. Inflammation of the eyelid margins occurs, with redness, thickening, and often the formation of scales and crusts or shallow marginal ulcers. Ulcerative blepharitis is caused by bacterial infection (usually staphylococcal) of the lash follicles and the meibomian glands.

Risk Factors

Chronic diseases such as diabetes, gout, anemia, and rosacea
History of sties and chalazia
Infections of the mouth and/or throat
Risk is often difficult to isolate
Seborrheic dermatitis or allergies

Clinical Manifestations

Seborrheic blepharitis	*General:* Foreign-body sensation
	Eyelids and lashes: Red lid margins, flaking and scaling around lashes, itching and burning sensation, loss of lashes
	Cornea and conjunctiva: Light sensitivity, conjunctivitis, possible cornea inflammation
Ulcerative blepharitis	*General:* Foreign-body sensation
	Eyelids and lashes: Crusts on the eyelids, leaving a bleeding surface

when removed; small pustules
develop in lash follicles; shallow
ulcers may develop; eyelids become
"glued" together during sleep
by dried drainage
Cornea and conjunctiva: Light sensitivity, conjunctivitis, possible
corneal inflammation

Complications

Condition may become chronic if not properly treated.

Diagnostic Tests

Clinical evaluation with characteristic manifestations
Detailed history to locate possible source
Possible laboratory isolation of causative agent

Therapeutic Management

Surgery	None
Drugs	*General:* use of seborrheic dermatitis medicated shampoos
	Ulcerative: antibiotic agents both topical and systemic
General	Blepharitis is stubborn to treat and is often resistant to various therapies
	Eyelid hygiene consists of scrubbing the lid margin daily with a cotton swab dipped in a diluted solution of baby shampoo.

bone cancer, primary

Skeletal malignancy arising from osseous, cartilaginous, fibrous, or reticuloendothelial tissues of the bone

Etiology and incidence: Etiology is unknown. Primary bone tumors are rare, accounting for only 0.2% of all malignancies in the United States. The tumors affect primarily children and adolescents (Ewing's sarcoma, osteosarcoma) and adults over age 65 (fibrosarcoma, chondrosarcoma, reticulum cell sarcoma).

Pathophysiology: Osteosarcomas are the most common primary bone tumor. Cancer cells originate in the mesenchyma of the medullary cavity of the bone (usually long bones around or in the knee) and proliferate rapidly, absorbing normal bone and promoting tissue destruction. The bone becomes sclerotic or lytic, or both, and an aggressive periosteal reaction ensues, accompanied by a soft tissue mass. The lungs are the most common metastatic site; spread to regional lymph nodes is rare. Fibrous tumors are similar in character to osteosarcomas.

Risk Factors

History of Paget's disease, fibrous dysplasia, or enchondromatosis
History of prior radiation

Clinical Manifestations

An initially painless mass is the most common presenting sign. Pain or swelling (or both) at the affected site is also common.

Complications

Pathological fractures occur with progressive destruction of normal bone tissue. Survival rate is about 50% with combination therapy and early treatment.

Diagnostic Tests

X-rays and bone scans of the involved bone allow visualization of the tumor. The definitive diagnosis is made through biopsy of the tumor. MRI is conducted to visualize tumor size and location and enhance resection abilities.

Therapeutic Management

Surgery	En bloc resection and reconstruction of affected limb, amputation of affected limb
Drugs	Systemic chemotherapy with methotrexate, intraarterial perfusion with doxorubicin as an adjunct before surgery
General	Radiation used with Ewing's sarcoma, rehabilitation after amputation, gait training, fitting of prosthesis

brain abscess

An intracerebral infection consisting of an encapsulated collection of pus

Etiology and incidence: Causes include extension of existing cranial infection (e.g., ear infection, sinusitis, mastoiditis, osteomyelitis, periodontal infection); penetrating head wounds; blood-borne transmission from a distant infection (e.g., bacterial endocarditis, abdominal/pelvic infections, bronchiectasis); IV drug abuse; or immunodeficiency. The incidence is highest in individuals with sinusitis or ear or pulmonary infection. The number of abscesses is increasing with the rise in immunodeficiency disorders and IV drug abuse.

Pathophysiology: The brain produces a poorly localized inflammatory response to the invading pathogen. Brain tissue subsequently liquefies and necroses, producing a cystic mass, which is encapsulated by glia and fibroblasts. As this mass enlarges, it increases intracranial pressure, causing signs and symptoms similar to those of a brain tumor.

Risk Factors

Blood-borne infections (e.g., bacterial endocarditis, peritonitis)
Immunodeficiency infections
Infections of the face and head (e.g., otitis media, sinusitis, mastoiditis, acne, or abscesses of teeth or gums)
IV drug use
Open head injury

Clinical Manifestations

Headache, nausea, vomiting, seizures, altered mental status, nuchal rigidity, and low-grade fever can occur. The duration of symptoms varies considerably, from hours to weeks.

Complications

The illness is progressive and usually fatal if left untreated. With treatment, the mortality rate is 30%, and more than half of survivors suffer some neurologic sequelae.

Diagnostic Tests

Clinical evaluation	Above manifestations and predisposing conditions
Lumbar puncture	*Contraindicated*
CT scan/MRI	Visualization of abscess

Therapeutic Management

Surgery	Biopsy, drainage and evacuation of abscess through stereotaxic techniques or craniotomy
Drugs	IV antibiotics as initial choice, depending on suspected organism and probable source of infection; later choices made from culture and sensitivity, along with Gram's stain results; steroids to reduce brain edema and intracranial pressure (ICP); anticonvulsants to control seizure activity
General	Serial-order CT scans to monitor progression; monitoring for hyponatremia, inappropriate antidiuretic hormone secretion; prevention of complications of extended bed rest (e.g., antiembolism stockings, ROM exercises, turning); early, aggressive rehabilitation to prevent or reduce neurological sequelae
Prevention	Prevention of brain abcess through prompt treatment of infections of face and head

brain cancer

See Brain Tumor, Primary.

brain tumor, primary

An expanding, intracranial lesion that may be either benign or malignant. However, since both types can be lethal if inaccessible or left untreated and malignant tumors rarely metastasize beyond the central nervous system, the distinction serves mainly to describe the rate of growth and invasiveness. Tumors are divided into six classes, according to their origin: (1) skull, (2) meninges, (3) cranial nerves, (4) neuroglia, (5) pituitary/pineal body, and (6) congenital.

Etiology and incidence: The etiology is unknown. Brain tumors are diagnosed in about 10,000 persons per year in the United States. Undiagnosed brain tumors are found in about 2% of all routine autopsies. They can occur at any age but are most prevalent between ages 30 and 50. The overall occurrence is evenly divided between the genders. Common childhood tumors include cerebellar astrocytomas, medulloblastomas, gliomas, ependymomas, and assorted congenital tumors. Common adult tumors include meningiomas, schwannomas, and cerebral astrocytomas.

Pathophysiology: As the tumor grows, the surrounding brain tissue is compressed or infiltrated (or both), causing focal disturbances. The flow and absorption of cerebrospinal fluid (CSF) are altered and/or obstructed, causing increased intracranial pressure (ICP). Blood vessels are compressed, altering or obstructing blood flow and resulting in tissue necrosis and seizures. If tumors arise in certain locations, brain tissue can shift, leading to herniation, infarction, and hemorrhage in the pons and midbrain.

Clinical Manifestations

The signs and symptoms depend heavily on the tumor's location, size, and rate of growth. Slow-growing tumors are often asymptomatic until they have grown quite large.

General   Headache, nausea, vomiting, impulsivity, diminished judgment, memory impairment, depression, seizures, drowsiness, lethargy, psychotic episodes, papilledema

Focal | *Frontal lobe:* Hemiplegia, expressive aphasia, ataxia, visual field defects, focal seizures
Parietal lobe: Focal sensory seizures, impaired position sense and two-point discrimination, hemianopsia, apraxia, anosognosia, speech disturbances, denial of illness
Temporal lobe: Convulsions, aphasia/dysphasia, olfactory aura preceding seizures
Occipital lobe: Hemianopsia, flashing light aura preceding seizures
Brainstem: Hemiplegia, hemianesthesia

Complications

Herniation of the brain can occur when intracranial pressure is expanded beyond compensatory levels. Prompt intervention is required, or the individual will die. Benign tumors that cannot be excised because of their size or location (or both) are generally fatal.

Diagnostic Tests

Clinical evaluation	Any of above manifestations, particularly headaches and recent onset of seizure activity
Neurological examination	Focal manifestations, impairment of mental status
CT scan/MRI/positron emission tomography (PET)	To detect tumor, midline shifts, and changes in ventricle size
Eye examination	To test visual fields and acuity and detect papilledema
Audiometry	To test hearing

Therapeutic Management

Surgery	Tumor excision, shunting
Drugs	Corticosteroids to reduce cerebral edema, anticonvulsants to control seizure activity, chemotherapeutic agents as adjunctive therapy or to treat recurrence
General	Radiation for tumor or residual tumor, rehabilitation for neurological sequelae

breast cancer

Ductal carcinomas account for 75% of all breast cancer; lobular and nipple carcinomas account for most of the remaining 25%.

Etiology and incidence: The cause of breast cancer is unknown although estrogen is thought to play some role. More than 50% of women diagnosed with the disorder show none of the known risk factors (see Risk Factors).

Breast cancer is the most common cancer among women in the United States, with more than 182,000 new cases diagnosed each year. The incidence is twice as high for women over age 65 as for those in the 45-to-64 age group. The incidence is rising, particularly among black women and women in their 20s and 30s; however, the mortality rate has remained stable at about 46,000 deaths per year. It is the second leading cause of cancer death in women.

Pathophysiology: Ductal carcinomas originate in the lactiferous ducts, where the cancer cells form a dense fibrotic core with radiating tentacles that invade surrounding breast tissue. The tumor mass is generally solid, nonmobile, irregularly shaped, poorly defined, and unilateral. Lobular carcinomas originate in the breast lobules and are bilateral. Nipple carcinomas originate in the nipple complex and often occur in conjunction with invasive ductal carcinomas. The lungs, bones, brain, and liver are common sites of breast cancer metastasis.

Risk Factors

Early menarche (before 11)/late menopause (after 52)
Excessive alcohol consumption
Exposure to ionizing radiation (particularly if exposure occurs before age 35)
Familial history of breast cancer (risk is increased if relationship is mother or sister, if disease is bilateral, or if disease developed before menopause)
High-fat diet
Nulliparity or first child after age 30
Personal history of atypical hyperplasia
Personal history of cancer (breast, colon, ovarian, endometrial, thyroid)

Radial scarring noted on tissue examination after a benign breast biopsy

Clinical Manifestations

The most common presenting sign is a lump in the breast. About 50% are found in the upper outer quadrant. Nipple discharge may be present. Pain, tenderness, changes in breast shape, dimpling, and nipple retraction rarely occur until the disease reaches an advanced stage.

Complications

The prognosis dims markedly as the number of involved lymph nodes increases. Pleural effusion, ascites, pathological fracture, and spinal compression can occur with advanced disease. Women treated with stage I tumors and no lymph node involvement have a 10-year survival rate of 80%. Women with stage II tumors have a 10-year survival rate of 60%.

Diagnostic Tests

A mass detected by breast self-examination, physical examination, or mammogram needs further follow-up. Definitive diagnosis is made by incisional, excisional, or needle biopsy of the mass.

Therapeutic Management

Surgery	Treatment of choice is resection of the lump with removal of a varying amount of surrounding healthy tissue, ranging from a margin of breast tissue to the entire breast, axillary lymph nodes, mammary lymphatic chain, and pectoral muscles; breast reconstruction
Drugs	Adjunct systemic multidrug chemotherapy used primarily for premenopausal node-positive women; adjunct hormone therapy (estrogens, androgens, progestins) used primarily for postmenopausal node- or receptor-positive women; antiestrogen therapy (Tamoxifen) as first line therapy

General   Radiation used as adjunct after surgery and for palliation in advanced disease; counseling for altered
                 body image; recovery support groups; instruction in breast self-examination

bronchiectasis

An irreversible dilation of the tracheobronchial tree, with destruction of the bronchial walls.

Etiology and incidence: Bronchiectasis is caused by conditions that repeatedly damage the bronchial walls and interfere with clearance of bronchial secretions, such as cystic fibrosis, immunodeficiency diseases, repeated respiratory tract infections, tuberculosis, inhalation of noxious gases, repeated aspiration pneumonia, and complications of measles and pertussis. Rare congenital anomalies may also be a cause. The incidence has declined dramatically since the introduction of antibiotics. Children are most vulnerable, and the incidence is highest among Alaskan Native Inuit and New Zealand Maori populations of the world.

Pathophysiology: Repeated inflammatory and infectious processes slowly alter the structure of the bronchial walls, diminishing cilia and impairing the ability to clear secretions, increasing mucus production, reducing elasticity and muscular response, and causing permanent dilation of various areas in the tracheobronchial tree.

Risk Factors

Smoking
Respiratory irritation
Repeated upper respiratory infections
Underlying disease (e.g., cystic fibrosis, immune deficiency,
    tuberculosis)

Clinical Manifestations

The individual is often asymptomatic early in the disease. A chronic cough with sputum production is the most common presenting sign. Hemoptysis and recurrent pneumonia are also common, as are dyspnea, wheezing, and fatigue.

Complications

Pulmonary hypertension, right ventricular failure, and cor pulmonale are common complications with long-standing disease.

Diagnostic Tests

Clinical examination	Chronic cough, mucopurulent sputum, hemoptysis, moist rales, rhonchi
Sputum	Foamy with sediment; large number of WBCs
Radiology	Chest x-ray shows increased markings, honeycombing, tram tracking
Bronchography	Definitive diagnosis made with visualization of bronchiectatic areas

Therapeutic Management

Surgery	Bronchial resection for confined disease unresponsive to conservative therapy
Drugs	Mucolytics to clear secretions; antibiotics to treat bacterial infection; bronchodilators to reduce dyspnea; influenza and pneumonia vaccines for prophylaxis
General	Chest physiotherapy with postural drainage to clear secretions; increase fluids and use vaporizer to liquefy secretions
Prevention	Avoid respiratory infections and air pollution; smoking cessation

bronchiolitis

Acute viral infection of the lower respiratory tract causing respiratory distress

Etiology and incidence: The major viral pathogens are respiratory syncytial virus and parainfluenza-3 virus. This disease generally affects children under age 2 and often is epidemic in nature. Each year 11 of every 100 children under 12 months of age are affected. Of these, 5% are hospitalized. The disease is transmitted through direct contact with respiratory secretions. The virus may live for hours on tissues, dishes, and countertops.

Pathophysiology: The infecting virus spreads to the medium and small bronchioles in the lower airway and attacks the epithelial cells. This causes edema of the ciliated cells, which protrude into the lumen, losing cilia and fusing with adjacent cells to form a giant cell. These cause edema of the bronchial mucosa and production of exudate, resulting in partial obstruction and trapping of air in the alveoli.

Clinical Manifestations

The illness is usually preceded by an upper respiratory infection, followed by rapid onset of respiratory distress with tachypnea, tachycardia, and a hacking cough. As the disease advances, deepening chest retractions and audible wheezing, lethargy, vomiting, and dehydration develop.

Complications

Atelectasis and pneumonia are common complications. Respiratory failure is also possible.

Diagnostic Tests

Definitive diagnosis is made by isolating the virus or by immunofluorescence or enzyme-linked immunosorbent assay (ELISA).

Therapeutic Management

Surgery	None
Drugs	None
	Ribavirin is experimental; a vaccine is in clinical trials
General	Oxygen mist, vaporizer, adequate fluid intake, rest

bronchitis, acute

A self-limited inflammation of the tracheobronchial tree.

Etiology and incidence: The condition is caused either by irritants (e.g., dust, noxious fumes, or smoke) or by a viral or bacterial infection. It often occurs in conjunction with other disease processes such as influenza, bronchiectasis, emphysema, or tuberculosis. It is more common in the winter months and is generally mild.

Pathophysiology: Congestion of the mucous membranes is followed by desquamation and edema of the submucosa. This interferes with the functioning of the cilia, phagocytes, and lymphatics, resulting in production of a sticky exudate that lines the tracheobronchial tree until it is coughed up. The exudate is an excellent medium for secondary infection.

Risk Factors

Chronic respiratory irritation
Repeated upper respiratory infections
Smoking
Underlying disease (e.g., emphysema, bronchiectasis, influenza, tuberculosis)

Clinical Manifestations

Acute bronchitis is often preceded by an upper respiratory infection. The most common presenting sign is a dry, hacking cough that increasingly produces viscous mucus.

Complications

Pneumonia is the most common complication. Acute respiratory failure occurs in some individuals with underlying pulmonary disease.

Diagnostic Tests

The diagnosis is usually made from the type of cough and sputum. Chest x-rays are taken to rule out other disorders. Arterial blood gases are monitored when underlying chronic disease is present, and sputum is cultured for evidence of superimposed infection.

Therapeutic Management

Surgery	None
Drugs	Antiinfective drugs with concomitant chronic obstructive pulmonary disease (COPD) or superimposed infection; antipyretics for fever
General	Rest, increased fluids, steam vaporizer

bronchitis, chronic

An obstructive pulmonary disorder characterized by a chronic and recurrent productive cough

Etiology and incidence: Bronchial irritants (e.g., cigarette smoke) in conjunction with a genetic predisposition are thought to be the chief cause. More than 14 million cases of chronic bronchitis are reported annually in the United States. Most of these cases occur in those under age 45, and the incidence is higher in women, those living in the South, and those living in heavily polluted areas. More than 3000 deaths from chronic bronchitis occur each year.

Pathophysiology: Chronic irritation leads to hypersecretion and hypertrophy of the bronchial mucous glands and an increase in the size and number of goblet cells. These cells invade the terminal bronchioles, damaging cilia, increasing sputum and bronchial congestion, and narrowing the bronchial lumen. As the disease progresses, leukocytes invade the secretions, aggravating the edema and eventually causing tissue necrosis. Granulated squamous epithelium replaces ciliated epithelium and fibroses, leading to tissue scarring, stenosis, airway obstruction, and a severe ventilation-perfusion imbalance.

Risk Factors

Chronic bronchial irritants
Improper or nonuse of respirators in occupational settings
Occupational exposure to airborne particulates

Clinical Manifestations

Chronic bronchitis may be asymptomatic for years. A productive cough and exertional dyspnea are typical presenting signs. The cough becomes increasingly progressive and the sputum production copious; several attacks per year are common. Chest retractions, wheezing, tachypnea, and cyanosis may also be present.

Complications

Cor pulmonale, pulmonary hypertension, right ventricular hypertrophy, and respiratory failure are common complications.

Diagnostic Tests

Clinical evaluation	Any of the above manifestations; history of chronic lung irritation (e.g., smoking, occupational exposure)
Radiology	Increased markings, hyperinflation
Pulmonary function	Residual volume increased, forced vital capacity and forced expiratory volume decreased, compliance and diffusion normal
Arterial blood gases	Pao_2 decreased, $Paco_2$ increased
Sputum	Culture of multiple microorganisms and neutrophils

Therapeutic Management

Surgery	None
Drugs	Antiinfective drugs for any infection; bronchodilators to reduce dyspnea; corticosteroids to reduce inflammation; flu and pneumonia vaccines for prophylaxis
General	Removal of irritant; chest physiotherapy to loosen secretions; vaporizer and increased fluids to liquefy secretions; oxygenation for hypoxia; consistent exercise to improve ventilatory and cardiac function; smoking cessation

bulimia nervosa

Eating disorder characterized by recurrent episodes of binge eating followed by purging, which is brought about through self-induced vomiting or use of laxatives, emetics, or diuretics. Most individuals maintain a normal or near-normal body weight.

Etiology and incidence: The etiology is unknown, but societal focus on dieting and thinness and associated negative images of obesity are thought to play a role. The incidence of bulimia is highest among adolescent females in affluent circumstances. The estimated prevalence in the United States is 5% of all young women in high school and college. The disorder is also more often seen in individuals whose occupation requires stringent weight control (e.g., jockeys, amateur wrestlers, models, actresses, and ballerinas). Persons with bulimia are highly resistant to treatment.

Pathophysiology: Vomiting causes fluid and electrolyte imbalances, which lead eventually to renal damage and cardiac arrhythmias.

Risk Factors

Adolescence/young adulthood
Affluent households
Female gender
Occupations that require stringent weight control

Clinical Manifestations

Excessive concern about weight, evidence of eating binges, evidence of purging activities (e.g., smell of vomit, laxatives, emetics, and diuretics in residence), rapid weight fluctuations, hypokalemia, swollen parotid glands, dental erosion, esophagitis, scars on knuckles from inducing vomiting.

Complications

Esophageal stricture and rupture and hemorrhage are common complications. Aspiration pneumonia is possible, particularly in concert with use of alcohol and recreational drugs. Sudden death from ventricular dysrhythmia is possible.

Diagnostic Tests

The diagnosis is made by reconstructing a clinical history of binge-purge behavior that occurs at least twice a week for at least 3 months.

Therapeutic Management

Surgery	Treatment of esophageal stricture/rupture
Drugs	Antidepressants
General	Psychotherapy

burns

Tissue injury, protein denaturation, edema, and loss of intravascular fluid resulting from exposure to or contact with a causative agent such as heat, electricity, chemicals, or friction.

Etiology and incidence: Causes include (1) exposure to, contact with, or inhalation of the products of thermal agents such as fire, radiation, or hot liquids; (2) contact with an electrical current; or (3) contact with or inhalation or ingestion of chemical agents (e.g., acids, alkalis, phenols, cresols, mustard gas, or phosphorus). In the United States, more than 2 million persons are burned each year; 15% require hospitalization, and 5% sustain a life-threatening burn. Burns are the second leading cause of death among young children.

Pathophysiology: Thermal and chemical injury disrupts the normal protective function of the skin, causing local and systemic effects. The extent of these effects depends on the type, duration, and intensity of exposure to the causative agent. With electrical burns, heat is generated as the electrical current passes through body tissues, causing thermal burns along the path taken by the current. Local damage is marked by histamine release and severe vasoconstriction, followed in a few hours by vasodilation and increased capillary permeability, which allows plasma to escape into the wound. Damaged cells swell and platelets and leukocytes aggregate, causing thrombotic ischemia and escalating tissue damage. Systemic effects, which are caused by vascular changes and tissue loss, include hypovolemia, hyperventilation, increased blood viscosity, and suppression of the immune system. The severity of the burn determines the extent of local and systemic effects. Severity is judged by the depth of the burn and the quantity of tissue involved. The depth of the burn is classified by degree. First-degree (superficial) burns affect the epidermis only; second-degree burns (split thickness) affect the epidermis and dermis; third-degree burns (full thickness) affect all skin layers and extend to subcutaneous tissue, muscle and nerves; fourth degree burns involve all skin layers plus bone. The percentage of body surface area (BSA) system of the American Burn Association classifies quantity as follows:

- *Minor burns:* Full thickness burns over less than 2% of BSA, partial thickness burns over less than 15% of BSA

- *Moderate burns:* Full thickness burns over 2% to10% of BSA, partial thickness burns over less than 15% to 25% of BSA
- *Major burns:* Full thickness burns over 10% BSA, partial thickness over 25% BSA
- *Any burn* to face, head, hands, feet, or perineum; inhalation and electrical burns; burns complicated by trauma or other disease processes

Clinical Manifestations

The following signs and symptoms can be expected within the first 24 hours:

Local	*First degree:* Wound is red, sensitive to touch, painful, and moist; surface blanches to light pressure
	Second degree (split thickness): Blistering likely
	Third degree (full thickness): Surface is white and pliable with no blanching, or black, charred, and leathery; hypoesthetic or anesthetic; hairs are easily dislodged from follicles
Systemic	Hypovolemic shock, dehydration, hypothermia, hyperventilation
	With inhalation injury: Respiratory obstruction or respiratory failure, or both

Complications

Infection, pneumonia, and respiratory failure are the most common causes of death with severe burns. The prognosis depends largely on the severity and location of the burns and the expertise of the burn management team.

Diagnostic Tests

Clinical examination	To determine the severity of the injury (degree, BSA) and the causative agent
Baseline laboratory studies	CBC, serum electrolytes, blood urea nitrogen, creatinine, arterial blood gases, bilirubin, alkaline phosphatase, urinalysis
Bronchoscopy	To determine extent of upper airway damage

Therapeutic Management

First- and second-degree burns, < 20% BSA

Surgery   None

Drugs   Analgesics for pain, prophylactic antibiotics to prevent infection, tetanus toxoid for immunization, topical antiinfective drugs

General   Cleaning with soap and cold water; débridement of blisters, splinting and positioning of involved joints, elevation of affected area

Third-degree burns, > 20% BSA

Surgery   Surgical débridement; escharotomy to relieve constrictures caused by scarring; fasciotomy with some electrical burns; skin grafting; amputation of severely burned extremities; reconstructive and plastic surgery to correct deformity

Drugs   IV narcotic analgesics; tetanus immunization, topical antiinfective drugs, IV antibiotics

General   Airway maintenance, humidification, and oxygen in inhalation injuries; IV fluid replacement; cleansing of wound; urinary catheter; nasogastric tube; central venous line; mechanical débridement; hydrotherapy; dressing changes; dietary calories, protein increased; parenteral nutrition; physiotherapy; hypertrophic scar management with pressure garments; long-term psychological support; vocational counseling; instruction for long-term adaptations

bursitis

An acute or chronic inflammation of a bursa

Etiology and incidence: The etiology of most bursitis is unknown, although trauma, overuse, arthritis, gout, and infection have been implicated.

Pathophysiology: Exposure to an etiologic agent causes irritation of the bursal sac, which becomes inflamed, edematous, enlarged, and tender.

Clinical Manifestations

Localized pain, redness, heat, swelling, and tenderness around a bony prominence (most often the shoulder) accompanied by limited ROM.

Complications

Repeated inflammation leads to a chronic condition marked by adhesions and calcifications in the bursal sac, permanent muscle atrophy, adhesion capsulitis, and reduced ROM.

Diagnostic Tests

The diagnosis depends on clinical evaluation and a pattern of the aforementioned symptoms or a history of trauma, repetitive motion, gout, or arthritis. With chronic bursitis, x-rays may show calcifications.

Therapeutic Management

Surgery	Needle aspiration of fluid in sac, excision of calcium deposits, removal of bursal sac
Drugs	Nonsteroidal antiinflammatory drugs (NSAIDs) for pain and inflammation, corticosteroid injections into bursa and surrounding tendons
General	Rest and immobilization of joint, passive ROM exercises as pain subsides

cancer

A cellular malignancy in which the affected cell displays unregulated growth and division and lack of differentiation as it invades adjacent tissues and proliferates. The altered cells, which form solid or diffuse tumors, are classified by the tissue from which they arise and are described according to a histogenetic system. (Specific malignancies are listed in alphabetical order by body site.)

Etiology and incidence: The transformation of normal cells into cancer cells (carcinogenesis) appears to be a multistep process involving many factors. Thus far, no single theory of causation has satisfactorily explained this process. Causative agents have been identified for some forms of cancer, and others are being investigated. Cancer is the second leading cause of death in the United States. Each year, more than 540,000 persons die of cancer, and 1.25 million new cases are diagnosed. Although various forms of cancer strike different societal subgroups, it is a universal disease seen across cultural, racial, gender, age, and socioeconomic groups.

Pathophysiology: Cancer occurs when certain cells proliferate without organization and with little or no differentiation. It has been theorized that certain stimuli, as yet to be definitively identified, initiate this proliferation by overpowering the normal mechanisms controlling growth. The result is uninhibited growth, uncontrolled function, and rapid motility, permitting spread of the cancerous cells to other parts of the body through invasion of adjacent tissue or migration via the blood or lymph system. The migration process is commonly called *metastasis*. The primary site of a malignancy (cancer cell growth) is the site of original growth; a secondary site is created when cells migrate to and colonize an additional body site.

Clinical Manifestations

The American Cancer Society lists seven warning signs of cancer that require immediate attention from a physician: (1) a change in bowel or bladder habits; (2) a sore that does not heal; (3) unusual bleeding or discharge; (4) a thickening or lump in the breast or elsewhere; (5) indigestion or difficulty swallowing;

(6) an obvious change in a wart or mole; and (7) a nagging cough or hoarseness.

Complications

The prognosis generally declines as the disease stage advances (with evidence of lymph node involvement or metastasis). If the condition goes untreated, the cancer cells continue to proliferate, and eventually death results. Cardiac tamponade, pleural effusion, and paraneoplastic syndromes, which are all complications that can occur with various malignancies, are oncological emergencies.

Diagnostic Tests

Cancer screening is an important tool in the early detection and diagnosis of cancer. The following chart summarizes the American Cancer Society's screening recommendations for asymptomatic individuals of average risk.

Examination	Gender	Age	Frequency
Sigmoidoscopy	M/F	>49	3 to 5 years
Stool blood test	M/F	>49	Annually
Digital rectal examination	M/F	>39	Annually
Prostate examination and prostate-specific antigen test	M	>49	Annually
Pap smear and pelvic examination	F	Sexually active or by age 18	Annually
Endometrial tissue sample	F	Menopause or high-risk individual*	Menopause
Breast self-examination	F	>19	Monthly
Clinical breast examination	F	>20-39	Every 3 years
		>39	Annually
Mammography	F	40 to 49	1-2 years
		>49	Annually

Health counseling and cancer check-up†	M/F	20 to 40 >40	Every 3 years Annually

C

*History of infertility, obesity, failure to ovulate, abnormal uterine bleeding, or estrogen therapy
†Counseling on use of tobacco, sun exposure, diet, risk factors, sexual practices, and environmental and occupational exposures

If screening techniques and the clinical examination indicate the possibility of cancer, a definitive diagnosis is made through histopathological examination of tissue obtained by aspiration cytological techniques or by excisional, endoscopic, or bone marrow biopsy. If an unequivocal diagnosis is made, staging is done for prognostic information and to guide treatment decisions. A comprehensive system known as the TNM system has been developed. It involves assessment of three basic components: the size of the primary tumor (T); whether regional lymph nodes (N) are involved; and whether distant metastases (M) are present.

Therapeutic Management

Surgery	Removal of primary tumor with or without lymph nodes and adjacent structures; palliative procedures to relieve symptoms
Drugs	Chemotherapeutic agents, hormones to reduce size of tumor and induce remission; immunotherapy or biologic response modifiers to strengthen immune function
General	Radiation therapy to reduce size of tumor and check metastasis; bone marrow transplant

See the following:

Bladder Cancer	*Lung Cancer*
Bone Cancer (Primary)	*Lymphoma (Non-Hodgkin's)*
Brain Tumor (Primary)	*Myeloma (Multiple)*
Breast Cancer	*Oral and Oropharyngeal Cancer*
Cervical Cancer	*Ovarian Cancer*
Colorectal Cancer	*Pancreatic Cancer*
Esophageal Cancer	*Prostate Cancer*

Hodgkin's Disease

Kaposi's Sarcoma

Kidney Cancer (Renal Cancer)

Leukemia

Liver Cancer (Primary)

Skin Cancer

Stomach Cancer (Gastric Cancer)

Testicular Cancer

Thyroid Cancer

Uterine Cancer (Endometrial Cancer)

cardiac tamponade

An acute and rapid collection of blood in the pericardial sac causing compression of the heart and decreased cardiac output

Etiology and incidence: Cardiac tamponade occurs when blood or fluid accumulates around the heart within the pericardial sac. Although not common, this occurs secondary to trauma to the heart, chest, or diseases such as pericarditis. The onset may be sudden or slow, but in either case, it is life threatening.

Pathophysiology: Normally, the pericardial sac holds 30 to 50 ml of fluid. In cardiac tamponade, fluid or blood fills the pericardial space causing compression and pressure on the heart. As the blood or fluid accumulates, the excessive extracardiac volume restricts blood flow in and out of the ventricles, causing decreased cardiac output and eventual systemic cardiac compromise.

Risk Factors

Blunt or penetrating trauma to the chest or heart
Acute pericarditis
Cardiac surgery

Clinical Manifestations

General	Anxiety, restlessness, and feeling of fullness in the chest; change in mental alertness
Cardiovascular	Muffled and distant heart sounds, tachycardia, decreasing blood pressure or pulses; pulses paradoxus, narrowed pulse pressure, jugular venous distention, elevated cardiovascular pressure (CVP), shock
Respiratory	Dyspnea, shortness of breath

Complications

Cardiopulmonary arrest

Diagnostic Tests

There are no specific diagnostic tests. History and clinical evaluation are diagnostic for therapeutic intervention of this life-threatening condition.

Therapeutic Management

Surgery	*Emergency intervention:* Immediate needle aspiration of pericardial fluid or blood (pericardiocentesis) is the only nonsurgical method to rapidly decompress the pericardial space. Thoracotomy is the definitive surgical treatment to correct the underlying problem.
Drugs	No specific drugs; treat underlying cause
General	Cardiac monitoring, especially during the pericardiocentesis

cardiomyopathy

Any structural or functional abnormality of the ventricular myocardium that results in enlargement or ventricular dysfunction and is not attributable to pressure or volume overload or to segmental loss of muscle function secondary to ischemia. The three major classifications are dilated (congestive) cardiomyopathy, hypertrophic cardiomyopathy, and restrictive cardiomyopathy.

Etiology and incidence: Cardiomyopathy is idiopathic in origin. However, underlying disease processes and factors may produce symptoms of cardiac involvement that simulate cardiomyopathy and as such, are important to consider. These processes include coronary artery disease (CAD); infections of all types (bacterial, viral, parasitic, fungal, rickettsial, spirochetal, helminthic); granulomatous diseases (sarcoidosis, giant cell myocarditis, granulomatosis); metabolic disorders (beriberi, kwashiorkor, thyrotoxicosis, myxedema); neoplasms; connective tissue disorders; hereditary autosomal dominant disorders, pheochromocytoma, acromegaly, neurofibromatosis; amyloidosis, fibroelastosis, Gaucher's or Löffler's disease; and toxins or drugs (alcohol, cocaine, cobalt, catecholamines, cyclophosphamide, psychotherapeutics, radiation, carbon monoxide, arsenic, immunosuppressive drugs).

Pathophysiology: Dilated cardiomyopathies are characterized by abnormal systolic pump function, gross dilation of the heart, and damage to the myofibrils. The cardiac valves and coronary arteries remain grossly normal. Hypertrophic cardiomyopathies are characterized by disordered diastolic function and reduced distensibility, as well as a marked pattern of distinctive hypertrophy involving thickening of the interventricular septum and a reduction in the size of the ventricular cavities. The ventricular walls become rigid and increase the resistance to blood flow from the left atrium. Ventricular outflow is obstructed, impeding ventricular ejection during systole. Restrictive cardiomyopathy is marked by abnormal diastolic filling and excessively rigid ventricular walls. Contractility is relatively unimpaired, and systolic emptying is normal.

Clinical Manifestations

Dilated type	Exertional dyspnea, fatigue, peripheral edema, neck vein distension, rapid pulse, narrowed pulse pressure, and crackles (symptoms usually are chronic)
Hypertrophic type	Chest pain, syncope, palpitations, exertional dyspnea, fatigue
Restrictive type	Exertional dyspnea, fatigue, edema, narrowed pulse pressure, distended neck veins

Complications

Complications include mural thrombus formation, pulmonary embolus, severe heart failure, and sudden death. The prognosis is poor in all categories of disease.

Diagnostic Tests

Chest x-ray	*Dilated:* Enlarged cardiac silhouette, prominent left ventricle, pleural effusions
	Hypertrophic: Enlarged cardiac silhouette
	Restrictive: Mild cardiac enlargement
Electrocardiography	*Dilated:* Left ventricular (LV) hypertrophy, sinus tachycardia, atrial and ventricular dysrhythmias, ST segment and T-wave changes, conduction disturbances
	Hypertrophic: LV hypertrophy, ST segment and T-wave changes, Q waves in inferior and precordial leads, atrial and ventricular dysrhythmias
	Restrictive: Low-voltage; conduction disturbances
Echocardiography	*Dilated:* LV dilation, abnormal diastolic mitral valve motion, decreased ejection fraction
	Hypertrophic: Narrow LV outflow tract, thickened septum, systolic ante-

rior motion of mitral valve, decreased LV chamber

Restrictive: Increased LV thickness and mass, pericardial effusion

Radionuclide studies
Dilated: LV dilation, hypokinesis, reduced ejection fraction

Hypertrophic: Hyperdynamic systolic function, reduced LV volume, increased muscle mass, ischemia

Restrictive: Myocardial infiltration

Cardiac catheterization
Dilated: LV enlargement and dysfunction, mitral and tricuspid regurgitation, elevated diastolic filling pressures, reduced cardiac output

Hypertrophic: Decreased LV compliance, mitral regurgitation, hyperdynamic systolic function, LV outflow obstruction

Restrictive: Decreased LV compliance, elevated diastolic filling pressures, normal systolic function

Therapeutic Management

Surgery
Dilated: Cardiac transplantation

Hypertrophic: With septal myopathy, myectomy

Restrictive: Excision of fibrotic endocardium

Drugs
Dilated: Symptoms direct intervention (e.g., diuretics or digitalis with congestive heart failure, anticoagulants to prevent mural thrombus formation, antidysrhythmics for dysrhythmias)

Hypertrophic: Beta-adrenergic blockers and calcium antagonists to decrease ventricular contractility and increase ventricular volume and outflow; with mitral valve regurgitation, antiinfectives as prophylaxis against endocarditis

Restrictive: Drugs to treat underlying disorders

General
Hemodynamic or cardiac monitoring, cardioversion for atrial fibrillation, intraaortic balloon pump to sustain severely depressed ventricular function, restriction of fluid and sodium intake, oxygen therapy, rest, exercise restrictions

carpal tunnel syndrome

Tingling sensation and decreased functioning in the wrist, hand, and fingers resulting from compression of the median nerve

Etiology and incidence: The exact cause is unknown, but highly repetitive flexing motions of the wrist are strongly implicated. Conditions that cause edema (e.g., diabetes, pregnancy, congestive heart failure, and renal failure) also have been suggested as causes. One theory links carpal tunnel syndrome to a vitamin B_6 deficiency in conjunction with repetitive movements. The incidence of carpal tunnel syndrome has increased dramatically over the past decade; it is one of the three leading occupational-related conditions in the United States and occurs most often in women.

Pathophysiology: The median nerve in the volar aspect of the wrist is compressed between the longitudinal tendons of the forearm muscles that flex the hand and transverse superficial carpal ligament. This causes paresthesias in the thumb, forefinger, middle finger, and half of the ring finger.

Clinical Manifestations

Pain, weakness, clumsiness, heaviness, numbness, burning, and tingling in one or both hands are the usual manifestations. The pain may be worse at night and lessen during the day unless the person's activities require repetitive wrist flexion. The pain may radiate to the shoulder and forearm.

Complications

If left untreated, carpal tunnel syndrome can cause permanent nerve damage with loss of sensation and movement.

Diagnostic Tests

Clinical evaluation with characteristic signs such as inability to make a fist; positive Tinel's sign (tingling and burning produced by light tapping over the tendon sheath on the ventral surface of the wrist); positive Phalen's sign (pain or numbness after 30 seconds of wrist flexion); wasting around fingernails; history of repetitive use; underlying disease; last trimester of pregnancy; weakened muscle response on electromyogram.

Therapeutic Management

Surgery	Release of carpal ligament for decompression of nerve if conservative measures are ineffective
Drugs	Local corticosteroid injections into tendon sheath to reduce inflammation
General	Restriction of repetitive wrist flexion, cock-up splints at night to reduce nerve pressure and relieve pain
	Cold laser treatments that reduce inflammation and improve circulation are pending Food and Drug Administration (FDA) approval.

cataract

A congenital or degenerative opacity of the lens that leads to a gradual loss of vision

Etiology and incidence: Cataracts are associated primarily with aging (senile cataracts) and chemical changes in lens proteins. Trauma, toxins, systemic disease, and intraocular inflammation are also causes. Congenital cataracts, which are rare, are the result of inborn errors of metabolism, exposure of a first-trimester fetus to rubella or toxins, and congenital anomalies. Cataracts are the third leading cause of blindness in the United States, and virtually everyone would develop cataracts if they lived long enough. More than 60% of those over age 65 and 90% of those over age 85 demonstrate lens opacities.

Pathophysiology: Senile cataracts form as a result of a chemical change in the gelatinous lens protein encapsulated behind the iris. As a result, the protein coagulates, the lens gradually clouds, and normal lens fibers swell and migrate within the lens. Because of these changes, a blurred image is cast on the retina. If the condition goes untreated, the opacity eventually becomes complete and blindness results.

Clinical Manifestations

Symptoms include progressive, painless blurring and distortion of objects, glare from bright lights, and gradual loss of vision. Signs include a gray or white coloring on the pupil and myopia.

Complications

The primary complication is blindness.

Diagnostic Tests

Cataracts are identified by ophthalmoscopic or slitlamp examination.

Therapeutic Management

Surgery	Intracapsular (rare) or extracapsular removal of the lens; follow-up laser surgery to remove secondary membrane that often forms
Drugs	Topical antiinfective drugs, mydriatic-cycloplegics, and hyperosmotic agents are used preoperatively; corticosteroids and mydriatics are used post-operatively
General	Corrective lenses, lens implants, and eyeglasses to correct farsightedness

cellulitis

A diffuse, spreading, acute inflammation and infection of the skin and subcutaneous tissues

Etiology and incidence: The most common cause of cellulitis is infection with *Streptococcus pyogenes* or *Staphylococcus aureus* after a break in the skin. It also can be caused by infection of gram-negative bacilli associated with diabetic foot ulcers or various bacteria introduced by animal or insect bites.

Pathophysiology: A break in the skin caused by trauma, ulceration, or lymphedema is invaded by a pathogen, setting up an inflammatory and infectious process. The infection spreads because the pathogen produces enzymes capable of breaking down the cellular components that usually wall off and contain the inflammation.

Clinical Manifestations

Local redness, swelling, and tenderness, usually of the lower extremities, are the most common presenting symptoms. The skin is hot to the touch and may have an orange peel–like appearance and texture. Red streaks may extend from indistinct borders, and purulent discharge may be present. Occasionally systemic manifestations develop, such as chills, fever, headache, and tachycardia.

Complications

Rare complications include severe necrotizing subcutaneous infection with gangrene and permanent damage to the lymphatic system.

Diagnostic Tests

The diagnosis is made by clinical examination.

Therapeutic Management

Surgery	Incision and drainage of abscesses, débridement of necrotic tissue

Drugs	Antiinfective drugs to treat infection, analgesics for pain
General	Immobilization and elevation of affected area to reduce edema; cool, wet dressings to relieve pain

C

cerebral aneurysm

A localized dilation of the wall of a cerebral artery. Most ruptured aneurysms (95%) are classified as saccular (berry) aneurysms. Other categories include fusiform and mycotic aneurysms.

Etiology and incidence: Cerebral aneurysms come from congenital defects in the vessel wall coupled with secondary factors such as atherosclerosis, head trauma, arterial hypertension, infection, and polycystic disease. It is the fourth leading cerebrovascular disorder in the United States, with 24,000 new cases diagnosed annually. The peak incidence is between ages 35 and 60, and women are affected slightly more often than men.

Pathophysiology: *Saccular aneurysms* are small, berrylike sacs that protrude outward in a pouch formation on cerebral arteries, primarily at bifurcations or branches of major arteries in the circle of Willis. A weakness in the vessel wall allows the intima to bulge outward, creating a sac that fills with blood to the point of rupture. Rupture occurs when pulse pressure creates a hole in the sac, leading to subarachnoid hemorrhage and irritation of the cranial nerves and underlying cortex. The damage depends on the severity of bleeding.

A *fusiform aneurysm* involves the entire circumference of the artery. It develops over time as the elastic fibers undergo degenerative changes, smooth muscle is replaced by fibrous tissue, and cholesterol deposits build up on the intima. These aneurysms usually form at the trunk of the basilar artery and rarely rupture. *Mycotic aneurysms,* which are rare, occur as a result of a systemic infectious process that causes arterial necrosis and leads to the formation of multiple aneurysms along the distal branches of the anterior or middle cerebral arteries.

Clinical Manifestations

Most aneurysms cause no symptoms until they rupture. At that point, typical symptoms include severe, abrupt-onset headache; stiff neck; nausea; vomiting; steadily increasing neurological deficits; seizures; and loss of consciousness. The extent of the symptoms depends on the location of the aneurysm and the severity of the bleeding. Ruptures are divided into five grades. Grade I ruptures involve minimal bleeding, no neurological deficit, and no loss of consciousness. The person is alert, and the only symptoms may be a slight headache and a stiff neck. Grade II ruptures involve mild bleeding, and the person displays mild neurological deficits (e.g., weakness) in addition to headache and nuchal rigidity. With grade III (moderate) bleeding, the person is confused or drowsy (or both) and has a severe headache, nuchal rigidity, and mild focal neurological deficits. Grade IV (severe) bleeding produces stupor, mild hemiparesis, and possibly decerebrate posturing. Grade V bleeding produces coma and decerebrate posturing.

Complications

Rupture often leads to residual neurological deficits, a permanent vegetative state, or death.

Diagnostic Tests

CT scan/MRI	To detect blood in subarachnoid space and displaced cerebral structures
Angiography	To determine whether aneurysm is intact
Lumbar puncture	Contraindicated with any sign of increased intracranial pressure (ICP)
Skull x-rays	Calcification of aneurysm wall
EEG	Shifts in cerebral structures

Therapeutic Management

Surgery	Resection, clipping, ligating, or wrapping of intact or remaining aneurysm after bleeding; ventriculostomy to treat increased ICP; ventriculoatrial shunt to treat hydrocephalus; evacuation of blood clots
Drugs	Anticonvulsants to control seizures, antihypertensives to control elevated blood pressure, corticosteroids to reduce cerebral edema; drugs to control vasospasms, stool softeners to prevent constipation and straining, analgesics for pain, chlorpromazine for shivering, antifibrinolytic agents to prevent bleeding in individuals who are not candidates for surgery
General	Ventilatory support; seizure precautions; antiembolic stockings; monitoring of neurological, cardio-

vascular, and hemodynamic systems; safety precautions; prevention of disuse syndrome; rehabilitation for residual neurological deficits or coma stimulation; instruction in how to avoid straining at stool

cerebral palsy

A broad classification encompassing nonprogressive motor disorders caused by prenatal, perinatal, or postnatal central nervous system damage and characterized by impaired voluntary movement and possible perceptual, intellectual, and language deficits and convulsive seizures. The four major categories of cerebral palsy (CP) are spastic, dyskinetic, ataxic, and mixed CP.

Etiology and incidence: A variety of prenatal, perinatal, and postnatal factors, alone or together, contribute to the development of CP. Prenatal causes, which are implicated in 44% of cases, include genetic factors, chromosomal abnormalities, teratogens, malformations in the brain, intrauterine infection, and fetal or placental transport malfunction. Perinatal causes (27% of cases) include prematurity, preeclampsia, sepsis, birth trauma, and asphyxia. Postnatal causes (5% of cases) include meningitis, head injury, and toxins. The cause is unknown or not readily apparent in 24% of diagnosed cases.

Among infants and children in the United States, the incidence of CP is about 2:1000. CP is the most common cause of permanent disability in children, and the incidence is rising.

Pathophysiology: CP has no characteristic pathological picture. Neurological damage varies widely and is manifested in a number of ways. Anoxia seems to play a major role, but that role is ill defined. Spastic syndromes (70% of cases) involve the upper motor neurons. Dyskinetic syndromes (20% of cases) involve the basal ganglia. Ataxic syndromes (10% of cases) involve the cerebellum or cerebellar pathways, or both.

Clinical Manifestations

Clinical signs and symptoms evolve as the damaged nervous system matures; the signs and symptoms vary according to the location and severity of the neurological damage.

General	Gross motor delays, abnormal motor performance, alteration of muscle tone, poor head and trunk control, poor balance, excessive docility or irritability, persistence of primitive reflexes

Spastic type	Weakness, paralysis, muscle wasting, and spasticity involving one to four limbs; scissors gait; toe walking; weakness of oral and lingual muscles with dysarthria, tongue thrusting; difficulty swallowing; abnormal posture; sudden, rigid extension of body while sitting; opisthotonic posturing
Dyskinetic type	Slow, involuntary writhing movements of the trunk, mouth, and limbs that increase with stress and cease during sleep; abrupt, jerky movements of distal extremities; severe dysarthria; drooling; choking and coughing while feeding
Ataxic type	Weakness; incoordination; intention tremor; wide-based, ataxic gait; rapid, repetitive movements; disintegration of movement in upper extremities when reaching
Associated problems	Intellectual, hearing, and visual impairments; language deficits; seizures; hyperactivity; short attention span

Complications

Aspiration and aspiration pneumonia may occur because of swallowing and choking with feeding. Hip dislocations, scoliosis, and joint contractures may occur because of hypertonicity or tone imbalance. Dental problems (e.g., malocclusion, gingivitis, caries, enamel defects) occur secondary to drooling, spasticity, and inadequate oral hygiene. Constipation is common. Skin breakdown and pathological fractures can result from disuse syndrome.

Diagnostic Tests

Because the clinical signs of CP emerge as the neurological system matures, it is rarely possible to detect CP in early infancy. Specific categorization of the syndrome may be impossible before age 2, and other progressive neurological disorders must be ruled out. A thorough neurological examination and history are the primary diagnostic tools in CP. Gross motor delays; motor abnormalities; and altered muscle size, function, and tone are crucial diagnostic indicators. Moro reflex persisting after age 4 months and tonic neck reflex persisting after age 6 months are also useful indicators. High-risk children should be monitored closely.

Therapeutic Management

Surgery	Correction of hip displacement, release of contractures, lengthening of heel cord to prevent tiptoe stance, spinal instrumentation for scoliosis, implantation of intrathecal pump to deliver medication for spasticity, dorsal rhizotomy (rare) to control spasticity
Drugs	Muscle relaxants and antianxiety agents to reduce spasticity and facilitate movement, anticonvulsants for seizure activity, stool softeners or suppositories for constipation
General	Long-term medical monitoring by neurologists, orthopedists, and pediatricians
	Physical therapy to reduce spasticity; maintain ROM; prevent contractures; promote head and trunk control; and improve balance, sitting, standing, and ambulation
	Occupational therapy to improve oral motor skills (sucking, chewing, swallowing) and facilitate activities of daily living (ADLs)
	Speech therapy to improve language and communication skills
	Adaptive equipment to assist mobility (wheelchairs, braces, scooter boards, standers); communication (communication boards, computers, switch controllers, power pads); recreation (adapted toys); and ADLs (bath aids, environmental control units, feeding aids)
	Counseling for child and family to adapt to disability

Education under provisions of the Americans with Disabilities Act (ADA)

Case management to provide support and to coordinate efforts by health care team

Respite care to aid primary caregiver

C

cerebrovascular accident (stroke)

Impairment of one or more vessels in the cerebral circulation, caused by thrombosis, embolus, stenosis, or hemorrhage, which interrupts the blood supply and results in ischemia of brain tissues

Etiology and incidence: A cerebrovascular accident (CVA) is caused by occlusion of a cerebral vessel. Most cerebrovascular occlusions occur secondary to atherosclerosis or hypertension, or a combination of the two. Other risk factors are diabetes mellitus, myocardial infarction (MI), bacterial endocarditis, rheumatic heart disease, aneurysms, head trauma, sick sinus syndrome, and a history of previous stroke or transient ischemic attacks (TIAs). CVA is the second most common cause of neurological disability and the third most common cause of death in the United States. More than 3 million persons are diagnosed with CVA each year, and of those diagnosed, there are more than 160,000 deaths. The incidence increases with age, with adults age 65 or older at greatest risk.

Pathophysiology: The general pathophysiology of a CVA involves occlusion of a cerebral vessel, which leads to ischemia of the brain tissue supplied by that vessel. If the obstruction is not removed, the affected tissue infarcts and dies, causing permanent neurological deficit or death. The severity of the CVA depends on the location and extent of the obstruction, the degree of collateral circulation, and the promptness of diagnosis and treatment.

Thrombotic strokes account for approximately 40% of ischemic cerebrovascular disease. The occlusion develops slowly over time as the atherosclerotic plaque builds up in the large-vessel walls. A TIA is a common precursor. Symptoms often evolve over hours or even days and are noticed when the person awakens in the morning. Damage from a CVA is generally extensive because of the large vessels involved and the likelihood that collateral circulation is diminished or absent.

Emboli, which cause 30% of strokes, arise when platelets, cholesterol, fibrin, or other miscellaneous hematogenous material break off from the arterial walls or the heart and travel to and block a cerebral vessel. The onset of symptoms is generally sudden and usually occurs in small distal cortical vessels, affecting cortical functions.

Lacunar strokes, which account for 20% of all CVAs, occur where small perforating arterioles branch off large cerebral vessels in the basal ganglia, internal capsule, and brainstem. The small subcortical arterioles are exposed to the constant high-pressure flow of the large branch arteries. Over the years the smaller vessels become thickened, thrombosed, and then obstructed. The resulting damage is distinctive, and these strokes are often labeled "pure motor" or "pure sensory" strokes.

Intracerebral hemorrhage accounts for 10% of all strokes and is the most catastrophic type. The onset is sudden, often occurs during exertion, and is triggered by bleeding that obstructs and ruptures the small subcortical arterioles in the deep brain. The pathology of the bleeding is not well understood, although some research indicates that it may be precipitated by microaneurysms that cause arteriolar necrosis.

Risk Factors

Underlying disease processes such as hypertension, diabetes, cardiovascular disease, blood dyscrasias

Personal history of previous CVA, aneurysm, rheumatic fever, or heart valve replacement

Familial history of arteriovenous malformation

Elevated serum cholesterol, lipoproteins, and/or triglycerides

Use of medications such as anticoagulants or oral contraceptives

Use of tobacco products

High-fat, high-cholesterol diet

Lack of exercise

Clinical Manifestations

The signs and symptoms of a stroke depend on the site and size of the obstruction. They typically include altered mental status, hemiparesis or hemiplegia, receptive or expressive aphasia, dysarthria, dysphagia, apraxia, hemianopsia, urinary incontinence, and emotional lability. Headache, seizures, stupor, and marked hypertension may also be present.

Complications

Coma and death are the most severe consequences of CVA. Permanent neurological deficits (e.g., paralysis, impaired intellectual capability, speech defects, loss of short-term memory, impaired judgment and problem-solving abilities, reduced impulse control) are common residual complications.

Diagnostic Tests

Clinical evaluation	Any of the above clinical manifestations, particularly in individuals with identifiable risk factors, decreased carotid pulse, or carotid bruit
CT scan/MRI	To identify area of infarct or bleeding
Ultrasonography	To identify diminished blood flow in vessels
Angiography	To detect occlusion of large vessels
Electroencephalopathy	To detect focal slowing around a lesion
Brain scan	To detect diminished blood flow, infarction, blood clots or arteriovenous malformation

Therapeutic Management

Surgery	Evacuation of hematoma or clot; placement of intracranial pressure (ICP) monitor; endarterectomy to remove atherosclerotic plaques; cerebral artery bypass surgery to increase blood flow to the brain; balloon angioplasty with intraarterial shunt to open stenosed vessels
Drugs	Thrombolytic enzymes such as tissue plasminogen activator (TPA), streptokinase, or urokinase to break up the thrombus or embolus and help restore blood flow to the brain
	Drugs must be given within 4 (TPA) to 8 (urokinase) hours of the incident. These drugs are not used for hemorrhagic strokes.
	Anticoagulants during stroke evolution to prevent further thrombosis; antihypertensives to control blood pressure; diuretics to reduce edema in the brain; anticonvulsants to control seizures; long-term aspirin therapy to prevent future stroke

General   Monitoring and support of vital functions; prevention of decubitus ulcers, thrombosis, and pneumonia; rehabilitation (e.g., occupational therapy for adapting activities of daily living, physical therapy to increase strength, range of motion and endurance; gait training to improve ambulation; cognitive therapy to improve memory and problem solving; speech therapy to improve communication; counseling for post-stroke depression and altered sexual functioning; vocational retraining

cervical cancer

Cancer of the cervix, predominantly squamous cell carcinoma (90% of cases). The remaining 10% are adenocarcinomas and are thought to be related to in utero exposure to diethylstilbestrol.

Etiology and incidence: Cervical cancer is now generally considered a sexually transmitted disease (STD). Probable agents are the human papilloma viruses, with the herpes simplex virus a possible cofactor. Cancer of the cervix is the third most common malignancy of the female reproductive tract, with more than 15,800 cases of invasive cervical cancer diagnosed annually in the United States; in addition, 65,000 cases of carcinoma in situ (preinvasive) are diagnosed each year. Incidence is higher in minority women (e.g., black, Hispanic, and Native American). More than 4,800 deaths from cervical cancer occur annually in the United States. Cervical cancer is the leading cause of cancer death in underdeveloped nations, particularly Latin America, Africa, India, and Eastern Europe.

Pathophysiology: Cervical cancer begins as a neoplastic change in the cervical epithelium and eventually involves the full thickness of the epithelium. An invasive tumor forms in a cauliflower shape, with a friable texture and a hard, nodular edge. The bladder, rectum, and lungs are common sites of invasion and metastasis.

Risk Factors

Onset of intercourse before age 20
Multiple sex partners
Teenage and/or multiple pregnancies
Smoking
History of genital warts or other sexually transmitted diseases
History of immune deficiency disease
Deficiency in vitamins A, C, and folic acid

Clinical Manifestations

Cervical cancer has no characteristic or typical symptoms. Bleeding, which begins as a blood-tinged discharge and progresses to spotting and frank bleeding, is the only significant sign. The bleeding is caused by ulceration of the epithelial surface; however, some tumors spread without ulceration and thus without bleeding. Other possible indicators include prolonged menstrual periods or an increase in number of periods and bleeding immediately after intercourse.

Complications

The prognosis with carcinoma in situ and noninvasive tumors is excellent, with survival rates approaching 100%. The prognosis with advanced disease has been poor (5-year survival is 58%), and complications arise from spread to the bowel, bladder, and pelvis and metastasis to the lung. Recent clinical trials using a combination of chemotherapy and radiation in advanced disease have improved the 5-year survival rates to 73%.

Diagnostic Tests

If a Pap smear of the cervix reveals atypical cells, a definitive diagnosis is obtained by colposcopy or biopsy. Cervicography may aid in staging of the tumor.

Therapeutic Management

Surgery	Conization, cryotherapy, electrocautery, or laser ablation to treat carcinoma in situ; hysterectomy to treat tumors with no parametrial invasion; pelvic exenteration to treat advanced disease
Drugs	Chemotherapy (cisplatin, 5-flourouracil) in combination with internal radiation for treatment of advanced disease
General	Combination of chemotherapy and radium implants to treat invasive disease and recurrences, external radiation as a palliative measure, counseling for body image and changes in sexual functioning
	Pap smear annually for early detection

chickenpox

An acute, viral, communicable disease characterized by clusters of maculopapular skin eruptions that become vesicular and produce a granular scab

Etiology and incidence: The cause is the varicella-zoster virus, which invades the body through the respiratory membranes. Chickenpox is a common childhood illness, with susceptibility typically extending from age 6 months to the time the disease is contracted. Epidemics occur in the winter and early spring in 3- to 4-year cycles. Immunity is produced after a course of the disease. More than 120,000 cases are reported annually in the United States. Case numbers are projected to drop with increases in immunization.

Pathophysiology: The virus enters the body by means of direct droplet contact through the respiratory system. The incubation period is 2 to 3 weeks before localized and systemic signs and symptoms appear. The person is considered infectious from the time of exposure until the final lesions crust over. After recovery, the virus is believed to remain in the body in a dormant or latent state in the dorsal root ganglia. Reactivation of the infection in adulthood manifests itself as shingles.

Clinical Manifestations

The first signs and symptoms are mild headache, low-grade fever, malaise, and anorexia, which occur about 24 hours before the first rash appears. The initial rash, which is maculopapular, appears on the head and mucous membranes and evolves within hours to itching, teardrop-shaped vesicles containing a clear fluid. The vesicles break and crust over within 6 to 8 hours. New lesions erupt in successive crops on the trunk and in sparse sprinkles on the extremities. The acute phase of the disease lasts 4 to 7 days, and new lesions seldom appear after the fifth day. All lesions are generally healed in 2 to 3 weeks.

Complications

The disease may be severe in adults, or in individuals whose T-cell immunity is depressed or who are taking corticosteroids or undergoing chemotherapy. Complications include conjunctival ulcers, encephalitis, meningitis, thrombocytopenia, secondary abscesses, cellulitis, pneumonia, sepsis, Guillain-Barré syndrome, and Reye's syndrome. Scratching of the lesions may cause scarring and disfigurement.

Diagnostic Tests

Diagnosis depends primarily on clinical examination of the characteristic lesions. Giemsa-stained scrapings from the lesions will show multinucleated giant cells, and a culture of vesicular fluid will grow the varicella-zoster virus.

Therapeutic Management

Surgery	None
Drugs	Antihistamines, topical steroids to relieve itching; acyclovir or zoster immune globulin after exposure in high-risk individuals; vaccine for prevention; *no salicylates* (aspirin-containing drugs)
General	Baking soda paste or calamine lotion on lesions to relieve itching, isolation until lesions crust, trimming of nails and use of mittens to prevent scratching of lesions, cool room and distractions to lessen focus on itching
Prevention	Varicella vaccine after first birthday

Chlamydia trachomatis infections

A constellation of sexually transmitted infections comprising urethritis, cervicitis, salpingitis, and lymphogranuloma venereum

Etiology and incidence: The cause is the *C. trachomatis* bacterium, which is transmitted during intercourse with an infected individual. Newborns of infected mothers may contract associated otitis, conjunctivitis, and pneumonia during passage through the birth canal. In countries with endemic areas, the disease can be spread through close contact within households. More than 4.5 million persons in the United States contract chlamydial infections each year, and these infections are the most common source of sexually transmitted diseases (STDs) world-wide. Chlamydial infections also are the leading cause of infant blindness in underdeveloped countries.

Pathophysiology: After intimate contact with an infected individual, the *Chlamydia* bacterium attaches to and is then ingested by the columnar epithelial cells in various receptacle sites, where it multiplies in the host cell. Common sites are the urethra and prostate in men and the urethra and cervix in women. The rectum and pharynx are sites for both genders. Sites for infants and children include the conjunctivae and respiratory tract.

The pathogenesis after this point is unclear, but most likely an immune response is triggered, producing a patchy, inflammatory response in the submucosa. This is spread by the lymphatics to such sites as the epididymis in men and the fallopian tubes in women. Inflammatory exudate is eventually replaced by fibrous tissue, leading to strictures in the urethra, epididymis, and fallopian tubes and scarring of the conjunctivae.

Lymphogranuloma venereum produces a localized, nodular lesion that spreads regionally via the lymph system (primarily the inguinal nodes), producing other nodular lesions, which mat together and form large abscesses. If the condition is left untreated, abscesses form throughout the lymph system and often rupture through epithelial surfaces, creating draining sinuses and fistulas.

Risk Factors

Unprotected sexual contact (vaginal, anal, oral) with an infected
  partner
Multiple sexual partners
Direct contact with mucous membranes of infected person
Vaginally delivered infants of infected mothers

Clinical Manifestations

Manifestations vary, depending on the mucous membrane
initially involved and the infecting strain of *C. trachomatis.*

Urethritis/cervicitis	Often asymptomatic; urinary pain and frequency; scanty mucoid urethral discharge (men), mucopurulent vaginal discharge (women); pain in scrotum with epididymitis; flank tenderness with salpingitis
Lymphogranuloma	Early sign is lesion on penis, labia, vagina, cervix, or rectum; men then have lymphadenopathy; systemic signs include fever, chills, severe headache
Pharyngeal infection	Asymptomatic or sore throat; red, dry tongue
Rectal infection	Bloody diarrhea, purulent discharge
Trachoma and conjunctivitis	Purulent discharge from eyes

Complications

Complications from untreated disease include urethral and
rectal strictures, pelvic inflammatory disease, sterility, fistulas,
elephantiasis, blindness, and pneumonia.

Diagnostic Tests

The primary diagnostic tools are a clinical examination with a
history of exposure to an infected partner or multiple partners,
and a culture of exudate that tests positive for *C. trachomatis.*

Therapeutic Management

Surgery	None
Drugs	Antiinfective drugs sensitive to *C. trachomatis* following treatment guidelines for type and dosage issued by the Centers for Disease Control and Prevention (CDC)
General	Cautioning patient to refrain from sexual activity until he or she is free of disease and to trace all potentially exposed sex partners, screening of high-risk populations to treat infected individuals and reduce the reservoir, information about STDs

cholecystitis, cholelithiasis, and choledocholithiasis

Acute or chronic inflammation of the gallbladder (cholecystitis) usually associated with gallstones (cholelithiasis), which lodge in the cystic duct. Choledocholithiasis is obstruction of the common bile duct by gallstones.

Etiology and incidence: Chronic cholecystitis is caused by repeated acute episodes. The cause of cholelithiasis is not clear, although abnormal metabolism of cholesterol and bile salts plays a crucial role. Most cases of acute cholecystitis (95%) are caused by gallstones lodged in the cystic duct. Five percent of cases are associated with trauma, burns, infection, prolonged anesthesia, or critical illness. Choledocholithiasis results when gallstones lodge in the common bile duct.

An estimated 35 million people in the United States have cholelithiasis, and 1 million new cases are diagnosed each year. Gallstones occur more often in women and in certain ethnic groups such as Native Americans. The incidence increases with age.

Pathophysiology: Gallstone formation begins with supersaturation of bile with an insoluble solute such as cholesterol or calcium bilirubinate. Rapid precipitation of cholesterol crystals occurs through some as-yet-unexplained process involving mucin glycoproteins. The precipitates grow under static conditions (i.e., reduced gallbladder motility or contractility) and form macroscopic stones. When the stone obstructs a cystic duct, the gallbladder distends and the wall becomes edematous and compresses capillaries and lymphatic channels, producing inflammation of the mucosa. The inflamed, ischemic mucosa allows reabsorption of bile salts, which sets up further damage. If the condition goes unchecked, the wall becomes friable and necrotic and is susceptible to perforation. When a stone obstructs the common bile duct, it often causes extrahepatic obstructive jaundice, infection, pancreatitis, or liver disease.

Risk Factors

High-calorie, high-cholesterol diet
Obesity
Lack of exercise

Underlying disease processes such as diabetes mellitus, regional enteritis, or blood dyscrasias

Use of medications such as birth control, estrogen supplements, and/or cholesterol-lowering drugs

Multiple pregnancies

Familial history of gallbladder disease

Clinical Manifestations

Acute cholecystitis	Colicky pain in right upper quadrant and right lower scapula; nausea, vomiting; low-grade fever
Chronic cholecystitis	Anorexia, flatulence, nausea, fat intolerance, episodic or diffuse abdominal pain, heartburn
Cholelithiasis	Asymptomatic
Choledocholithiasis	Asymptomatic; jaundice and pain

Complications

Necrosis and perforation of the gallbladder with generalized peritonitis, cholangitis with or without septic shock, pancreatitis, biliary cirrhosis, and bowel obstruction with perforation and peritonitis are all complications of biliary disease.

Diagnostic Tests

Ultrasonography	To visualize gallstones
Biliary scintigraphy	If common bile duct is obstructed, gallbladder cannot be visualized on scan
Transhepatic cholangiography	To visualize stones in common bile duct

Therapeutic Management

Surgery	Laparoscopic cholecystectomy to remove gallbladder, endoscopic procedure to remove stones by balloon or basket, sphincterotomy to release ductal stones into intestine, laparotomy with cholecystectomy and T-tube placement in some cases when other methods are not appropriate

Drugs   Oral urodisol to dissolve stone, methylterbutyl ether instilled directly into gallbladder via percutaneous transhepatic catheter to dissolve stone, antiinfective drugs, analgesics

General   Lithotripsy delivers external shock waves to pulverize stones

Prevention   Low-fat diet, exercise program

chronic fatigue syndrome (immune dysfunction syndrome)

A poorly understood illness characterized by pervasive, chronic, and incapacitating fatigue

Etiology and incidence: The etiology is unknown, although popular theories propose a viral link or an overactive immune system. Chronic fatigue syndrome is a relatively new phenomenon and is most often associated with professionals in their 20s and 30s. The syndrome is diagnosed in women twice as often as in men. Cases are now being increasingly diagnosed in children.

Pathophysiology: The cause is unknown, but a viral infection (e.g., herpesvirus, retrovirus, or enterovirus) in interaction with a dysfunctional immune response is suspected.

Clinical Manifestations

The primary symptom is persistent or relapsing debilitating fatigue that does not respond to bed rest and that reduces normal activity levels by 50% or more for 6 months or longer. Other signs and symptoms include low-grade fever; sore throat; pharyngitis; painful, palpable cervical or axillary lymph nodes; myalgia; arthralgia; sleep disturbances; depression; and inability to concentrate.

Complications

None known

Diagnostic Tests

No definitive test exists. A clinical evaluation that includes the primary symptom plus six to eight other signs and symptoms is the most reliable indicator. Tests to rule out other disorders (e.g., leukemia, lymphoma, or underlying psychiatric disorders) are important.

Therapeutic Management

Surgery	None
Drugs	Investigational antiviral drugs and immune modulators are under study in clinical trials
General	Supportive measures, balanced regimen of exercise and rest cycles, counseling for depression, support groups for coping

chronic obstructive pulmonary disease

An umbrella term encompassing a cluster of diseases, including asthma, bronchitis, bronchiectasis and emphysema, in which recurrent obstruction of airflow is a prominent feature. (See also asthma, bronchitis, bronchiectasis, and emphysema.)

Etiology and incidence: Causes are discussed under the specific disease processes; however, smoking, air pollution, and industrial exposure are major risk factors. More than 30 million persons in the United States are estimated to have some type of chronic obstructive pulmonary disease (COPD). This disease constellation is the fourth leading cause of death in the United States with more than 106,000 deaths reported annually.

For Pathophysiology, Clinical Manifestations, Diagnostic Tests, and Therapeutic Management, see the specific disease.

cirrhosis

A chronic, degenerative disease of the liver characterized by destruction of the hepatic parenchymal cells, which are replaced by regenerative nodules surrounded by fibrotic tissue. (See also esophageal varices.)

Etiology and incidence: The etiology is not fully understood, but several factors play important roles, including alcohol abuse; malnutrition; infectious processes (e.g., hepatitis, schistosomiasis, syphilis); toxins (e.g., arsenic, carbon tetrachloride, phosphorus); drugs (e.g., chlorpromazine, methyldopa, methotrexate, tolbutamide, isoniazid, amitriptyline); genetic disorders (e.g., galactosemia, Wilson's disease, alpha-antitrypsin deficiency); congenital malformations (e.g., biliary atresia); and vascular disorders (e.g., portal vein thrombosis, Budd-Chiari syndrome, chronic heart failure). Other factors remain unknown.

In the United States, most cirrhosis develops secondary to alcohol abuse and is the tenth leading cause of death, with more than 25,000 deaths reported annually. The most rapidly growing type of cirrhosis is occurring secondary to hepatitis C infections. In Africa and Asia, cirrhosis secondary to chronic viral hepatitis B is a major cause of death.

Pathophysiology: Cirrhosis is the end-stage disease that begins with one of the many etiologic factors. The development and progression of cirrhosis are tied to the severity of the injury and the liver's response. A severe, acute injury may be involved, as in hepatitis, or a moderate chronic injury may be the cause, as in alcohol abuse. When an injury causes destruction of parenchymal cells, the initial response is fibrosis, as the liver attempts to repair itself. Fat-storing cells proliferate and are transformed into myofibroblasts, which alter the secretion, synthesis, and degradation of collagen. This results in deposition of excessive connective tissue, which alters normal lobular structures, interferes with cellular nutrition, obstructs hepatic blood flow, and forms anastomotic channels that shunt arterial blood away to efferent hepatic veins. The regenerative attempts continue as long as an injury is present. The resulting changes in the intrahepatic circulatory pathways make the system less efficient and eventually lead to an increase in portal vein pressure. The change in or destruction of lobular architecture interferes with various liver functions, such as metabolism, detoxification, storage, and blood and bile formation.

Risk Factors

Excessive chronic alcohol ingestion
Malnutrition
History of infectious diseases (e.g., hepatitis, schistosomiasis, syphilis); biliary disease; vascular disorders (e.g., portal vein thrombosis, Budd-Chiari syndrome, chronic heart failure) genetic disorders (e.g., galactosemia, Wilson's disease, alpha-antitrypsin deficiency)
Use of hepatotoxic drugs
Exposure to hepatotoxic chemicals or toxins

Clinical Manifestations

Early	Often asymptomatic; otherwise, abdominal pain, diarrhea, nausea, vomiting, fatigue, fever
Midcourse	Chronic dyspepsia, constipation, anorexia, weight loss, pruritus, easy bruising, bleeding gums, nosebleeds, upper gastrointestinal bleeding, enlarged liver
Late	Telangiectasis, spider angiomas, enlarged breasts, testicular atrophy, jaundice, impotence, enlarged spleen, depression, abdominal vein distention, ascites, encephalopathy, peripheral neuropathy

Complications

Complications include bleeding esophageal varices, which can lead to massive hemorrhage; hepatorenal syndrome, which leads to renal failure; and hepatic encephalopathy, which leads to coma and death.

Diagnostic Tests

Liver biopsy	Definitive histological changes
Serum albumin	Decreased
Prothrombin time	Prolonged
CBC	Evidence of anemia, leukopenia, thrombocytopenia

Blood glucose	Decreased
Ultrasonography	Hepatosplenomegaly, enlarged portal veins
Liver scans	Reduced liver uptake

Therapeutic Management

Surgery	Liver transplantation for advanced disease, portal systemic shunt to treat resistant esophageal varices, peritoneovenous shunt for ascites
Drugs	Diuretics to reduce edema, digestants to promote fat digestion, supplemental vitamins; stool softeners
General	Elimination of toxic agents such as alcohol or drugs; diet high in protein, carbohydrates, and calories and low in sodium; blood and blood products, gastric lavage, esophageal balloon for bleeding varices
	Transjugular intrahepatic portosystemic shunt (TIPS) to divert portal blood from liver
	Variceal sclerosis via endoscopy to treat esophageal varices
	Abdominal paracentesis for ascites
	Renal dialysis for renal failure

cold, common (upper respiratory infection)

A self-limiting, acute viral infection of the upper respiratory tract. The resulting inflammation involves the nasal passages, throat, sinuses, trachea, and bronchi.

Etiology and incidence: The common cold can be caused by one of many viruses. The rhinovirus group causes about 40% of cases. Spring and summer colds are often caused by picornaviruses, fall colds by parainfluenza viruses, and winter colds by coronaviruses. The mechanisms of spread are not clearly defined and may vary somewhat by viral type. Direct contact is implicated in rhinovirus colds; airborne infection by droplet is probably the mechanism in other viral strains. Colds are the leading cause of acute morbidity in the United States. Sixty-one million cases are reported annually.

Pathophysiology: The pathogenesis of colds is still sketchy. The virus is deposited in the nasopharynx, where it moves to the adenoids and a rich bed of viral receptors. An inflammatory reaction is evoked, resulting in vasodilation, mucus production, coughing, and sneezing about 16 hours after initial infection. The virus spreads to the ciliated epithelial cells in the nasal passages, and symptoms continue for 4 to 10 days. The virus is active for about 3 weeks and may affect the trachea and bronchi, particularly in individuals with chronic respiratory disease.

Clinical Manifestations

Typical symptoms include nasal congestion and discharge, sore throat, sneezing, coughing, headache, and fatigue. Febrile reactions occur in infants and young children but are uncommon in older children and adults.

Complications

The most common complications are the secondary overlay of a bacterial infection with purulent sinusitis or otitis media and the triggering of bronchospasms in persons with asthma.

Diagnostic Tests

The diagnosis is made by clinical examination, while ruling out secondary bacterial sinusitis, otitis media, and streptococcal pharyngitis.

Therapeutic Management

Surgery	None
Drugs	Acetaminophen analgesics for headache, nasal sprays for decongestion, saline gargle or topical anesthetics for sore throat, *no aspirin for infants or children, no antibiotics*
General	Rest for comfort and to minimize spread, proper handwashing and careful handling of items in the environment to minimize viral contact by others, adequate fluids for hydration

colorectal cancer

C

Most colorectal tumors (95%) are adenocarcinomas, which originate as benign, adenomatous polyps in the rectum or colon.

Etiology and incidence: No definitive etiologic factors have been identified, although environmental and dietary factors have long been suspected. The incidence of colon cancer in the United States ranks behind breast and lung cancer in women and prostate and lung cancer in men. Each year colorectal cancer is diagnosed in more than 138,000 persons, and it is the second leading cause of cancer deaths, with an overall rate of more than 55,000 deaths annually. In 93% of cases, the disease is diagnosed after age 50, and the incidence is equally distributed across gender lines, although women more often have cancer of the colon and men cancer of the rectum.

Pathophysiology: Over a period of 5 years or longer, the adenomatous polyps degenerate into malignant tumors, which are most often located in the rectum or lower colon. The tumor spreads by direct extension through the bowel wall and by intraluminal, hematogenous, and regional lymph node metastases. The liver and lungs are common sites of distant metastasis.

Risk Factors

Familial history of colorectal cancer and/or polyposis syndromes

Personal history of inflammatory bowel disorders and/or bowel polyps

History of cholecystomy

Diet high in animal fat and red meat (fried or broiled) and low in fiber, calcium, and vitamin D

Alcohol abuse

Smoking

Clinical Manifestations

Cancer of the bowel is largely asymptomatic during the early stages. The most common presenting sign is rectal bleeding on defecation. Changes in bowel patterns, excessive gas, bloating, and cramping may also occur. Pain is unlikely until advanced stages of the disease.

Complications

The chance of survival falls below 50% for patients with regional node involvement, and more than half of these individuals have node involvement at the time of diagnosis. Bowel obstruction or perforation, paralytic ileus, hemorrhage, and liver failure occur with advancing disease.

Diagnostic Tests

A history of risk factors, positive result on occult fecal blood test, or palpable lesion on rectal examination indicates a need for follow-up. Visualization of a lesion by colonoscopy or barium enema examination or an elevated carcinoembryonic antigen level indicates the need for tissue biopsy, which is the only definitive mode of diagnosis.

Therapeutic Management

Surgery	Excision of well-differentiated rectal tumors, resection of the colon around the tumor with removal of the associated lymphatic drainage system, colostomy, laser or bypass surgery for inoperable obstructing tumors
Drugs	Adjunct systemic chemotherapy of 5-fluorouracil (5-FU) and levamisole for colon tumors; 5-FU and metronidazole for rectal tumors
General	Radiation plus chemotherapy when four or more positive nodes are found and for palliation, instruction in ostomy care and support groups, counseling for altered body image

congestive heart failure

A complex clinical syndrome that results when the heart is unable to pump an adequate supply of blood to meet the body's metabolic needs, leading to inadequate tissue perfusion; vascular, cardiac, and pulmonary congestion; and diminished functional capacity.

Etiology and incidence: Congestive heart failure (CHF) can have a number of causes, which can be classified as either decreasing myocardial motility or increasing myocardial workload. Causes that decrease motility include coronary artery disease, myocarditis, cardiomyopathy, tumors, lupus erythematosus, and scleroderma, as well as drugs such as beta-blockers and calcium antagonists. Hypertension, valvular heart disease, intracardiac shunting, anemia, hyperthyroidism, and arteriovenous fistulas increase workload. Pericarditis, tamponade, and cardiac dysrhythmias interfere with ventricular filling. The incidence of CHF is increasing as the population ages. It is estimated that 2.5 to 3 million persons in the United States have CHF, and it is the most common hospital discharge diagnosis for individuals over age 65.

Pathophysiology: When the heart is unable to pump a sufficient supply of blood to meet the body's demands, three primary compensatory mechanisms attempt to maintain cardiac function: (1) the sympathetic nervous system response increases, with increased catecholamine discharge, in an effort to increase myocardial contractility, which in turn causes vasoconstriction that increases peripheral resistance and cardiac workload; (2) cardiac fluid volume increases in an effort to stretch the fibers in the ventricles and increase the force of the contraction; and (3) the myocardium hypertrophies in an attempt to increase the amount of contractile tissue available and thus increase contractility.

When these compensatory mechanisms are insufficient or when they are active over extended periods, they become ineffective and eventually contribute to failure of the pump. Pump failure usually begins with the left ventricle and progresses to the right ventricle. It may be either acute or chronic, depending on the cause.

Clinical Manifestations

Left ventricle failure	Tachycardia, fatigue, and dyspnea on exertion; intolerance to cold; cough; blood-tinged sputum; restlessness; paroxysmal nocturnal dyspnea; insomnia; crackles and wheezes in the lungs; ventricular and atrial gallops
Right ventricle failure	Fatigue, fullness in the neck and abdomen, ankle swelling, distention of neck veins, weakness, anorexia, nausea, liver enlargement, nocturia, ascites, tricuspid murmur

Complications

Acute pulmonary edema occurs with acute heart failure and is manifested as extreme dyspnea, cyanosis, hyperpnea, and plunging oxygen saturation. Death occurs if the condition is not treated immediately. Myocardial infarction and renal failure are other complications of CHF.

Diagnostic Tests

Blood chemistry	Elevated blood urea nitrogen (BUN), creatinine, and glucose; decreased potassium and sodium; elevated aspartate aminotransferase, bilirubin; prolonged partial thromboplastin time
Arterial blood gases	Decreased oxygen saturation
CBC	Decreased Hgb and Hct with anemia
Chest x-ray	Cardiomegaly; engorged pulmonary vasculature
Echocardiography	To visualize increased or decreased chamber dimensions, decreased wall motion
Cardiac catheterization	Definitive diagnosis of cause and extent of damage

Therapeutic Management

Surgery	Heart transplantation for end-stage failure, intraaortic balloon pump to provide circulatory assistance, left ventricular assistive device for those awaiting transplantation
Drugs	Diuretics to reduce edema and ventricular filling volume; vasodilators, antihypertensives, or alpha-adrenergic blocking agents to dilate vessels and reduce venous filling pressure and peripheral resistance; inotropics (digitalis) to increase contractility; angiotensin-converting enzyme inhibitors to reduce angiotensin II in individuals with advanced CHF
General	Bed rest with head elevated; oxygenation; low-salt diet; fluid restriction; monitoring and support of vital functions; prevention of thrombosis, pneumonia, and skin breakdown; stress reduction

conjunctivitis

An inflammation or infection of the conjunctiva of the eye

Etiology and incidence: Causes include viruses, bacteria, airborne or contact allergens, and environmental irritants (e.g., sun, wind, dust, smog, smoke, and noxious gases). Conjunctivitis is common and is easily spread when bacterial or viral in nature.

Pathophysiology: The severity varies by exposure and cause. The etiologic agent comes in contact with and irritates the conjunctiva, setting up an inflammatory response. Recurrent inflammation leads to thickening of the conjunctival layer and lid margins.

Clinical Manifestations

Bacterial type	Purulent drainage, lid swelling, moderate discomfort, redness of conjunctiva
Viral type	Clear discharge, swollen preauricular node, tearing, redness, moderate discomfort, light sensitivity
Allergen or irritant	Clear discharge, profuse tearing, feeling of something in the eye, intense itching (allergen), severe swelling of the lid, generalized redness of the eye, moderate burning feeling

Complications

If left untreated, infection may spread from conjunctiva to cornea and cause ulceration, perforation, and blindness.

Diagnostic Tests

Smears and cultures of discharge are done to determine if viral or bacterial agent is present. Conjunctival scrapings are used to rule out inclusion conjunctivitis, trachoma, and vernal conjunctivitis. Vision, intraocular pressure, cornea, iris, pupil, and pupillary response are all normal.

Therapeutic Management

Surgery	None
Drugs	Topical antiinfective drugs for bacterial cause, topical antivirals for viral cause, topical corticosteroids for allergens
General	Saline irrigation for discharge and comfort, warm compresses for inflammation and cool compresses for itching

corneal ulcer

A local necrosis of corneal tissue that ultimately leads to scarring and reduced visual acuity

Etiology and incidence: The most common cause is infection after trauma or contact lens overwear. Other causes include herpes simplex infection, chronic blepharitis, conjunctivitis, gonorrhea, trachoma, chemical burns, prolonged exposure to air in the absence of a blink reflex, and severe vitamin A or protein depletion resulting from malnutrition.

Pathophysiology: The cornea usually becomes infected or inflamed through an outside agent or chronic irritant, and a dull, grayish lesion forms and then necroses and suppurates, creating an ulcer. The ulcer may or may not infiltrate deeper layers of tissue. The deeper the penetration, the more severe the signs, symptoms, and complications. As the ulcer heals, it is replaced by fibrous tissue, which causes opaque scarring and reduced vision.

Clinical Manifestations

Pain, tearing, and photophobia are the most common manifestations. Bloodshot eyes and pus in the anterior chamber behind the cornea may be present in chronic cases.

Complications

Perforation of the cornea, with a prolapse of the iris and eventual destruction of the eye, is the major complication.

Diagnostic Tests

A fluorescein stain turns green and readily delineates the ulcerated area. A slitlamp examination allows inspection of the eye's surface and the deeper layers of the cornea to determine the extent of ulceration. Cultures identify the infectious organism.

Therapeutic Management

Surgery   Repair of any laceration or removal of foreign object; removal of prolapsed tissue; corneal transplantation for severe scarring or perforation

Drugs   Topical anesthetics for pain; topical and systemic
         antibiotics, antifungals, and antivirals to treat
         infection; topical steroids to treat inflammation;
         mydriatics to dilate pupil with increased
         intraocular pressure; cycloplegics to restrict
         eye movement and reduce pain

General Warm compresses for lid swelling; irrigation to
         cleanse eye; bilateral pressure dressings to aid
         reepithelialization; dark glasses for photophobia

coronary artery disease

A disorder that impedes the blood-flow in the arteries serving the myocardium of the heart. (See also angina and myocardial infarction.)

Etiology and incidence: The primary causes of coronary artery disease (CAD) are arteriosclerotic and atherosclerotic processes, which narrow and occlude the vessel lumen and thicken the arterial walls.

Vascular disease (CAD and cardiovascular accident [CVA]) is the leading cause of death in the United States. The incidence of CAD increases with age, with men up to five times as susceptible as women, until menopause, when risk equalizes for men and women. CAD is much more prevalent in western societies than in other areas of the world.

Pathophysiology: The exact pathological mechanisms that induce atherosclerosis are not well understood. Current hypotheses are (1) the lipid hypothesis, in which an elevation of plasma low-density lipoprotein penetrates the arterial wall and causes a lipid buildup in the smooth muscle cells, and (2) the endothelial injury hypothesis, which suggests that a mechanical or chemical injury to the endothelial barrier sets up a tissue response, with platelet adhesion and aggregation. In either case, atherosclerosis is marked by changes in and thickening of the intimal lining of the arterial vessel. Lipids, smooth muscle cells, and connective tissue form a plaquelike substance on the lining. This process is slow and may occur over a lifetime. Arteriosclerosis causes hypertrophy and subintimal fibrosis, resulting in intimal thickening and loss of elasticity of the vessel wall, which widens the pulse pressure and increases the systolic pressure. Atherosclerotic processes reinforce this loss of elasticity. Arterial lumens become increasingly narrow and may become obstructed, causing ischemia of the myocardium. The plaque may harden, calcify, and undergo fissure or rupture, simulating a thrombosis or embolus that is rapidly occluding a lumen.

Risk Factors

Underlying disease processes (e.g., hypertension or diabetes)
Familial hyperlipidemia
Gender (males ages 35 to 55, females after menopause)

High serum cholesterol and triglyceride levels
Smoking
High-fat diet
Sedentary lifestyle
Obesity
Stress
Use of birth control pills or estrogen in women under age 50

Clinical Manifestations

CAD is asymptomatic until myocardial ischemia occurs. The two major manifestations of ischemia are chest pain (angina) and myocardial infarction. See Angina and Myocardial Infarction for diagnosis and treatment options.

Crohn's disease (regional enteritis)

A nonspecific chronic inflammatory disease of the gastrointestinal system most commonly affecting the distal ileum and the colon

Etiology and incidence: The etiology is unknown, and research examining the causal role of immune factors, infectious agents, and dietary factors has proved fruitless. An estimated 30 to 50 cases occur per 100,000 persons, and the incidence is rising in underdeveloped countries, among blacks and Hispanics, and in Western and Northern European and Anglo-Saxon populations. The disease is equally distributed across gender lines, is most common among the Jewish population, and occurs primarily between ages 15 and 30.

Pathophysiology: Crohn's disease begins with lymphedema in the GI submucosa and microscopic focal ulcerations of the mucosa. The inflammation spreads slowly and progressively, involving all layers of the intestinal wall, which thicken with extensive fibrosis and granulomas as patchy ulcerations form on the mucosa. This process creates a characteristic cobblestone appearance of the mucosa. As the disease progresses, the mesentery becomes edematous and thickens, and mesenteric fat extends onto the serosal surface of the bowel, causing serositis with adhesion of bowel loops to one another. Mesenteric lymph nodes enlarge, and abscess and deep sinus tracts and fissures are formed. Eventually the lumen of the intestine severely narrows or becomes obstructed. This process often affects one segment of the intestine, skips over normal tissue, and then repeats the obstructive process in another segment (i.e., forming skip lesions).

Clinical Manifestations

Symptoms may be abrupt or insidious in onset and are characterized by exacerbations and remissions. The most common presenting features are chronic diarrhea with urgency and incontinence; abdominal pain and cramping, often in the lower right quadrant; fever; anorexia; and weight loss. However, some individuals have acute abdominal pain resembling that caused by appendicitis.

Complications

Complications of Crohn's disease can be either intestinal or systemic. An anal fistula or perianal abscess caused by chronic diarrhea is the most common complication. Other fistulas may form to the bladder, vagina, or skin. Malabsorption, obstruction, perforation, and cancer of the colon are other intestinal complications. Systemic complications include arthritis, episcleritis, stomatitis, erythema nodosum, pyoderma gangrenosum, ankylosing spondylitis, sacroiliitis, uveitis, and sclerosing cholangitis.

Diagnostic Tests

Barium series	Linear ulcerations, skip lesions, thickening of wall, narrowing of lumen
Colonoscopy	Cobblestone mucosa
Biopsy	To aid in differentiation of disease
Laboratory studies	Nonspecific; may include decreased Hgb and Hct, serum albumin, and folic acid; elevated erythrocyte sedimentation rate

Therapeutic Management

Surgery	Bowel resection with failure to respond to conservative therapy, colectomy with ileostomy when disease is limited to colon, strictureplasty to open obstructions
Drugs	Sulfasalazine, corticosteroids, and metronidazole to treat inflammation and ulceration; anticholinergics for diarrhea; fat-soluble vitamins, folic acid, iron, calcium magnesium, and zinc for replacement; immunosuppressive agents for retractive disease
General	Adequate rest; nutrition; NPO in acute phase to rest bowel, followed by total parenteral nutrition or restricted diet low in fiber; emotional support for anxiety and depression; referral to source of information and support group

croup

A general term applied to an acute viral symptom complex characterized by inflammation of the upper and lower respiratory tracts, hoarseness, a "barking" or "brassy" cough, respiratory distress, or stridor most commonly heard on inspiration

Etiology and incidence: Croup is a common respiratory disease seen most commonly in children between 6 months and age 3. The disease peaks in 2 year olds. Most often, croup is seen seasonally beginning in late fall and peaking during the early winter months. Males are considered to be more susceptible than females.

Pathophysiology: The parainfluenza viruses, especially type 1, are the common pathogens. Other less common viral causes of croup include the respiratory syncytial virus (RSV) and influenza A and B viruses. The infection causes inflammation of the larynx, trachea, bronchi, bronchioles, and the lungs themselves. Airway obstruction, if it occurs, is in an area of the trachea just below the glottis (the subglottic region). As airway obstruction increases, the work of breathing and breathing distress increase and the child tires.

Clinical Manifestations

The child often has an upper respiratory infection but can have no symptoms at all. The child is put to bed and awakens with respiratory distress including a "barking" or "metallic" cough, hoarseness, noisy inspirations, and restlessness. Often, the child is frightened and anxious. Fever may or may not be present. The child's fright and alarm on the part of the parents only make the child more anxious and make the symptoms worse. Most commonly with symptom management and calm parents, the attack subsides within a few hours and by the next day, the child appears well. Hospitalization is necessary for 1% to 15% of children with croup.

Complications

Significant airway swelling and respiratory distress may result in subepiglottic narrowing. There may be decreased breath sounds with atelectasis and hypoxemia. Hypercapnia may or may not be present. Of the children who are hospitalized with croup, 1% to 5% require intubation to ensure adequate blood and tissue oxygenation.

Diagnostic Tests

Most important to the care and treatment of croup is its correct identification. Croup must be differentiated from the following:

Epiglottitis	A rapid and progressive bacterial disease that requires prompt identification, airway protection, and antibiotics. This disease is characterized by rapid onset, high fever, drooling, and stridor.
Acute tracheitis	This bacterial infection has a similar rapid onset to croup. Differentiating characteristics include purulent secretions, high fever, and a left shift of the WBC count.
Foreign body	This may also mimic croup. Differentiating characteristics include no preceding upper respiratory infection, no fever, and confirmation of a foreign object on x-ray.

Therapeutic Management

Surgery	None
Home therapy	Mildly ill children (no stridor at rest) may be managed at home
Drugs	None
General	The child should be kept comfortable and well hydrated. Rest is important. Crying and agitation may cause fatigue and increased respiratory distress.
	Use cold-steam vaporizers or humidifiers with fine mist. If a vaporizer or humidifier is not available, the parent may take the child into the cool night air, in front of an open freezer, or into a cool basement.
Hospital therapy	Hospital admission may be necessary because of respiratory distress and resulting hypoxemia.

Drugs   Although controversial in the past, today's therapy for children hospitalized with croup generally includes steroid treatment.

General   Cool mist humidification; rest; fluids; humidified oxygen if PaO_2 is less than 60 mm Hg. Endotracheal intubation and ventilatory support may be necessary if the child's $PaCo_2$ is greater than 45 mm Hg.

Cushing's syndrome (hypercortisolism)

C

Hypersecretion of glucocorticoids by the adrenal gland, which produces a characteristic constellation of clinical abnormalities, including a moon face and truncal and neck fat pad deposits. It is classified into adrenocorticotropic hormone (ACTH)-dependent (75%) and ACTH-independent (25%) forms. ACTH-dependent forms are also referred to as *Cushing's disease*.

Etiology and incidence: An ACTH-secreting tumor causes ACTH-dependent Cushing's syndrome. The tumor may be a pituitary adenoma or an ectopic tumor. The causes of ACTH-independent Cushing's syndrome include adrenal cancer, adrenal adenoma, micronodular adrenal disease, and factitious or iatrogenic factors. Overall incidence of Cushing's syndrome is rare and is most common in women of childbearing age. Iatrogenically induced cases are on the increase.

Pathophysiology: Increased glucocorticoid production is triggered by one of the causal agents. The increased glucocorticoids act as a sort of antianabolic, creating a mediated antagonism in insulin action that results in biochemical energy deprivation. This leads to protein wasting, glucose intolerance, fragility of the vascular system, and reduced effectiveness of the immune system.

Clinical Manifestations

General	Muscle weakness and wasting; fragile, thinned skin; purple striae; easy bruising; poor wound healing; moon face; buffalo hump; heavy trunk; thin extremities; back pain; kyphosis; edema; hypertension; mood swings
Children	Precocious puberty, cessation of linear growth
Women	Masculinization (hirsutism, atrophy of breasts, clitoral enlargement, deepening voice, temporal baldness); menstrual irregularities
Men	Feminization (breast enlargement, higher voice, lighter beard); impotence

Complications

Potential complications include osteoporosis, pathological fracture, peptic ulcer, diabetes mellitus, congestive heart failure, and psychoses.

Diagnostic Tests

24-hour urine	Increased urinary-free cortisol >250 μg/day
Dexamethasone suppression	Dose of dexamethasone is given at night; positive test result shows reduced plasma cortisol levels next morning (<50% of baseline)
Metyrapone, ACTH stimulation, corticotropin-releasing hormone tests	To determine etiology
CT/MRI	To detect adrenal tumors

Therapeutic Management

Treatment is directed at the underlying cause.

Surgery	Transsphenoidal pituitary resection of the tumor; resection of ectopic tumors, adrenal adenomas, adrenal carcinoma; bilateral adrenalectomy for treatment-resistant pituitary tumor and micronodular adrenal disease
Drugs	Glucocorticoid and mineralocorticoid lifelong replacement when bilateral adrenalectomy is performed, adrenal inhibitors or ketoconazole used when ectopic tumor cannot be removed, chemotherapy with mitotane for inoperable adrenal carcinomas
General	Irradiation of the pituitary when surgery cannot be tolerated in treating a pituitary tumor, education that recovery can require a year or longer and that treatment initially makes the patient feel worse

cystic fibrosis

An inherited disease of the exocrine glands that results in multisystem involvement primarily by affecting the respiratory and gastrointestinal systems. It typically is characterized by chronic obstructive pulmonary disease (COPD), abnormally high loss of electrolytes through the sweat glands, and pancreatic enzyme insufficiency, leading to digestive impairments and malabsorption syndrome.

Etiology and incidence: Cystic fibrosis (CF) is caused by defective genes that are inherited from both parents as an autosomal recessive trait. One gene is responsible for encoding a membrane-associated protein called *cystic fibrosis transmembrane conductance regulator (CFTR)*. The exact function of CFTR is unknown, but research shows that it is closely tied to chloride transport. Current research focuses on the causes of seemingly unrelated multisystem effects.

CF is the most common lethal genetic disease among white children and young adults in the United States, with an incidence of one in 2500 to 3500 live births. Blacks also are affected, but the rate is about one in 17,000 births. CF is rare in Asians and Native Americans.

Pathophysiology: In CF, the exocrine glands are affected in one of three ways: (1) they produce and become obstructed by thickened, sticky mucus; (2) they produce excess normal secretions; or (3) they secrete excess sodium and chloride. The lungs are normal at birth, but bronchioles and bronchi soon become clogged with thick mucous plugs, leading to associated opportunistic infections and overinflation of the lungs. Bronchial walls thicken and airways remain filled with purulent secretions, leading to fibrosis and atelectasis. Chronic hypoxemia leads to hypertrophy of the pulmonary arteries, which leads to pulmonary hypertension and right ventricular hypertrophy. The pancreatic ducts also become clogged with mucous plugs, which interfere with pancreatic enzyme activity. Digestive enzymes fail to reach the small intestine, and as a result, digestion and absorption of nutrients are markedly impaired, leading to excess fat and protein in the stools. The biliary tracts in the liver become plugged with mucus and fibrose over time. Salivary glands and bile ducts may also become clogged. Sweat glands secrete abnormal levels of sodium and chloride, leading to excessive loss of these electrolytes.

Clinical Manifestations

Signs and symptoms vary widely, involve several systems, and change as the disease progresses. Some children show manifestations at birth, whereas others do not develop symptoms for years. Manifestations range from mild to life threatening. The earliest sign is a meconium ileus, seen at birth in about 10% of infants with CF. All children display sweat gland abnormalities, 85% to 90% have pancreatic and GI tract involvement, and 50% show respiratory involvement.

Sweat glands/skin	Salty-tasting skin; salt crystals on nose, forehead, and hairline; dehydration; alkalosis in heat or with fever
Pancreas/GI tract	Meconium ileus with cramps, nausea, vomiting, and abdominal distention; frequent, bulky, oily, and foul-smelling stools; normal or voracious appetite; weight loss; failure to thrive; pot belly; wasted buttocks; thin extremities; sallow skin; anemia; easy bruising; rectal prolapse
Respiratory tract	Wheezing; dry cough; rhinitis; gagging; dyspnea; intercostal retractions; use of accessory muscles to breathe; barrel chest; digital clubbing; cyanosis; repeated episodes of upper respiratory infection (URI); bronchial pneumonia
Reproductive system	Delayed onset of puberty; amenorrhea; viscous cervical secretions that block sperm entry in women; sterility in men

Complications

Complications are numerous and can include biliary cirrhosis, esophageal varices, portal hypertension, diabetes mellitus, pneumothorax, cor pulmonale, congestive heart failure, peptic ulcer, intestinal obstruction, intussusception, pancreatitis, cholecystitis,

and cardiac arrhythmias. CF is a terminal disease. However, the
median death rate has climbed from 7.5 years in 1966 to 28 years
in 1993. A few individuals have survived to age 50.

Diagnostic Tests

Clinical evaluation	Any of the above manifestations, particularly salty skin; failure to thrive; and frequent URIs; family history
Quantitative pilocarpine	Sodium or chloride concentration over 60 mEq/L
Iontophoresis sweat test	To obtain definitive diagnosis

Therapeutic Management

Surgery	Heart-lung or liver transplantation with advanced disease; treatment of complications (e.g., resection of bowel obstructions, cholecystectomy, portal shunt for esophageal varices)
Drugs	Antibiotics to treat pulmonary infections; amiloride HCl (aerosol) to inhibit sodium and water reabsorption in the lungs; DNase and other drugs to thin mucus; alpha-antitrypsin to reduce inflammation; pancreatic enzyme replacements (e.g., pancrelipase); bronchodilators to aid breathing
General	Diet therapy with 50% increase in normal caloric and protein intake, high fat intake, multivitamins, water-miscible vitamin E, sodium supplements, enteral supplementation in severe cases
	Prophylaxis against respiratory infection with pertussis, measles, influenza, and pneumonia vaccines
	Chest physiotherapy to increase movement of mucus from lungs (postural drainage, percussion, vibration, and assisted coughing; oxygen therapy for hypoxia; exercise to stimulate mucus movement)
	Long-term psychological counseling for individual and family, genetic counseling for parents, support groups, home care and respite care

cystitis

See Urinary Tract Infection.

cysts (dermoid, epidermal, sebaceous)

A slow-growing, benign cystic tumor found in the subcutaneous tissue below the skin or in the intradermal tissue of the skin

Etiology and incidence: Cyst formation is commonly caused by inflammation, internal rupture of an acne pustule or whitehead, impaired localized circulation, or trauma. Some individuals may be genetically predisposed to cyst formation.

Pathophysiology: Cysts contain a soft, yellow-white, cheesy substance that is often fetid and that forms when a hair follicle becomes obstructed. The type of cyst determines the contents of the cyst. Dermoid cysts are located deep in the subcutaneous tissue; have walls of keratinizing epidermis containing sweat glands, hair follicles, and sebaceous glands; and are often present at birth. Epidermal cysts (e.g., acne cysts) are found in the epidermis on the face, scalp, neck, and back; they contain laminated layers of keratin. Sebaceous cysts, or wens, occur primarily on the scalp and contain soft keratin, epidermal debris, and greasy material.

Clinical Manifestations

Cysts are found on or under the skin, are generally less than 3 cm in diameter, and are round, firm, globular, and movable to the touch. They are nontender unless infected. Cysts, particularly sebaceous type, can grow as large as a grapefruit.

Complications

Cysts may become infected.

Diagnostic Tests

A characteristic lesion is seen on clinical examination.

Therapeutic Management

Surgery	Excision of the cyst and cyst wall, incision and drainage of infected cysts
Drugs	Antibiotics for infected cysts
General	Instruction not to touch, squeeze, or pick lesions, since this may lead to infection

decubitus ulcer

See Pressure Sore.

depression

Depression is an abnormal mood state in which a person characteristically has a sense of hopelessness, helplessness, worthlessness, despair, morbid thoughts, and psychomotor retardation or agitation.

Etiology and incidence: Many adults have experienced "blue" days and feelings of depression. This depression is often situational, and soon, everything feels right again. However, clinical depression is a mood state that lasts longer and causes the individual to become dysfunctional. It is the most frequently occurring psychiatric condition in the general population. The onset of depression occurs usually in the twenties, but it may begin in infancy, childhood, or later-stage adulthood.

The American Psychological Association DSM-IV categorizes depression as *major depressive disorder, single episode* (severe symptoms of depression lasting every day for most of the day for at least 2 weeks); *major depressive disorder; recurrent* (two or more major depressive episodes with a separation between episodes of at least 2 months); and *dysthymic disorder* (a chronic, milder depressive disturbance almost every day for most of the day for at least 2 years). It is estimated that the prevalence of major depression in women ranges from 20% to 25% and in men from 5% to 12%. Dysthymic depression is found in approximately 6% of the general population. The suicide rate secondary to depression is approximately 15%.

Pathophysiology: The two subsets of clinical depression are exogenous or reactive, and endogenous. *Reactive depression,* also referred to as *secondary depression,* is precipitated by something outside the person such as loss of a loved one, environmental catastrophe, divorce, or a serious medical condition. *Endogenous* depression is primary or biological. It arises within the individual and may be caused by genetic or biochemical factors such as neurotransmitter functioning. Of the two, endogenous depression is often more severe and difficult to treat. All types of major clinical depression cause changes and abnormalities in the body's biochemical functioning including corticotropin, acetylcholine, dopamine, noradrenaline, and gamma-aminobutyric acid. Changes occur in structural brain images and reduced metabolism in the frontal cortex. Forty to sixty percent of outpatients and 90% of inpatients have abnormalities in sleep EEGs and alterations in the neurotransmitters.

D

Risk Factors

Women are commonly at a 2:1 higher risk
Biological relative with depression
Girls and women in traditional roles that reinforce dependency and passivity
Lack of job, change in social situation, divorce, change in financial status
Isolation
Chronic illness

Clinical Manifestations

Mild depression	Unpleasant feeling about self; self-sacrificing, especially in relation to giving in to others; inhabition of normal pleasurable activities or spontaneous behavior; difficulty concentrating; preoccupation with trivial things; pessimistic outlook toward life; irritability toward self for not living up to an ideal standard; dependence on others for gratification; somatic symptoms
Severe depression	Utter despair and hopelessness, sense of emptiness, unrelieved sense of guilt and feelings of worthlessness, severe immobility or agitated behavior, catatropic expectations and outlook, lack of interest in self and environment, retarded thought process, retarded bodily processes, preoccupation with self, delusional thinking, loss of contact with reality

Complications

Mild depression if not treated may migrate into recurrent major depression or a dysthymic disorder. If the depression is major or severe, the individual may be at risk for suicide.

Diagnostic Tests

Clinical evaluation	Interviewing, history taking, and clinical evaluation are important forms of diagnostic evaluation of depression.
Suicide screening	If the individual is clearly depressed, suicide screening and potential for lethality should be determined.
Blood tests	Conduct tests to screen for general medical causes and to rule out problems such as thyroid abnormalities.
Drug screens	Drug screening and drug levels should be obtained if the individual has been taking any antidepressants and/or other psychotropic agents.
Electrocardiogram	Cardiopathology should be ruled out before initiating antidepressant medications.

Therapeutic Management

Surgery	None
Drugs	Antidepressants as indicated
	Combined with antipsychotics for psychotic depression
General	*Mild:* Establish trusting, supportive relationship, therapy, and/or support group; assess strengths and coping strategies; encourage occupational and recreational therapy; provide education and support to family.
	Severe: Assess for suicidal thoughts and self-destructive behaviors; provide protective environment as indicated; establish trusting, supportive relationship; assess strengths and coping strategies; encourage occupational and recreational therapy; provide education and support to family.
	Electroconvulsive therapy may be indicated *only* if the individual does not respond to other therapies.

dermatitis (eczema)

A superficial inflammation of the skin with redness, edema, vesicles, crusting, scaling, and sometimes itching. Common types include atopic, contact, nummular, or seborrheic dermatitis, all of which may be acute or chronic in nature.

Etiology and incidence: The cause of atopic dermatitis is unknown, but the condition is often associated with other atopic diseases such as allergic rhinitis, asthma, or hay fever. These individuals have high serum levels of IgE antibodies. The response is thought to be hereditary, and it is seen in infants, children, and adults. Contact dermatitis, which can be irritant or allergic in nature, is caused by contact with various biological or chemical irritants, such as acids, alkalis, dyes, detergents, latex, metals, plant oils, and solvents. The etiology of nummular dermatitis is unknown, but the condition is associated with increased stress and winter weather and is most commonly seen in middle age. The cause of seborrheic dermatitis is also unknown; this condition is associated with hereditary factors and underlying neurological disease and can be seen in neonates and children, as well as adults.

Pathophysiology: The histological agent causes inflammatory changes in the skin, including vasodilation, edema, mononuclear cell infiltration into the dermis and epidermis, and breakdown of the epidermal cells. This leads to the visible changes on the skin's surface (e.g., redness, swelling, oozing, crusting, scaling, and itching). If the process is repeated over a period, the epidermis thickens, producing hyperkeratosis and a chronic scaly appearance.

Clinical Manifestations

Atopic type	Constant itching that sets up an itch/scratch/rash/itch cycle; red, scaly papules that coalesce into plaques that ooze and crust; common sites are hands, face, and flexural areas
Contact type	Transient redness to bulla formation; itching is common; weeping, crusting

Nummular type	Sharply circumscribed, moist, oozing discoid plaques that later become dry and scaly
Seborrheic type	Dry, diffuse scaling of scalp; oozing, crusted, red-yellow scalp lesions or scaly plaques that recur; may be found in external ear canals, eyebrows, and nasolabial folds and on sternum

Complications

Secondary infection is the most common complication. Chronic dermatitis, which appears on the hands or feet, can restrict function and become crippling.

Diagnostic Tests

Clinical evaluation with characteristic manifestations; detailed history to locate possible source of contact rash; patch test may isolate allergens; immunofluorescence shows elevated IgE in atopic dermatitis.

Therapeutic Management

Surgery	None
Drugs	Antipruritics for itching; topical/systemic cortico-steroids to relieve inflammation; topical kerato-lytics to reduce scaling
General	Oils on affected areas; removal of irritant in contact dermatitis; daily use of seborrheic shampoos; humidification; cool, wet cloths on open lesions

diabetes insipidus

A transient or permanent disturbance of water metabolism that results in excretion of excessive quantities of diluted urine. It may be pituitary (central), renal (nephrogenic), or intake regulated (primary) in nature.

Etiology and incidence: Central diabetes insipidus (DI) is the result of a lack of antidiuretic hormone (ADH), which can be caused by brain injury from head trauma, neurosurgery, irradiation of the pituitary, hypothalamic tumors, or infiltrative metastatic diseases. More than half of diagnosed cases are idiopathic. Nephrogenic DI results when the body is unable to respond normally to ADH. The condition is inherited as an X-linked recessive disorder or acquired in association with disorders such as renal disease, sickle cell disease, fibrosarcoma, granuloma, polynephritis, metabolic disease, polycystic disease, or pregnancy, or with toxic agents that reduce glomerular filtration. Primary DI results from excessive water intake caused by psychogenic disorders (e.g., schizophrenia) or dipsogenic disorders (e.g., multiple sclerosis, meningitis, encephalitis, neurosarcoidosis, or tuberculosis).

Pathophysiology: Central DI begins when some form of brain injury reduces the amount of ADH. This leads to a decrease in the hydroosmotic permeability of the distal collecting tubes in the kidney, allowing the dilute urine formed in the proximal nephrons to be excreted unchanged. The result is a slight dehydration effect, an increase in plasma osmolality, and stimulation of the thirst mechanism. The individual drinks more, and as a result input and output are balanced and osmotic pressure in the body stabilizes at an above-normal level. In nephrogenic DI the kidneys are rendered ADH resistant and hydroosmotic permeability is reduced, with the same end result as in central DI. Primary polydipsia is caused by excessive water intake, either because of a severe cognitive dysfunction or because the thirst regulator has been disrupted by disease or trauma. Plasma osmolality is reduced, which causes a decrease in the production of ADH and dilutes the urine, and excretion rises to meet intake. As intake and output are balanced, plasma osmolality stabilizes at below-normal levels.

Clinical Manifestations

The most common presenting signs and symptoms are unquenchable thirst, polydipsia, frequency of urination, polyuria, nocturia, dry skin, slight dehydration, and constipation.

Complications

A prolonged increase in urine volume and flow can lead to hydroureter and hydronephrosis. An individual who has no thirst mechanism may experience severe dehydration and circulatory collapse.

Diagnostic Tests

Fluid deprivation test	*Central and nephrogenic DI:* Urine osmolality remains low
	Primary DI: Osmolality increases
Vasopressin administration after fluid deprivation	*Central DI:* Osmolality rises
	Nephrogenic and primary DI: Osmolality is unchanged

Therapeutic Management

Surgery	None unless related to underlying disease
Drugs	*Central DI:* Synthetic vasopressin or chlorpropamide to increase urine osmolality
	Nephrogenic DI: Thiazide diuretics to reduce urine volume
General	Identification and treatment of any underlying organic cause for DI, reduction of sodium and caffeine in diet for central DI and nephrogenic DI, monitoring for hypoglycemia if chlorpropamide is prescribed, information about long-term hormone replacement therapy

diabetes mellitus

A disease complex characterized by persistent hyperglycemia caused by insufficient insulin production or resistance to the metabolic action of insulin. Diabetes mellitus (DM) is generally classified as insulin-dependent (IDDM, type I), non–insulin-dependent (NIDDM, type II), or secondary DM.

Etiology and incidence: The precise causal mechanisms in DM are unknown, although genetics and a faulty autoimmune response are thought to play major roles in type I diabetes. Genetics and obesity are risk factors for type II diabetes. Secondary diabetes is caused by an array of underlying primary pathological abnormalities such as pancreatic disease, liver disease, muscle disorders, endocrine dysfunction, genetic system defects, or as a result of drug side effects. DM has been diagnosed in more than 8 million persons in the United States, and an estimated 7 million undiagnosed cases are suspected. DM is the leading cause of irreversible blindness and chronic renal failure, and is the seventh leading cause of death in the United States. It plays a large role in cardiovascular disease and stroke. Diabetes is found worldwide, and the incidence is increasing rapidly. Type I accounts for 10% to 15% of cases, and the age of onset is primarily childhood or adolescence. Type II accounts for 85% to 90% of cases, and onset generally occurs after age 40. A small number of cases are secondary DM, and the age of onset varies according to the cause of the underlying primary pathological condition.

Pathophysiology: Diabetes occurs if the body cannot produce insulin (type I), or if it is unable to use the insulin produced (type II); in either case, the ultimate result is hyperglycemia and impaired glucose transport. Type I diabetes is characterized by a genetic predisposition manifested in one of several human leukocyte antigens. Recent research suggests that the genetic predisposition, coupled with an unknown factor, triggers an ongoing autoimmune process that systematically destroys the beta-cells in the pancreas, thereby interfering with the body's ability to produce insulin. Type II diabetes involves either a defect in the insulin release sites in the pancreas or a resistance to the action of insulin stemming from a decrease in the number of receptor sites in the peripheral tissues. This type of DM is often associated with obesity.

In both types of DM, the result is interference with glucose transport across cell membranes in peripheral muscle and adipose tissue, leading to faulty oxidation and energy production. Metabolism of fat, carbohydrate, and protein is impaired, as are storage of glycogen in the muscle and liver and storage of fatty acids and triglycerides in adipose tissue. Amino acid cell transport is disrupted. Unrestrained gluconeogenic and glyco-genolytic processes in the liver cause overproduction of glucose. As the blood glucose level rises, renal tubules fail to reabsorb all the glucose; this produces glucosuria and osmotic diuresis, with water and electrolyte loss through the urine. Hyperglycemia also damages myelin nerve coverings, leading to neuropathy. Glyco-sylation (attaching of glucose to protein molecules) in the capillaries causes thickening of the capillary membrane and microangiopathy. Atherosclerotic processes are accelerated, and vessel elasticity diminishes.

Clinical Manifestations

Type I	Abrupt onset with polyuria, polydipsia, polyphagia, weight loss, weakness, fatigue, dehydration
Type II	Usually asymptomatic in early stages, with pruritus vulvae a common presenting symptom in women; later manifestations include skin infections, cold extremities, fatigue, blurred vision, delayed healing, and polyuria

Complications

Diabetic ketoacidosis is a common acute complication in type I diabetes. If left untreated, it leads to coma and death. Nonketotic hyperglycemic-hyperosmolar coma is an acute com-plication in type II diabetes. It is often accompanied by seizure activity and has a mortality rate of about 50%. Systemic chronic complications include cardiovascular and peripheral vascular disease, retinopathy, nephropathy, neuropathy, dermopathy, and impotence.

Diagnostic Tests

Fasting blood sugar	Greater than 126 mg/dl on two occasions
Glucose tolerance test	>200 mg/dl for 2-hour sample and one other sample after administration of 75 g of glucose
Hemoglobin A_1C	Used to measure blood glucose levels cumulatively over a 3-month period A value greater than 7% is abnormal. This test is also used to monitor control of DM.
Blood insulin	Absent in type I, normal or elevated in type II
Plasma C-peptide	Absent in type I, normal or elevated in type II

Therapeutic Management

Surgery	Recommended only for chronic complications such as coronary artery grafts and eye surgery Pancreas transplant surgery in conjunction with renal transplant surgery is experimental for Type I cases.
Drugs	Insulin for type I, oral hypoglycemics for type II, thiazolidinediones (Resulin) used to resensitize the system to insulin
General	Dietary control aimed at maintaining stable body weight; distributing caloric intake into small, evenly spaced loads; avoiding high-fat, high-sugar foods; weight reduction with obesity; regular monitoring of blood sugar; education about disease, complications, medications, and diet; counseling and support for adaptation to long-term disease
Prevention	Healthy adults over age 45 should be tested for DM every 3 years.

diarrhea

A change in bowel habits marked by frequent passage of loose, watery, unformed stool. Diarrhea may be an acute or a chronic condition.

Etiology and incidence: Diarrhea can be caused by a wide range of factors such as sugar intolerance, use of antacids that contain poorly absorbed salts, laxative abuse, ingestion of large amounts of certain sugar substitutes, bacterial toxins, viral infections, bile acids, drugs, fat, carbohydrate malabsorption syndromes, mucosal disease, and bowel surgery that alter intestinal transit and strictures. Diarrhea is a common symptom that may be transient or may indicate underlying disease.

Pathophysiology: Diarrhea occurs when the amount of fluid absorbed by the body declines; when the amount of fluid produced increases, overwhelming the bowel's absorptive capacities; when motor disturbances affect bowel motility and secretory capacities; or when injury to the bowel mucosa produces blood and mucus in the stool.

Clinical Manifestations

The primary symptom is a change in normal bowel habits that results in frequent, loose, watery, unformed stools that are often accompanied by cramping, abdominal pain, and urgency.

Complications

Hypokalemia, dehydration, and vascular collapse are possible complications with severe or chronic diarrhea. Infants and small children are particularly prone to dehydration.

Diagnostic Tests

The diagnosis is made by clinical evaluation, history, and examination of the stool macroscopically and microscopically. Stool measurements, cultures, microscopic examination, and flexible sigmoidoscopy can help determine the cause.

Therapeutic Management

Surgery	None
Drugs	Antidiarrheal drugs that increase intestinal tone (paregorics), reduce peristalsis (anticholinergics), increase bulk (methylcellulose), and absorb fluid (pectin)
General	Treatment of underlying disorder, monitoring and replacement of fluid and electrolytes, perirectal skin care

diphtheria

An acute, highly communicable disease affecting the mucous membranes of the respiratory tract

Etiology and incidence: Diphtheria is caused by the gram-positive rod *Corynebacterium diphtheriae* and is spread by direct contact with an infected person, carrier, or contaminated articles or surfaces, particularly in crowded and poorly maintained environments. Effective immunization efforts have made this disease rare in many parts of the world. However, the incidence has been increasing since the early 1970s, especially in the Pacific Northwest, and children under 15 years of age are particularly vulnerable.

Pathophysiology: The pathogen invades and multiplies in the nasopharynx, producing a toxin that causes necrosis of the epithelial membrane and forms a patchy, grayish-green pseudomembrane composed of bacteria, fibrin, leukocytes, and necrotic tissue. The toxin is spread systematically by the bloodstream, and lesions form in distant organs, including the lungs, heart, kidneys, and central nervous system. The individual is communicable from exposure until the bacilli are no longer present (2 to 4 weeks). Cutaneous diphtheria, characterized by skin lesions, is also common.

Clinical Manifestations

The incubation period is 1 to 4 days; the first symptoms include a mild sore throat, nasal discharge, dysphagia, low-grade fever, cough, hoarseness, nausea, vomiting, and chills. A grayish-green membrane forms on the nasal mucosa, soft palate, nasopharynx, larynx, and tonsils. If a respiratory obstruction develops, dyspnea, stridor, retractions, hypoxia, and cyanosis may be evident.

Complications

Severe complications are common without prompt treatment; they include myocarditis, heart failure and sudden death, polyneuritis, encephalitis, renal failure, cerebral infarction, thrombophlebitis, pulmonary emboli, respiratory paralysis, pneumonia, and respiratory failure.

Diagnostic Tests

Clinical evaluation and characteristic clinical signs, particularly the membrane, are used for tentative diagnosis. Definitive diagnosis is made by culture of the causative agent.

Therapeutic Management

Surgery	Tracheostomy for airway obstruction
Drugs	Diphtheria-tetanus-pertussis immunization for all children, with periodic diphtheria-tetanus toxoid boosters through adulthood for prevention; immunization of close contacts, including health care personnel; diphtheria antitoxin given promptly on clinical diagnosis; antiinfective drugs to kill the causative gram-negative bacteria
General	Isolation, bed rest progressing to restricted activity, oxygen, fluid replacement if needed, cultures until three negative results are achieved, cultures of close contacts

diverticular disease

Inflammation of acquired, saclike projections (diverticula) that have formed in the gastrointestinal wall and have pushed the mucosal lining through the surrounding muscle; they may become infected, bleed, or rupture

Etiology and incidence: Diverticula are thought to be caused by an increase in intraluminal pressure in the bowel, which forms a pouch in weakened areas of the wall. The mechanism that weakens the wall is unclear. However, a highly refined diet lacking fiber is believed to be a contributing factor. Abnormal colonic motility patterns and spastic colon have also been implicated. The formation of diverticula is known as diverticulosis. An infection of the diverticula that causes inflammation is diverticulitis.

Diverticulosis and diverticulitis are most common in developed Western countries. The incidence of diverticulosis increases with age, and approximately one third to one half of those over age 60 have the disease; of those, 10% to 20% develop diverticulitis. Diverticulitis is more severe in those under age 50, and men are three times more likely than women to be affected in that age group.

Pathophysiology: Diverticulitis occurs when undigested food mixed with bacteria accumulates in a diverticulum, forming a hard mass called a *fecalith*. The fecalith diminishes the blood supply to the diverticulum and an infection ensues, followed by inflammation and a microperforation of the diverticular mucosa, submucosa, and adjacent serosa into the surrounding pericolic fat. A pericolic abscess forms, which may range from microscopic to a large mass. Repeated episodes of diverticulitis lead to scarring, fibrosis, stricture of the bowel wall, and continued narrowing of the lumen.

Clinical Manifestations

Complaints of pain and localized tenderness in the lower left abdominal quadrant with a low-grade fever are the typical presenting symptoms. Nausea, vomiting, and abdominal distention are also seen.

Complications

Intestinal obstruction, fistula formation, and perforation of the bowel with peritonitis and hemorrhage are possible complications of recurrent bouts of diverticulitis.

Diagnostic Tests

A history of diverticulosis, complaints of localized abdominal pain, and a possible palpable abdominal mass are highly suggestive. A flexible sigmoidoscopy may detect orifices of diverticula and thickening of bowel wall *(contraindicated during acute attack)*; a water-soluble contrast enema or CT scan is used to outline diverticula and display effacement of pericolic fat. Laboratory tests reveal a polymorphonuclear leukocytosis with an elevated sedimentation rate.

Therapeutic Management

Surgery	Bowel resection with or without colostomy to treat recurrent attacks or complications
Drugs	Analgesics for pain, antibiotics for infection, stool softeners
General	NPO with bed rest, nasogastric tube and IV hydration for acute attack, high-fiber diet after inflammation resolves, instruction about continuing diet with high-fiber content, colostomy care instructions

dysmenorrhea

Pain associated with menstruation

Etiology and incidence: The cause of primary dysmenorrhea is unknown, but the disorder is thought to be tied to uterine contractions and ischemia mediated by prostaglandin. The most common cause of secondary dysmenorrhea is endometriosis. Dysmenorrhea is a common gynecological complaint, occurring in 10% of adolescents and young adults. It declines in severity with age and childbirth.

Pathophysiology: It is thought that increased sensitivity of the myometrium to prostaglandin causes uterine contractions and ischemia of the uterine muscle, resulting in a cramping pain. Secondary dysmenorrhea is tied to an underlying pelvic disorder that produces similar cramping conditions.

Clinical Manifestations

An aching pain low in the abdomen may radiate to the lower back and legs. The pain begins with menses, peaks after 24 hours, and typically subsides within 2 days. Headache, nausea, diarrhea, and urinary frequency may also be present.

Complications

None

Diagnostic Tests

With secondary dysmenorrhea, a pelvic examination or laparoscopy or both to rule out underlying disorders is recommended.

Therapeutic Management

Surgery	Laser ablation of endometriosis, dilation and curettage (D&C), hysterectomy for underlying disorders, presacral neurectomy for primary dysmenorrhea that is unresponsive to medication
Drugs	Prostaglandin synthetase inhibitors (e.g., ibuprofen, naproxen sodium) to relieve pain; low-dose oral contraceptives if pain continues
General	Regular exercise, adequate rest, no tobacco use

Ebola virus

Ebola hemorrhagic fever is a severe, often fatal disease in humans and nonhuman primates (monkeys and chimpanzees) that has appeared sporadically since its initial recognition in 1976.

Etiology and incidence: The Ebola virus is named after a river in the central African nation of the Democratic Republic of the Congo. Until recently, only three outbreaks of Ebola virus have been identified in Zaire and Sudan. Persons in the United States are at risk only if they have close personal contact with persons in Zaire or Sudan who are infected with the Ebola virus. Although the exact origin of the Ebola virus remains unknown, researchers believe that the virus is animal-borne and is found in African animal hosts. Humans can transmit the virus to each other by direct contact with blood and/or secretions of an infected and unprotected person or by close, personal contact with health care workers working with infected persons.

Pathophysiology: Ebola is a viral hemorrhagic fever caused by the Ebola virus, a member of a family of ribonucleic acid (RNA) viruses known as filoviruses. The pathophysiology of this rare yet deadly disease remains speculative. Humans do not "carry" the virus. The manner in which the virus first appears in a human at the start of an outbreak has not been determined. It is thought that the first patient becomes infected through contact with an infected animal. The course of the disease remains inconsistent, some individuals recover and others die. It is speculated that those who die usually have not developed a significant immune response to the virus at the time of death.

Risk Factors

Exposure to diseased primates in Zaire or Sudan
Providing care for a diseased individual and not wearing full protective clothing
Contact with an unprotected health care provider who is caring for a diseased individual

Clinical Manifestations

Incubation period	Two to four days from exposure

Early

Within a few days	*Most patients:* High fever, headache, muscle aches, stomach pain, fatigue, diarrhea
	Some patients: Sore throat, hiccups, rash, red and itchy eyes, vomiting blood, bloody diarrhea

Late

Within a week of infection	*Most patients:* Chest pain, shock, and death
	Some patients: Blindness, bleeding

Complications

Cardiopulmonary collapse and death are possible complications.

Diagnostic Tests

Clinical examination	History of contact with primates or infected individual, red and itchy eyes and skin rash
Laboratory	CBC; antigen-capture enzyme-linked immunosorbent assay (ELISA) testing; IgG ELISA; polymerase chain reaction (PCR); blood cultures for malaria and virus isolation; stool culture

Therapeutic Management

Currently no standing treatments exist for Ebola hemorrhagic fever. If the fever is suspected, local and state health departments should be immediately advised.

Surgery	None
Drugs	Electrolyte replacement, antibiotics for secondary infections

Diagnostic Tests

Clinical evaluation	History of exposure, nuchal rigidity, positive Kernig's sign, pathological reflexes, muscle weakness, paralysis
Cerebrospinal fluid	Elevated pressure; WBCs, proteins slightly elevated; glucose normal; occasional isolation of the virus (mobile ameobae can be seen on wet mount)
Serology	Increase in antibody titer early in disease
Immunofluorescent stain of biopsy brain tissue	Positive for specific viruses

Therapeutic Management

Surgery	None
Drugs	Antiinfective drugs for ameobic infections: acyclovir for herpes infections, sedatives for restlessness, anticonvulsants for seizure activity, mannitol and corticosteroids to reduce cerebral edema and inflammation
General	Maintenance of fluid and electrolytes; maintenance of the airway: may need mechanical ventilation; oxygen to maintain blood gases; maintenance of nutritional status: may need nasogastric tube; seizure precautions; rest; neurological assessments; secretion precautions to prevent transmission of some viral agents; prevention of spread through mosquito-ant-tick control

endocarditis (infective endocarditis)

An inflammation and infection of the endothelial layer of the heart and cardiac valves

Etiology and incidence: Endocarditis is caused by staphylococcus, streptococcus, pneumococcus, enterococcus, and gonococcus organisms. Fungi and diphtheroids have also been implicated. Men are more susceptible, and the mean age is about 55 years. The overall mortality rate is about 25%, but it rises to as high as 70% in elderly patients.

Pathophysiology: The bacterial agent travels to the heart via the bloodstream after a transient bacteremia. They are attracted to and colonize a fibrin-platelet vegetation that forms from previous endothelial damage. The pathogens are resistant to normal host defense mechanisms because the vegetation prevents access of the defense mechanisms to the microorganisms.

Risk Factors

Personal history of rheumatic heart disease, valvular disease, or congenital heart defect
Individuals with prosthetic valves, pacemakers, or arteriovenous shunts
Recent history of invasive cardiac procedures or cardiac surgery
IV drug abusers
Immunosuppressed individuals
Multiple body piercing and tattoos
Recent history of dental or periodontal work
Use of an intrauterine device

Clinical Manifestations

Subacute bacterial endocarditis (SBE)	Onset is insidious with malaise, night sweats, chills, aching, anorexia, weight loss, intermittent fever, headache, and dyspnea over several weeks.
	When embolization occurs, petechiae of the skin and mucous membranes, splinter hemorrhages of the fingernails, macules on the palms and soles, retinal

hemorrhage, and neurological sequelae are also present.

Late signs include clubbing of the fingers and splenomegaly.

Acute bacterial endocarditis (ABE)	Rapid onset of high fever, chills, and severe aching; rapid course with embolization and manifestations of various complications

E

Complications

The course of endocarditis is progressive and fatal without treatment. Complications include stroke, congestive heart failure, renal failure, meningitis, subarachnoid hemorrhage, and heart failure.

Diagnostic Tests

Clinical evaluation	History of symptoms, risk factors, heart murmur
CBC	Anemia, leukocytosis, elevated erythrocyte sedimentation rate
Blood cultures	To identify causative agent
Echocardiography	To detect vegetations, abscesses, damaged valves, regurgitation
Urinalysis	Proteinuria, hematuria with renal involvement
Rheumatoid factor	Positive in 50% of individuals with SBE of at least 6 weeks' duration

Therapeutic Management

Surgery	Removal of thrombi, valve replacement in cases of uncontrollable sepsis
Drugs	Antiinfective drugs targeted at causative agent; aspirin for fever, aches
General	Rest, forcing fluids during temperature elevation, high-calorie supplements, monitoring for complications

endometriosis

Growth of endometrial tissue outside the uterine cavity, associated with infertility, abnormal uterine bleeding, and pain

Etiology and incidence: The cause of endometriosis is unclear, but the prevailing hypothesis suggests dissemination and implantation of endometrial cells at local ectopic sites via retrograde menstruation through the fallopian tubes and distant sites via the bloodstream or lymphatics. Sites can be anywhere in the body, but pelvic structures are most common. Another hypothesis suggests transformation of coelomic epithelium into endometrium-like glands. Approximately 25% of women can expect to develop endometriosis. It is seen most commonly during the childbearing years.

Pathophysiology: After implantation of endometrial cells, primarily on pelvic structures (e.g., the ovaries, ligaments, oviducts, and peritoneal surface of the uterus), the cells grow to form lesions. These lesions are subject to hormonal cycles and bleed during menstruation, causing irritation and inflammation of the surrounding tissue, leading to fibrosis and adhesions.

Risk Factors

Familial history
Late childbearing or nulliparity
Müllerian duct abnormalities
Cervical or vaginal atresia

Clinical Manifestations

The major symptom is secondary dysmenorrhea, although many individuals are asymptomatic. Other symptoms are abnormal uterine bleeding, dyspareunia, infertility, lower abdominal pain, nausea and vomiting, and pain associated with a full bladder or with defecation.

Complications

The primary complication is infertility or spontaneous abortion.

Diagnostic Tests

Laparoscopy with biopsy allows visualization and histological confirmation of the lesions.

Therapeutic Management

Surgery	Laparoscopy to remove or vaporize lesions, hysterectomy with bilateral salpingo-oophorectomy for intractable pain and/or extensive disease
Drugs	Gonadotropin-releasing hormone agonists, progestins, and antigonadotropic agents to inhibit ovarian function and suppress endometrial growth; prostaglandin synthase inhibitors to relieve dysmenorrhea; estrogen replacement and calcium supplement after removal of ovaries
General	Emotional support for depression, altered body image, and possible infertility

E

epididymitis

Inflammation of the epididymis of the testes. There are many causes, including different kinds of infections or trauma.

Etiology and incidence: The most frequent cause of epididymitis is a sexually transmitted disease (STD). Specifically, STDs caused by *Neisseria gonorrhoeae* and *Chlamydia trachomatis* among heterosexual men and *Escherichia coli* among homosexual men. Other causes include trauma, urological procedures, prostatitis, urethral structure disease, and seminal vesiculitis. It is the most common of all intrascrotal problems. An estimated 600,000 cases of epididymitis occur each year in the United States. Epididymitis accounts for 20% of all hospital inpatient admissions in military urology practices.

Pathophysiology: Epididymitis occurs most often unilaterally, when urine is mixed with bacteria or a virus, reflexus (flow back) from the posterior urethra, prostate ducts, or seminal vesicles. In the early stages, cellulitis associated with local pain and edema appears. As the condition progresses and becomes acute, the entire scrotum becomes erythematous and painful, often producing an inflammatory hydrocele. Late stages of the disease may cause peritubular fibrosis and occlusion of the epididymis that may result in sterility.

Risk Factors

STDs resulting in urethritis
Prostatitis
Urinary reflux or cystitis
Urological procedures
Strenuous activities

Clinical Manifestations

Scrotum	*Early stages:* Scrotal sac may be reddened, swollen, tender, or hot to touch; varicole.
	Late stages: Significant edema; redness; diffuse pain; overlying scrotal skin may be dry, flaky, and without the normal rugated appearance

Testis	The affected side may be enlarged and painful. A mass may be palpated.
Abdomen	Pain on the affected side lower quadrant may be present.
Nausea and vomiting	Pain and overall status may cause nausea and vomiting.

Complications

Orchitis is the most common complication of epididymitis. Infertility and sterility are serious long-term complications.

Diagnostic Tests

Blood tests	WBC count (elevated in acute episodes)
Urinalysis	Evidence of infection, culture may identify causative organism
Urethral discharge culture	Culture may identify causative organism, especially gonococcal or chlamydial urethritis
Prostatic secretion culture	Evidence of associated prostatitis
Doppler stethoscope and/ or testicular radio-nuclide scan	To rule out torsion of the testis

Therapeutic Management

Surgical	Rarely indicated
Drugs	Antibacterial or antiinfective agents as appropriate for identified organisms
	Analgesics for discomfort and pain management
	Antiemetics for nausea and/or vomiting
General	Bed rest; scrotal support either by positioning or by athletic support; Sitz bath, local heat, or ice packs may be used to decrease discomfort

epiglottitis (acute supraglottitis)

A severe, rapidly progressive infection of the epiglottis and surrounding tissues that causes obstructive airway inflammation

Etiology and incidence: The responsible organism for epiglottitis is usually *Haemophilus influenzae* type B. This uncommon yet serious disease is seen most often in children between ages 2 and 5 but can occur from infancy to adulthood.

Pathophysiology: The infection, acquired through the respiratory tract, moves and settles in the supraglottic region, causing inflammation, swelling, and cellulitis. The swelling is rapid and severe, resulting in mechanical obstruction of the airway. Breathing becomes difficult and as the airway swells shut, CO_2 retention and hypoxia result. Clearance of inflammatory secretions is also impaired.

Risk Factors

Children ages 2 to 5
No *H. influenzae* type B conjugate vaccine
Late autumn and winter months

Clinical Manifestations

Often the child starts with an upper respiratory infection, cold, sore throat. The common history is that the child goes to bed with slight cold-type symptoms and awakens later complaining of sore throat and pain on swallowing. The child has a fever and appears ill. As the airway swelling progresses, often quite rapidly, the child assumes a sitting position, leaning forward with chin thrust forward, mouth open, and tongue protruding outward. Drooling of saliva is common because of the inability to swallow. The child appears irritable, extremely restless, and frightened. The child is not hoarse, but because of the swelling, has a thick, muffled voice. The child's throat is red and inflamed and a distinctive, large, cherry-red edematous epiglottis is visible on careful inspection of the throat. *However, visualizing the throat should not be attempted if emergency airway equipment is not available.*

Complications

The most significant complication of epiglottitis is the loss of airway. Throat inspection should never be attempted unless the child is in the hospital and emergency airway equipment, including endotrachial intubation equipment, is available.

Diagnostic Tests

Direct visualization of the epiglottitis	Direct visualization of the epiglottitis is diagnostic, but as previously stated, manipulation of the airway may initiate sudden and potentially fatal airway obstruction.
X-ray	Lateral and anteroposterior neck x-rays may be used to differentiate between croup, bacterial tracheitis, and epiglottitis.

Therapeutic Management

Speed is vital	An adequate airway is vital and primary to all other care. Care should be taken not to upset the child. If at all possible, keep the parents with the child and keep the child in a sitting position.
Surgery	None, unless tracheostomy is needed for airway maintainance
Drugs	IV antibiotics for bacterial epiglottitis, corticosteroids may be used to reduce edema
General	Endotracheal intubation with airway support
Prevention	The American Academy of Pediatrics recommends that all children, beginning at 2 months of age, receive the *H. influenzae* type B conjugate vaccine. This vaccine is now part of the child's routine immunization schedule.

epilepsy

See Seizures.

epistaxis

Bleeding from the nose

Etiology and incidence: Epistaxis may be caused by a variety of factors such as irritation, trauma, underlying coagulation disorders, or localized or systemic infections. At least 10% of the population is thought to have suffered at least one episode of epistaxis. Children and men are more susceptible, and winter is the time of most common occurrence.

Pathophysiology: Bleeding results when damage interferes with the vascular integrity of the superficial vessels in the fragile mucosa of the nasal passages. Most bleeding originates in the anterior portion of the nose from Kiesselbach's plexus, a highly vascular network in the anterior nasal septum. Posterior bleeding usually originates from the turbinates or lateral nasal wall.

Clinical Manifestations

Bleeding from the nostrils

Complications

Pooled blood may cause sinusitis and otitis media. Large blood loss can cause anemia or interfere with cerebral and cardiopulmonary tissue perfusion. In individuals with an altered mental status, aspiration of blood is also a possible complication.

Diagnostic Tests

Inspection with a nasal speculum to determine the site of bleeding
Radiographs to locate fracture if trauma is the cause

Therapeutic Management

Surgery	Reduction and fixation of nasal fractures, ligation of the internal maxillary artery for uncontrolled posterior bleeding, split-thickness skin grafts to correct chronic bleeding in Rendu-Osler-Weber syndrome
Drugs	Analgesics for pain; if posterior chamber is packed, antiinfective drugs to prevent sinusitis and otitis

media; if a large amount of blood was swallowed, nonabsorbable antibiotics to prevent breakdown of blood and ammonia absorption

General   Upright position; pinching of the nose with thumb and forefinger for 5 to 10 minutes (anterior bleeding); cauterization of site if pressure fails; packing of nasal cavity to apply pressure (posterior bleeding); blood replacement if anemia is evident

E

esophageal cancer

Squamous cell carcinomas, which account for 60% of esophageal cancer, arise from the surface epithelium, most commonly in the middle and lower esophagus. Adenocarcinomas, which constitute the remaining 35%, arise from the gastric fundus and develop in the lower third of the esophageal tract.

Etiology and incidence: The etiology is not well defined but is associated with chronic esophageal irritation. The incidence is low in the United States, but the disease is endemic in central China and southeast Africa, with reports of 50 cases per 100,000. This cancer is most common in older adults, with blacks affected three times as often as whites and men three times as often as women.

Pathophysiology: A squamous cell carcinoma begins as a small mucosal patch that grows, ulcerates, and extends into the esophageal lumen and then the recurrent laryngeal nerve and tracheobronchial tree. Extension to the aorta and other adjacent structures also occurs. Metastasis to local and abdominal lymph nodes and to most body organs follows.

Risk Factors

Smoking and tobacco use (chewing)
Alcohol abuse
Drug abuse (e.g., morphine, opium)
Malnutrition
Environmental carcinogens (e.g., nitrosamines, silica, fungi)
History of cancer of the larynx or pharynx
History of chronic inflammation of esophagus, achalasia (failure of esophageal sphincter to relax), tylosis, or caustic burns to esophagus

Clinical Manifestations

Dysphagia is the most common presenting symptom. Regurgitation and weight loss may also occur.

Complications

The prognosis is poor, with less than 5% long-term survival. Complications of advanced disease include esophageal obstruction, hemorrhage, and perforation.

Diagnostic Tests

The tumor is diagnosed with visualization on esophageal x-ray followed by esophagoscopy with a brush biopsy.

Therapeutic Management

Surgery	Resection of tumor for palliation; esophagectomy with Dacron graft replacement; esophageal dilation to aid eating
Drugs	Preoperative systemic, cisplatin-based chemotherapy
General	Radiation for palliation and to control pain, head of bed propped up on 4-inch blocks to prevent reflux, treatment of esophagitis

esophageal varices

Dilated blood vessels in the esophagus

Etiology and incidence: The cause of esophageal varices is portal hypertension in association with cirrhosis, liver parenchymal disease, duodenal ulcer, or acute pancreatitis. About 50% of individuals with cirrhosis eventually develop bleeding esophageal varices.

Pathophysiology: Portal veins narrow and become obstructed as a result of the underlying disease process. As the lumen narrows, the venous blood returning to the right atrium from the intestine and spleen seeks new routes through collateral vessels. These collateral vessels enlarge and become tortuous, and the mucosa ulcerates.

Clinical Manifestations

Hematemesis and melena are common. However, bleeding may occur abruptly, with massive hemorrhage accompanied by blood coming out of the mouth.

Complications

Esophageal rupture, with massive hemorrhage and death, is the most common complication. With acute bleeding, the mortality rate is about 50%. Approximately 60% of individuals die within a year of the first episode of bleeding.

Diagnostic Tests

History of underlying disease, plus hematemesis or melena
Hemorrhage with varices is confirmed by an upper gastrointestinal series, and bleeding site is confirmed by endoscopy or mesenteric angiography.

Therapeutic Management

Surgery	Portacaval, splenorenal, or mesocaval shunt to relieve portal pressure; ligation of bleeders
Drugs	Vasopressin or beta-blocker to lower portal hypertension, antacids or histamine receptor antago-

nists to inhibit gastric acid, vitamin K, antibacterial agents

General   Control of acute bleeding through ice water lavage and esophageal tamponade techniques, blood transfusions, fluid replacement, sclerotherapy to thrombose varices, transjugular intrahepatic portal systemic shunting (TIPS) to divert portal blood flow from liver

E

esophagitis

See Gastroesophageal Reflux Disease.

fibrocystic breast disease

Single or multiple cysts in the breast

Etiology and incidence: The cause is unclear but is thought to be related to a hormonal imbalance, with an excess estrogen production and a progesterone deficiency during the luteal phase of the menstrual cycle. Fibrocystic disease is the most common breast condition, occurs primarily during the childbearing years, and is estimated to be present in at least half of all women. It accounts for half of all breast surgery.

Pathophysiology: The precise process of cyst formation is unknown. However, a wide variety of morphological changes occur in fibrocystic disease, including fibrosis, cyst formation, sclerosing adenosis, and ductal hyperplasia. The cysts may be nonproliferative, proliferative without atypia, or atypically hyperplastic.

Clinical Manifestations

Symptoms typically appear about 1 week before the onset of menstruation and subside about 1 week after menstruation stops. They include lumpy breast tissue; tender, burning, aching, heavy breasts; and nipple discharge.

Complications

Women with atypical hyperplasia have a greater risk of cancer. Infection is another possible complication.

Diagnostic Tests

Clinical evaluation with mammography or ultrasound
Definitive diagnosis made by biopsy and histological examination of tissue

Therapeutic Management

Surgery	Subcutaneous mastectomy for chronic disease
Drugs	Progestin/estrogen injections in second half of cycle to correct hormonal imbalance
General	Support bra, heat compresses to reduce breast pain; forgoing foods with methylxanthines (e.g., coffee, tea, chocolate), which increase metabolic breast activity

food poisoning

Enteric or neural intoxication after ingestion of bacterially contaminated food

Etiology and incidence: Food poisoning is caused by one of the following organisms: staphylococcal enterotoxins, *Clostridium botulinum, Clostridium perfringens, Vibrio parahaemolyticus,* or *Bacillus cereus.* The resulting illness is noncommunicable.

F

Pathophysiology: The causative organism multiplies in the food before ingestion; the pathogenesis is organism specific. Staphylococcal enterotoxins form in foods held at room temperature. They act on the gastric mucosa, producing hyperemia, erosion, petechiae, and purulent exudate. *C. perfringens* reproduces rapidly in cooled and reheated food and acts on the epithelial layer of the ileum, increasing absorption of fluid, sodium, and chloride and inhibiting glucose absorption. *V. parahaemolyticus* multiplies in uncooked seafood and invades the intestinal tissue, producing necrosis, ulceration, and granulocytic infiltration of the mucosa. *B. cereus,* an aerobic spore, multiplies in foods held at room temperature and attacks either the gastric or intestinal mucosa. *C. botulinum* forms a toxin in improperly processed foods in anaerobic conditions; it is a neurotoxin that impairs autonomic and voluntary neurotransmission and causes muscular paralysis.

Clinical Manifestations

The signs and symptoms depend on the causative agent.

Staphylococci	Symptoms appear within 7 hours of ingestion: weakness, acute nausea and vomiting, intestinal cramps, diarrhea
Enteric type (*C. perfringens, V. parahaemolyticus, B. cereus*)	Symptoms appear within 24 hours of ingestion: nausea, vomiting, abdominal pain, diarrhea
C. botulinum	Symptoms appear within 36 hours of ingestion: dry mouth, diplopia, loss of pupillary light reflex; nausea, vomiting, cramps, and diarrhea precede

dysphagia, dysarthria, and progressive descending muscular paralysis

Complications

The complication of enteric manifestations is dehydration, and
infants and small children are most susceptible. Botulism is fatal
in about 10% of cases, usually because of respiratory failure.

Diagnostic Tests

Cultures	Stomach contents, feces, or suspected food for causative organism
Serum	Positive for botulinal toxins

Therapeutic Management

Surgery	Tracheostomy if necessary for airway with botulism
Drugs	Trivalent botulinal antitoxin as soon as possible after onset of botulism
General	*Botulism:* Gastric lavage, mechanical ventilation if necessary, nasogastric tube feedings, fluid and electrolyte replacement, prevention of skin breakdown and contractures during paralysis, minimization of stimuli, precise communication because of altered vision and loss of speech, allaying anxiety about paralysis and treatment *Other causes:* Fluid and electrolyte replacement, instruction in prevention

frostbite

Localized cold injury

Etiology and incidence: Frostbite is caused by exposure to damp cold temperatures around freezing or to dry cold temperatures well below freezing. Susceptibility is increased by dehydration, exhaustion, hunger, substance abuse, impaired circulation, and impaired consciousness. Factors that promote heat loss (e.g., wet clothing, contact with wet metal, wind chill, radiation) increase the severity of injury, as does prolonged exposure to cold. The very young and the elderly are more prone to frostbite, as are those from warmer climates who are not acclimated to cold.

Pathophysiology: Cold exposure can cause cellular injury either by direct formation of ice crystals in the cells or by vascular spasm and occlusion, which result in inadequate tissue perfusion. Cell dehydration leads to vasoconstriction and increased blood viscosity, with sludge and thrombus formation. As thawing takes place, venous stasis occurs at the sites of injury, obstructing the vascular bed and causing edema and tissue necrosis. Tissue damage may range from superficial (skin and subcutaneous tissue) to deep (muscle, tendon, and neurovascular structures).

Clinical Manifestations

Superficial	Injured area is white, waxy, soft, and numb while still cold; as thawing occurs, area becomes flushed, edematous, and painful, and may become mottled and purple.
	In 24 hours, large blisters form and remain about 2 weeks before turning into a hardened eschar that remains for about a month before separating, leaving painful, sensitive new skin that often sweats excessively.
Deep	Injured part remains hard, cold, mottled, and blue-gray after thawing; edema forms in entire limb and may remain for months.
	Blisters may or may not form after a delay of several weeks; after several weeks, dead tissue blackens and sloughs off; a line demarcates dead from live tissue

Complications

Loss of digits, ears, nose, and extremities is possible, as is secondary infection.

Diagnostic Tests

Diagnosis is made by clinical examination plus a history of exposure to cold.

Therapeutic Management

Surgery	Escharotomy; sympathectomy for severe vaso-spasm; débridement after retraction of viable tissue (3 to 4 months after injury); amputation of nonviable extremities (several months after injury)
Drugs	Immunological agents (tetanus) and antiinfective drugs for prophylaxis; analgesics for pain; plasma expanders to reduce sludge and thrombus formation
General	Rapid rewarming by immersion in water (37.8° C to 43.3° C [100° F to 110° F]); fluid and electrolyte replacement; whirlpool baths; precautions with injured area to prevent dislodgment of eschar and further damage; counseling for altered body image from loss of limbs; exercise to prevent joint restriction

gastritis

An acute or chronic inflammation of the gastric mucosa

Etiology and incidence: Many factors can cause acute gastritis, including alcohol ingestion; drugs (e.g., aspirin, nonsteroidal antiinflammatory agents [NSAIDs], corticosteroids, cytotoxins, antimetabolites); ingested poisons (e.g., DDT, ammonia, mercury, or carbon tetrachloride); ingestion of corrosive agents; *Helicobacter pylori* infection; trauma; burns; and endotoxins. Acute gastritis occurs five times more often in those who abuse alcohol than in the general population. Chronic gastritis is associated with peptic ulcer disease, renal disease, alcoholic cirrhosis, ulcerative colitis, and diabetes mellitus. Chronic use of NSAIDs, radiation treatments, genetics, diet, prolonged emotional stress, and gastrectomy may also be predisposing factors in chronic gastritis. Type B chronic gastritis is caused by a specific infection with *Helicobacter pylori*.

Pathophysiology: In acute gastritis the stomach mucosa erodes because of hydrochloric acid and one or more predisposing factors, which serve as irritants. The erosions, which are caused by back diffusion of the hydrogen ion and mucosal ischemia, involve the granular layer and lead to submucosal hemorrhage and inflammation. Spontaneous remission occurs if the irritant is removed.

Chronic gastritis begins as an inflammatory infiltration of the lamina propria by plasma cells and leukocytes. The surface epithelial cells become flattened and necrotic in what is called the *superficial gastritis phase*. In the atrophic gastritis phase, the plasma cells and leukocytes also invade the fundic glands and intraglandular spaces, and the glands atrophy as mucous thickness decreases and the muscularis mucosae hypertrophies. Finally, in the gastric atrophy phase, the fundic glands lose the parietal and chief cells as metaplasia occurs, accompanied by thinned mucosa and minimum inflammation with marked gland loss. Type A is when chronic gastritis involves the fundus; type B is when it involves primarily the antrum with some fundic involvement.

Clinical Manifestations

Acute	Rapid onset of epigastric pain, indigestion, feeling of early fullness, anorexia, weight loss, cramping, nausea, vomiting, hematemesis, melena, general malaise
Chronic	Often asymptomatic; dyspepsia, flatulence, diarrhea, intolerance of spicy and fatty foods, no relief from antacids

Complications

Individuals who have gastric atrophy often develop pernicious anemia. Untreated gastric disease can lead to obstruction, perforation, and peritonitis. Individuals with metaplasia have a higher risk of gastric cancer.

Diagnostic Tests

Clinical evaluation	History of exposure to one or more predisposing factors or agents
Endoscopy with biopsy/cytology	To visualize lesions, erosions, and bleeding sites and to rule out carcinoma
Stool guaiac	Positive
Nasogastric aspiration	Frank blood
Serum gastrin	Elevated in type A chronic gastritis
Intrinsic factor antibodies	Present in type A
Antibodies to gastrin-producing cells	Present in type B

Therapeutic Management

Surgery	Partial or total gastrectomy, pyloroplasty, vagotomy for major uncontrollable bleeding associated with acute gastritis
Drugs	Antacids; histamine receptor antagonists and vasoconstrictors for acute gastritis; vitamins C and B_{12} in chronic gastritis with accompanying pernicious anemia; antibacterial agents for *H. pylori* infection

General   Removal of causative agents; ice water lavage to control bleeding; laser therapy by endoscopy; blood transfusions; with acute gastritis: NPO, then diet that eliminates irritants

gastroenteritis

A self-limiting, acute inflammation of the stomach and small intestine caused by ingestion of food, water, or feces contaminated with pathogenic agents, parasites, or toxins

Etiology and incidence: Causative agents include bacterial and viral pathogens, such as *Campylobacter coli, Escherichia coli, Salmonella* and *Shigella* organisms, Norwalk virus, and rotavirus; parasites, such as *Ascaris, Enterobius,* and *Trichinella* species; and toxins, such as poisonous plants or toadstools, arsenic, lead, and mercury. Inability to digest and absorb carbohydrates has also been implicated as a cause, although it is rare and the mechanism is poorly understood. Various forms of gastroenteritis are common manifestations worldwide and are often mistaken for food poisoning. Bacterial, parasitic, and viral types of gastroenteritis are infectious and can be transmitted directly or indirectly.

Pathophysiology: The pathological conditions depend on the causative agent. Toxigenic agents, such as some *E. coli* and *Shigella* strains, release an exotoxin that impairs intestinal absorption. Invasive pathogens, such as some *Shigella* and *Salmonella* species and *E. coli,* penetrate the mucosa of the small bowel, causing cellular destruction, necrosis, ulceration, bleeding, and exudation of protein-rich fluid. Pathogens such as rotaviruses attach to the mucosal wall and destroy cells in the intestinal villa, causing malabsorption of electrolytes. Parasites and toxins also interfere with intestinal functioning. The general result of all pathogenic agents is increased GI motility and increased secretion of fluids and electrolytes.

Clinical Manifestations

The onset is often sudden, with abdominal pain and cramping, nausea and vomiting, diarrhea with or without blood and mucus, anorexia, general malaise, and muscle aches. Dehydration, hypokalemia, and hyponatremia occur with persistent vomiting and diarrhea.

Complications

Dehydration, shock, vascular collapse, and renal failure, in rare instances leading to death, are complications of gastroenteritis.

Infants, small children, the elderly, and debilitated individuals are at greatest risk.

Diagnostic Tests

Diagnosis relies on identification of the causative agent through stool and blood cultures, Gram's stain, and direct swab rectal cultures.

Therapeutic Management

Surgery	None
Drugs	Antidiarrheal agents for all types; antiemetics, except for viral or bacterial gastroenteritis, in which impairment of GI motility is avoided; antiinfective agents for bacterial gastroenteritis with systemic involvement (not generally recommended for simple gastroenteritis, because these drugs may prolong the carrier state and contribute to the emergence of drug-resistant organisms)
General	Rest, increased fluid intake, electrolyte replacement, bland diet

gastroesophageal reflux disease

Esophageal, laryngeal, or pulmonary inflammation and injury related to repeated reflux of gastrointestinal contents. Esophageal inflammation is often called *esophagitis.*

Etiology and incidence: Reflux (backflow of gastric and intestinal contents into the esophagus) is the result of an incompetent lower esophageal sphincter. Factors that contribute to this incompetence include pyloric surgery; prolonged nasogastric tube intubation; drugs, alcohol, nicotine, or fatty foods, which lower intrinsic sphincter pressure; and conditions or positions (lying down) that increase intraabdominal pressure.

Pathophysiology: Hydrochloric acid and pepsin are belched back into the esophagus from the stomach. These gastric secretions attack intercellular junctions in the distal esophagus, causing patchy, superficial lesions, edema, and necrosis. When bile salts are also refluxed, they potentiate the corrosiveness of gastric secretions and attack the plasma membranes. As the disease progresses, the lesions spread to the entire esophagus. After the mucosal tissue necroses, the cells are replaced with a proliferation of basal cells, which cause a narrowing and branching of papillae, leading to hyperplasia of the esophagus. With chronic reflux, the normal squamous epithelium is gradually replaced by columnar epithelium (mucosal metaplasia). The esophagus eventually becomes scarred, develops strictures, and is shortened.

Clinical Manifestations

Early	Heartburn (particularly with spicy or fatty meals, exercise, and recumbent positions) that is relieved by antacids
Midcourse	Heartburn accompanied by high epigastric and substernal pain, regurgitation, dysphagia
Late	Bleeding, dysphagia, disappearance of heartburn

Complications

Complications include obstruction, hemorrhage, and tearing or esophageal perforation from strictures. If the gastric contents are refluxed and then aspirated, the larynx, trachea, and lungs are damaged. Repeated aspiration may lead to chronic pulmonary disease. Infants, children with brain injuries, and adults in a vegetative state are particularly susceptible to pulmonary complications from repeated reflux and aspiration. Individuals with long-standing disease have a greater risk of esophageal cancer.

Diagnostic Tests

Esophageal acidity test	To confirm reflux
Esophageal manometry	To determine sphincter competence
Acid perfusion test	To confirm esophagitis
Endoscopy with biopsy	To evaluate extent of disease

Therapeutic Management

Surgery	Fundoplication to eliminate reflux is performed in patients with severe complications, particularly recurrent aspiration pneumonia
Drugs	Antacids for pain, antisecretory drugs to reduce gastric secretions, gastrokinetics to stimulate salivation and improve sphincter pressure; *anticholinergics are contraindicated* because they lower sphincter pressure
General	Head of bed elevated; avoidance of food or drink that stimulates acid production (e.g., coffee, alcohol) or lowers sphincter pressure (e.g., smoking, chocolate, fats); many small meals; no food at least 2 hours before bedtime or remain upright 2 hours after eating; increased fluid intake; esophageal dilation to manage strictures; periodic endoscopic evaluation for cancer

G

genital warts

A sexually transmitted disease of the genitalia and perianal regions characterized by multiple fleshy, painless growths

Etiology and incidence: Genital warts are caused by various strains of the human papilloma virus (HPV) and are transmitted by sexual contact. Worldwide the incidence has been increasing rapidly over the past decade.

Pathophysiology: The virus invades superficial layers of the epidermis, infects cells in the stratum spinosum, and stimulates cell division, causing excessive cell proliferation and formation of the wartlike projections on the penis, vagina, cervix, vulva, perineum, rectum, and anus and in the perianal regions; they may also be seen on oral mucosa. Laryngeal warts have been seen in vaginally delivered infants born to infected mothers.

Clinical Manifestations

Soft, moist, fleshy pink-to-brown projections that appear in clusters on genital, perianal, or oral mucosa

Risk Factors

Unprotected sexual contact with an infected partner
Multiple sex partners

Complications

Secondary infections, giant condylomata that destroy large segments of penile tissue, and malignant transformation are all possible complications.

Diagnostic Tests

The diagnosis is made by clinical examination and confirmed by biopsy. Biopsy is also performed to rule out carcinoma and the condylomata seen in late-stage syphilis.

Therapeutic Management

Surgery	Removal by curette, cryotherapy, or electrosurgery
Drugs	Topical application of trichloroacetic acid/podophyllin/5-fluorouracil (5-FU) cream to warts
General	Refraining from sexual activity until clear of disease; examination and treatment of all potentially exposed sex partners; instruction about sexually transmitted diseases, the importance of completing treatment regimens, and the importance of regular examinations for genital and cervical carcinoma; instruction that treatment does not cure and relapse is common

G

glaucoma

A disorder in which increased intraocular pressure leads to eventual vision impairment and possible degeneration of the optic nerve. It may occur primary and secondary to other ocular disease. Glaucoma is classified as open or closed angle.

Etiology and incidence: The etiology of primary glaucoma is unknown, but predisposing factors include heredity, hyperopia, and vasomotor instability. It is estimated that 1.5% to 2% of Americans over 40 years of age have glaucoma, and more than 12% of newly diagnosed cases of blindness are attributable to glaucoma. African Americans and those with a family history are most susceptible. Ninety percent of primary glaucoma cases are the open-angle type, which occurs most often after age 65.

Pathophysiology: Increased intraocular pressure (IOP) is related to an imbalance in the production, inflow, and outflow of aqueous humor. Inflow occurs through the pupil and outflow through the meshwork at the juncture of the iris and cornea. In secondary glaucoma the meshwork becomes clogged by blood, fibrin, or inflammatory cells produced by an underlying ocular disorder. Primary open-angle glaucoma is marked by degenerative changes to the meshwork that block outflow. In primary closed-angle glaucoma, the anterior chamber is shallow, the filtration angle is narrow, and the iris obstructs the meshwork at Schlemm's canal. Sometimes dilation of the pupil or trauma pushes the iris forward, narrowing the angle and resulting in obstruction in an acute attack. Primary or secondary glaucoma may be congenital; the condition is hereditary (primary) or is caused by fetal defects in the ocular structure or underlying congenital systemic disorders (secondary).

Clinical Manifestations

Open-angle glaucoma	Often asymptomatic, frequent changes in prescription for glasses, mild headaches, vague visual disturbances, halos around lights, difficulty adjusting to darkness
Closed-angle glaucoma	Severe pain in and around eye, tearing, colored rainbow halos

around lights, recurring episodes
of blurring and impaired vision,
mild dilation of pupils, hazy
cornea, possible nausea and
vomiting

Complications

Untreated glaucoma leads to progressively diminishing vision,
degeneration of the optic nerve, and blindness.

Diagnostic Tests

G

Tonometry	To measure elevation in IOP
Visual field studies	To detect impairment in central and peripheral visual fields
Gonioscopy	To detect cellular debris or adhesions and differentiate open-angle from closed-angle type
Ophthalmoscopy	To visualize optic nerve

Therapeutic Management

In secondary glaucoma, treatment focuses on the underlying
disease process in conjunction with mydriasis.

Surgery	*Open-angle:* Laser/external trabeculoplasty to improve drainage if medications fail
	Placement of filtering devices if trabeculoplasty fails
	Closed-angle: Laser iridotomy/peripheral iridectomy to push iris back and increase angle
	Ocular implants for some complex forms of glaucoma
Drugs	*Open-angle:* Beta-adrenergic blockers and diuretics to reduce production of aqueous humor, miotics to reduce pressure, and adrenergics to increase aqueous outflow
	Closed-angle: Hyperosmotic agents, carbonic anhydrase inhibitors, and miotics to reduce pressure or abort acute attack; narcotic analgesics for pain

General   *Open-angle:* Avoidance of tobacco use, fatigue,
                 emotional upset, and ingesting large quantities
                 of fluid; instruction in instillation of eye
                 drops, and long-term use of medications and
                 their side effects.

Prevention   Glaucoma screening (annual tonometry) recom-
                 mended for adults over age 35 for early
                 detection

glomerulonephritis, acute

A primary or secondary autoimmune renal disease involving the glomerulus in the kidney and classified as postinfectious, rapidly progressive (crescentic), or immunoglobulin A (IgA) neuropathy. (See also Nephrotic Syndrome.)

Etiology and incidence: Postinfectious glomerulonephritis is caused by a bacterial, viral, or parasitic pathogen. Acute poststreptococcal glomerulonephritis (APSGN), the prototypic postinfectious disease, is caused by a streptococcal infection that occurs elsewhere in the body, such as in the respiratory tract or skin. The incidence of APSGN is dropping rapidly in developed countries. It is most common in boys ages 3 to 7 years but can occur at any age. It has a rapid onset and usually resolves spontaneously.

Rapidly progressive (crescentic) glomerulonephritis is either idiopathic, related to the production and deposition of the antiglomerular basement membrane antibody, or occurs as part of multisystem disease. This type of glomerulonephritis is rare and is most often seen in men. IgA neuropathy is idiopathic and is usually a primary disease, although it can be secondary. It is common in children and young adults, affects males six times as often as females, and is particularly prevalent in Asia.

Pathophysiology: Acute glomerulonephritis occurs when antigens from the etiologic agent provoke an antibody response, which results in antigen-antibody complexes that are deposited in the glomerular capillary walls. The deposits can be the continuous type or the more common discontinuous granular form. They cause a cascade of inflammatory changes in the glomeruli, resulting in vasoconstriction, a marked decrease in plasma flow, and a decrease in the filtering surface; this in turn reduces the glomerular filtration rate. A compensatory mechanism increases the synthesis of prostaglandins and the hydrostatic pressure in other glomeruli to increase flow and maintain the filtration rate. If acute glomerulonephritis is progressive, the compensatory mechanisms eventually induce glomerular damage through thickening and scarring of the filtration membrane.

Clinical Manifestations

APSGN	Onset of symptoms occurs 1 to 6 weeks after infection; symptoms include hypertension, headache, edema, oliguria, dark urine, reduced urine output, flank pain, weight gain, fever, chills, nausea, and vomiting; about half of cases are asymptomatic
Crescentic type	Similar to APSGN but the onset is more insidious and weakness, fatigue, and fever are the predominant symptoms
IgA neuropathy	Similar to APSGN but the onset usually occurs 1 to 2 days after upper respiratory infection or enteral illness and is often accompanied by hematuria

Complications

Complications include congestive heart failure, acute or chronic renal failure, and end-stage renal disease.

Diagnostic Tests

Urinalysis	Hematuria (microscopic or gross), proteinuria, sediment, RBC casts
Blood chemistry	Increased blood urea nitrogen (BUN), serum creatinine, and serum lipid; decreased serum albumin
Renal biopsy	Obstruction of glomerular capillaries
ASO titers	Positive in APSGN
IgA serum	Elevated in 50% of IgA nephropathy cases
IgA-fibronectin	Elevated aggregates with IgA nephropathy

Therapeutic Management

Therapy focuses on treating symptoms and preventing complications.

Surgery	Renal transplantation for end-stage renal disease
Drugs	Antihypertensives for hypertension, diuretics for edema, antiinfective drugs if infection is still

present, Kayexalate for hyperkalemia, phosphate-binding agents, corticosteroids with crescentic glomerulonephritis

General   Bed rest; fluid, potassium, and sodium restrictions; reduced protein intake if uremia is present; hemodialysis or peritoneal dialysis for renal failure

G

gonorrhea

An acute, sexually transmitted infection of the epithelium of the genitalia, perianus, and pharynx

Etiology and incidence: Gonorrhea is caused by *Neisseria gonorrhoeae*. The peak incidence occurs between 20 and 24 years of age. Infants born to mothers infected with the disease can contract gonococcal ophthalmia during the passage through the vagina.

Pathophysiology: After intimate contact, the gonococcus attaches to and penetrates the columnar epithelium, producing a patchy inflammatory response in the submucosa with resultant exudate. In men, affected areas include the urethra, prostate, Littre's and Cowper's glands, and seminal vesicles. In women, affected areas include the urethra, cervix, and Bartholin's and Skene's glands. The rectum, pharynx, and conjunctivae are vulnerable in both genders. Direct extension of the infection occurs through the lymphatics to the epididymis and fallopian tubes. The inflammatory exudate is replaced by fibroblasts, producing fibrous tissue and strictures of the lumen of the urethra, epididymis, or fallopian tubes.

Risk Factors

Unprotected sexual contact (vaginal, anal, oral) with an infected partner
Multiple sexual partners
Vaginally delivered infants of infected mothers
History of sexually transmitted diseases

Clinical Manifestations

Male genitalia	Urethral pain; dysuria, purulent discharge; urinary frequency and urgency
Female genitalia	Usually asymptomatic; urinary frequency
Pharynx	Sore throat; dry, red tongue
Perianal	Anal itching, burning, and bleeding; pain on defecation; diarrhea; rectal discharge
Conjunctivae	Purulent discharge

Complications

Complications arise with untreated disease and include pelvic inflammatory disease in women and epididymitis and urethral stricture in men. Both genders may have disseminated disease, with pustular skin lesions, septicemia, endocarditis, meningitis, and arthritis.

Diagnostic Tests

The primary diagnostic tools are the clinical examination, a history of exposure to an infected partner, and a culture of the exudate that is positive for the organism.

Therapeutic Management

Surgery	None
Drugs	Antiinfective drugs sensitive to the organism, following treatment guidelines of the Centers for Disease Control and Prevention
General	Instruction about sexually transmitted diseases and the importance of completing all treatment, refraining from sexual activity until free of disease, and tracing all potentially exposed sex partners

gout

A primary or secondary recurrent, acute arthritis of the peripheral joints, particularly the great toe

Etiology and incidence: The precise causal mechanism of gout is unknown. However, a host of factors act as precursors to overproduction or undersecretion of uric acid, including genetic factors (hyperactivity of hypoxanthine guanine phosphoribosyl transferase, superactivity of phosphoribosyl pyrophosphate, fructose intolerance); environmental factors (ethanol abuse, diuretic use, severe muscle exertion); underlying disease processes (diabetes mellitus, polycythemia, hypertension, renal disease, leukemia, sickle cell anemia); and the evolutionary absence of the enzyme uricase. Gout occurs most often in men. Gout is rare in women before menopause, and in postmenopausal women it is often linked to diuretic use. The incidence of gout is increasing in developed countries.

Pathophysiology: A factor triggers an overproduction or undersecretion of uric acid. The plasma becomes supersaturated with uric acid, and a crystal urate precipitate is formed and deposited in avascular tissues (e.g., cartilage, tendons, and ligaments of peripheral joints) and cooler tissues (e.g., the ears). Through an undefined mechanism, the crystals are released at various times, causing an acute inflammatory reaction in the joint with extension to the periarticular tissues. Repeated acute attacks lead to chronic arthritis and deformed joints.

Clinical Manifestations

Acute pain, redness, swelling, tenderness, and heat at the affected joint are typical presenting features. Fever, chills, and malaise may also be present. Limited motion is present in the affected joint or joints.

Complications

Complications include infection of ruptured deposits, renal involvement with formation of renal calculi, and secondary degenerative arthritis.

Diagnostic Tests

A tentative diagnosis is made by clinical examination and elevated serum uric acid levels and confirmed with needle aspiration of synovial fluid, which is positive for urate crystals.

Therapeutic Management

Treatment is aimed at terminating the acute attack and preventing future attacks by lowering uric acid levels and resolving existing deposits.

Surgery	Removal of large crystal deposits (tophi)
Drugs	Colchicine for long-term prophylaxis and to reduce inflammation in acute attack; nonsteroidal antiinflammatory agents to reduce inflammation in established gout; antihyperuricemic drugs for those with frequent attacks or chronic disease to reduce uric acid levels or increase excretion of uric acid (lifelong treatment); sodium bicarbonate to alkalize urine in patients who form calculi
General	Rest of joint; avoidance of alcohol and purine-rich foods, weight reduction if necessary to reduce wear and tear on joints, increased fluid intake, instruction in long-term use of medications and their side effects

G

Guillain-Barré syndrome

A rapidly progressive, acute inflammatory demyelinating polyneuropathy characterized by muscle weakness and paralysis of the extremities and possible respiratory paralysis with abnormal sensation and loss of reflexes.

Etiology and incidence: The cause is unknown, but Guillain-Barré syndrome (GBS) is hypothesized to be an autoimmune disorder involving sensitization of peripheral nerve myelin. It is thought to be connected to a previous nonspecific infection and has been associated with inoculation for swine influenza. The incidence of GBS in the United States is 1.7:100,000 individuals, and the disorder occurs across age and gender lines.

Pathophysiology: Mononuclear cells infiltrate the peripheral nervous system and set up an inflammatory response in the blood vessels of the cranial and spinal nerves. Demyelination of the peripheral nerves results, causing muscle weakness that begins in the lower extremities and ascends through the body in a symmetric fashion. Respiratory paralysis and facial weakness occur in 30% to 40% of cases. In some cases axonal destruction can cause atrophy in distal muscles and permanent neurological impairment.

Clinical Manifestations

The first sign is symmetric muscle weakness in the distal extremities accompanied by paresthesia. This weakness spreads upward to the arms and trunk and then to the face. This ascension usually peaks about 2 weeks after onset. Deep tendon reflexes are absent. Difficulty chewing, swallowing, and speaking may occur, and respiratory paralysis may develop. Bladder atony, postural hypotension, tachycardia, and heart block may be seen. Deep, aching muscle pain is also common.

Complications

About 5% of affected individuals die of respiratory failure. Another 10% have permanent residual neurological deficits. About 90% of survivors make a full recovery, but the recovery time may be as long as 3 years.

Diagnostic Tests

The diagnosis is based on the clinical presentation and cerebrospinal fluid samples, which show an increase in protein without an increase in lymphocyte count. Electromyography produces abnormal nerve conduction results.

Therapeutic Management

Surgery	Tracheostomy to provide ventilation in the event of respiratory failure
Drugs	Immunoglobulin given IV to counteract neurological defect, narcotic analgesics for pain, prophylactic antiinfectives
	Corticosteroids are generally contraindicated because they worsen the ultimate outcome; however, a trial dose of steroids may be used if disease progression is unrelenting.
General	Plasma exchange to speed recovery of neurological deficit, respiratory monitoring and mechanical ventilation for respiratory paralysis, cardiac monitoring for sinus tachycardia and bradyarrhythmia, communication systems if ventilator is used or with facial paralysis, passive range-of-motion exercises, turning to prevent contracture and skin breakdown, rehabilitation to aid neurological recovery, counseling and support of individual and family for long-term adaptation

Hantavirus

Hantavirus pulmonary syndrome (HPS) is a rare, yet potentially fatal pulmonary and systemic disease caused by contact with contaminated saliva or inhaled excreta aerosols of diseased rodents, especially the deer mouse.

Etiology and incidence: Hantaviruses are a part of the viral family *Bunyaviridae*. They represent one of the groups of zoonotic viruses, which can be transmitted from animals to humans. The human diseases associated with Hantaviruses are divided into two major groups: (1) HPS seen in North America and (2) Seoul hemorrhagic fever and renal syndrome viruses found mostly in Asia and Europe. HPS was first reported in 1993 in the Four Corners area of the southwest. Since its identification, HPS has been found in more than half of the United States. Rodents, especially the deer mouse, carry the Hantavirus that causes HPS. Infection occurs by being exposed to their droppings, specifically urine and feces. Aerosols from the urine and feces act as the transmission route for infection. Known Hantavirus infections in humans occur primarily in adults and are associated with domestic, occupational, or leisure activities that bring humans, usually in rural settings, in contact with infected rodents. Each specific Hantavirus appears to have preferential rodent hosts. Available data strongly suggest that the deer mouse is the primary reservoir of the HPS in the southwestern United States.

Pathophysiology: Rodents are the primary reservoir hosts of recognized Hantavirus. Human infection may occur when infective saliva or excreta are inhaled as aerosols produced directly from the animal. Transmission may also occur when dried materials contaminated by rodent excreta are disturbed, directly introduced into broken skin, introduced onto the conjunctivae, or possibly ingested in contaminated food or water.

Hantaviruses have lipid coverings that are susceptible to most disinfectants, or most general-purpose household disinfectants. The length of time these viruses survive after being shed in the environment is uncertain.

Risk Factors

Repeated exposure to rodent infested areas
Any activity that puts the individual in contact with rodent
  droppings, urine, or nesting materials
Use of infested trail shelters or camp in other rodent habitats
Exposure to crawl spaces under houses or in vacant build-
  ings that may have rodent populations
Houses, yards, or buildings infested with rodents

Clinical Manifestations

Incubation period	May be from 1 to 5 weeks from the time of exposure to the onset of symptoms
Early	100% of the time: fatigue; fever (lasting 3-5 days); muscle aches, especially large muscle groups such as thighs, hips, back, and shoulders.
	50% of the time: headaches; dizziness; chills; and/or abdominal problems such as nausea, vomiting, diarrhea, and abdominal pains
Late	Coughing; shortness of breath; fast breathing (26 to 30 times/min); feelings of suffocation.
	At this stage, the disease progresses rapidly, necessitating hospitalization and often ventilation within 24 hours

Complications

Within 24 hours of initial evaluation, most individuals develop some degree of hypotension and progressive evidence of pulmonary edema and hypoxia, usually requiring mechanical ventilation. Individuals with fatal infections progress to disseminated intravenous coagulation (DIC), pulmonary and cardiovascular collapse, and death.

Diagnostic Tests

Clinical evaluation	History of exposure to rodents or rodent-infested areas
Laboratory	Fall in serum albumin; rise in hematocrit; WBC count raised with shift to left; atypical lymphocytes; platelet count below 150,000; proteinuria; mild elevation of transaminase, creatine phosphokinase, amylase, and creatinine; prolonged prothrombin time and partial prothrombin time
Radiological	Characteristic radiological evolution is as follows: (1) minimal changes of interstitial pulmonary edema, (2) alveolar edema, and (3) pleural effusions

Therapeutic Management

Surgery	None
Drugs	Broad spectrum antibiotics; prompt corrective management of electrolyte, pulmonary, and hemodynamic abnormalities; vasopressors to maintain blood pressure
General	Supportive in nature; early intensive care management; careful monitoring; mechanical ventilation; severe cases may benefit from extracorporeal membrane oxygenation

hay fever

Hay fever, also called *allergic rhinitis*, is the most common seasonal acute hypersensitive reaction causing watery, itchy eyes, sneezing, nasal congestion, and clear watery nasal discharge.

Etiology and incidence: Airborne allergens or pollens from trees, weeds, or grasses are the cause. Spring reactions are mostly caused by tree pollens, summer reactions are due to grass and/or weed pollens, and fall reactions are caused by weed pollens. Occasionally, airborne fungal spores may cause allergic rhinitis. An estimated 40 million Americans have some type of allergic rhinitis. This makes hay fever among the top 10 most prevalent chronic conditions.

Pathophysiology: Susceptible persons exposed to a pollen or antigen react by producing an antibody, immunoglobulin E (IgE), which is directed at fighting the antigen. The IgE binds to mast cells (found in tissues) and basophils (found in the bloodstream) in the body. Both types of cells contain granules filled with histamine or other chemicals known collectively as mediators. When the antigen enters the body, it attaches to the IgE on the mast cells. The mast cells then break apart and release histamine. The histamine interacts with the receptors and irritates areas of the nose, eyes, and throat. Histamine release results in swelling of the nasal mucosa, runny nose, and itchy eyes. Persons who have hay fever are thought to have more IgE. This may contribute to overreaction of the immune system in hypersensitive individuals.

Risk Factors

Family history of hay fever
Known exposure to sensitive allergens

Clinical Manifestations

The nose, roof of the mouth, pharynx, and eyes begin to itch gradually or abruptly after exposure to allergens. Symptoms include watery, itchy eyes; sneezing; nasal congestion; and clear, watery nasal discharge. Pruritis may follow. Severe cases may manifest frontal headaches, irritability, anorexia, depression, and insomnia.

Complications

Secondary infections
Asthma
Perennial rhinitis

Diagnostic Tests

History and physical examination	Exposure to known allergens
	Previous seasonal history of similar signs
	Clinical findings as described above
Laboratory tests	CBC with WBC differential; sputum, nasal, and bronchial secretions may be evaluated for presence of eosinophils
Skin testing	Used to identify and/or confirm responsible pollens

Therapeutic Management

Surgery	None
Drugs	Antihistamines, decongestants, corticosteroid nasal inhalers, antipruritics
	Desensitization injections for severe cases that do not respond to episodic treatment
General	Allergen recognition and avoidance of exposure to allergens (e.g., pollens, dust, trees, weeds) responsible for the allergic response.

headache

Pain or aching of the head associated with various intracranial or extracranial factors. Headaches may be categorized as tension, vascular (cluster, migraine), or traction inflammatory.

Etiology and incidence: Although tension headaches are the most common type, their precise etiology is not well defined. However, most are related to muscle tension, minor trauma, increased stress or anxiety, food and environmental allergens, infection or lesions of the oral or nasal cavity, ear infections, or eye strain. Traction inflammatory headaches are either intracranial or cranial. Intracranial headaches may be caused by increased intracranial pressure stemming from an underlying process such as a brain tumor, abscess, or hematoma; meningitis; syphilis; tuberculosis; cancer; or subarachnoid hemorrhage. Cranial changes in the skull caused by neoplasms, temporal arteritis, or involvement of the sensory nerves of the scalp with a disease such as herpes zoster also can cause headaches. Vascular disturbances caused by exposure to toxic substances (e.g., alcohol, lead, arsenic, and carbon monoxide) are causes of headache. Some vascular headaches such as migraines and cluster headaches are idiopathic.

Each year approximately 30 million Americans seek medical treatment for recurrent headache. Tension headaches are most common and occur in adults across age and gender lines. Migraines affect about 5% of the general U.S. population, and women in their early childbearing years are the most susceptible, particularly just before or during menstrual periods. Cluster headaches are most common in men in their 30s and 40s.

Pathophysiology: Headache pain occurs when afferent pain fibers on the cranial nerves (V, VII, IX, or X) carry sensory stimuli to central nervous system tissue. The location and diffusion of the pain are dictated by the cause, the extent of tissue affected, and the cranial nerve or nerves involved. Pain can be highly localized and specific or diffuse and generalized. Involvement of the deep brain structure often causes referred pain.

Clinical Manifestations

Tension	Bilateral, dull, nonpulsatile ache, typically bifrontal or nuchal-occipital; transient or chronic

Migraine	Paroxysmal, throbbing, unilateral pain that lasts hours to days; cyclical pattern; possible nausea and vomiting; aversion to light and noise; may be preceded by an aura (shimmering visual manifestation) or prodromal behavioral alterations ranging from depression to euphoria or triggering food cravings
Cluster	Deep, agonizing, nonthrobbing pain often beginning during sleep and involving an eye, temple, cheek, and forehead on one side; lasts from 30 minutes to 3 hours, with several headaches occurring each day for several weeks; tearing and redness of affected eye
Traction	Deep, dull, steady ache that is worse in the morning and is aggravated by coughing or straining
Arteritis	Soreness of one or both temples that becomes a chronic, burning, well-localized pain; the affected scalp artery is prominent, tender, incompressible, and pulseless

Complications

Complications are usually associated with an underlying disease process rather than the headache itself. However, headaches associated with temporal arteritis, if left untreated, may cause blindness.

Diagnostic Tests

Diagnosis centers on classification of the head pain and identifying the potential cause. A neurological history and a physical examination, with identification of precipitating or underlying disease, are paramount. CT and MRI are useful in detecting intracranial lesions. Cerebral angiography may help detect vascular abnormality.

Therapeutic Management

Surgery	None
Drugs	*Tension:* Analgesics
	Migraine: Analgesics, ergot preparations, or sumatriptan for acute attacks; beta-blockers or

serotonin agonists for prophylaxis in chronic
retractable syndromes

Cluster: Prophylaxis with drugs such as valproic
acid, verapamil, or lithium carbonate is more
effective than administration of drugs during
acute attacks

General Treatment of any identified underlying disease,
application of cold or hot compresses, elimination
of food or environmental allergens, counseling,
stress management, biofeedback

H

hearing impairment (deafness)

Acquired or congenital diminished auditory capacity that may be classified as sensorineural, conductive, or central. Loss with no organic basis has been called *psychogenic, simulated,* or *functional.* Hearing loss ranges from partial to complete.

Etiology and incidence: Causes of sensorineural impairment include trauma, noise, infection, aging, exposure to certain toxins, and drugs. Conductive loss results from disorders of the middle and external ear, such as otitis media, otosclerosis, or perforation of the eardrum. Central hearing loss is induced when the brain's auditory pathways are damaged by such underlying disorders as cerebrovascular accident or a brain tumor. Congenital losses may result from fetal or neonatal anoxia; delivery trauma; fetal exposure to toxins, rubella, or syphilis; Rh incompatibilities; and bilirubin toxicity. Psychogenic loss has no traceable organic basis and is thus thought to be psychological in origin.

Pathophysiology: In sensorineural impairment, damage to the cochlea or cranial nerve VIII results in interference with bone conduction of sound waves from the inner ear. Conductive loss occurs when injury to the middle or external ear results in interference with air conduction of sound waves to the inner ear. Some individuals have both conductive and sensorineural impairment. Central impairments interfere with auditory brainstem pathways. There is no organic pathological condition in functional hearing loss.

Clinical Manifestations

The overriding manifestation is a reduced ability to distinguish sound. It is often progressive and may range from a mild loss to total deafness.

Complications

Permanent, nontreatable deafness is the central complication.

Diagnostic Tests

Weber tuning fork	Lateralization of sound to deaf ear in conductive loss and to better ear in sensorineural loss
Rinne tuning fork	Bone conduction heard longer than or as long as air conduction in conductive loss; air conduction heard longer in sensorineural loss
Schwabach test	Examiner hears longer than examinee in sensorineural loss and vice versa for conductive loss
Audiometry	To distinguish types and identify degree of impairment

Therapeutic Management

Surgery	Stapedectomy for loss caused by otosclerosis, cochlear implants in some cases to treat profound deafness
Drugs	None
General	Hearing aids for conductive loss; instruction in sign language, speech, and lip reading for the profoundly deaf; use of specialized assistive devices (e.g., amplified or typed-message telephones, low-frequency or flashing doorbells, closed-caption television decoders, flashing alarm clocks, alarm bed vibrators, flashing smoke detectors); counseling and support groups for adaptation

heat exhaustion

Exposure to high ambient air temperature that leads to excessive body fluid loss and eventual hypovolemic shock and electrolyte imbalance

Etiology and incidence: Heat exhaustion is caused by insufficient water intake, insufficient salt intake resulting in electrolyte imbalances, and a deficiency in the production of sweat. These result in fluid volume and electrolyte depletion.

Pathophysiology: The individual is in high, humid temperatures without adequate rest, and fluid and electrolyte replenishment. As fluid and electrolytes become depleted, blood vessels dilate, and the demand for cardiac output increases. Heat exhaustion then results. If not promptly or adequately treated, heat exhaustion may result in heat stroke (see Heat Stroke).

Risk Factors

Prolonged exposure to hot, humid environment
Loss of body fluids from sweating and failure to drink enough
  replacement fluids to ensure fluid and electrolyte balance
Older ages
Chronic diseases such as diabetes or blood-vessel diseases
Alcoholism or other drug abuse
Recent illness involving fluid loss from vomiting or diarrhea
Heavy or restrictive clothing
Poor acclimation to hot and humid weather

Clinical Manifestations

Dizziness; fatigue; faintness; headache; profuse sweating; pale, clammy skin; rapid, weak pulse; low blood pressure; fast, shallow respirations; muscle cramps; intense thirst; confusion with impaired judgment; malaise; and total body weakness are all indicators.

Complications

If not promptly and adequately treated, it may result in heat stroke.

Diagnostic Tests

Positive history and clinical evaluation

Therapeutic Management

Surgery	None
Drugs	Fluid and electrolyte replacement based on laboratory findings
	If there are no laboratory tests, offer electrolyte-rich fluids as soon as tolerable.
General	Place in a cool environment; undress to cool body; lie down either flat or head slightly lower than feet; apply cool compresses; use other comfort measures.

H

heat stroke

Extreme and prolonged hyperthermia of the body in which the core body temperature reaches 103° to 106° F [39.4° to 41.1° C] without the body attempting to cool off by sweating and with altered mentation

Etiology and incidence: This serious and potentially fatal problem occurs when the body's temperature soars and the body does not attempt to cool by sweating. It occurs most often when overexposure to extreme heat and a breakdown in the body's heat-regulating mechanisms occur. Sweating normally cools the body. When sweating ceases, the body's core temperature rises rapidly. Heat stroke occurs most often in older adults or individuals with diseases such as diabetes mellitus, chronic renal failure, and cardiovascular or pulmonary problems. Environmental conditions that may lead to heat stroke are prolonged periods of high temperature with accompanying high humidity. If heat stroke is not rapidly identified and treated, death may result.

Pathophysiology: The individual is in high humid temperatures without adequate rest and fluid and electrolyte replenishment. As fluid and electrolytes become depleted, blood vessels dilate and the demand for cardiac output increases. Eventually, the sweat glands stop functioning, When sweating ceases; the core body temperature rises rapidly. The skin becomes hot and dry, and an altered level of consciousness occurs. If not treated, cardiovascular collapse results.

Risk Factors

Prolonged exposure to hot, humid environment
Loss of body fluids from sweating and failure to drink enough
  replacement fluids to ensure fluid and electrolyte balance
Older ages
Chronic diseases such as diabetes or blood-vessel diseases
Alcoholism or other drug abuse
Recent illness involving fluid loss from vomiting or diarrhea
Heavy or restrictive clothing
Poor acclimation to hot and humid weather

Clinical Manifestations

Heat stroke is often preceded by heat exhaustion, with an elevated temperature (103° to 106° F [39.4° to 41.1° C]). Skin is reddish, flushed, and dry. Early manifestations include elevated blood pressure; bounding rapid pulse; rapid, irregular respirations; agitation; weakness; dizziness; and nausea and vomiting. Late manifestations are a decreased level of consciousness and coma.

Complications

The most common complication is cardiovascular collapse, leading to coma and death.

Diagnostic Tests

Positive history and clinical evaluation

H

Therapeutic Management

Medical care must be executed rapidly and aggressively. Heat stroke is an emergency. Transport victim to hospital as soon as possible. First aid before transport to hospital should include rescue breathing or CPR if needed. If the individual is conscious or semi-conscious, wrap him or her in cold, wet sheets or place the individual in cold bath water. Do not delay transport to initiate these first aid measures.

Surgery	None
Drugs	IV fluids with accurate replacement of fluids and electrolytes
	Sedatives or muscle relaxants as needed to control shivering or muscle twitching
General	Emergency management including airway maintenance with oxygenation and ventilation support if needed
	Invasive and rapid cooling of the body with constant monitoring
	Cooling methods include tepid water mist; fans; ice packs to the head, groin, neck, and axillae; or invasive cooling such as ice water lavage, cold water peritoneal dialysis, and cardiopulmonary bypass.
	Shivering should be avoided.
	Careful body temperature monitoring, cardiovascular and cardiac monitoring, and other supportive therapies as needed

hemophilia

A hereditary bleeding disorder characterized by impaired coagulability of the blood

Etiology and incidence: Hemophilia is caused by a deficiency of blood clotting factors VIII, IX, or XI, which are carried on genes on the X chromosome. Sons of men who are hemophiliacs are normal, whereas daughters are obligatory carriers. Sons of women who are carriers have a 50% chance of being hemophilic, and daughters have a 50% chance of being a carrier. Hemophilia is the most common X-linked genetic disease; it occurs in 1.25 of every 10,000 live male births in the United States.

Pathophysiology: Hemophilia A (absent factor VIII), hemophilia B (absent factor IX), and hemophilia C (absent factor XI) are the most common types. The absence of the clotting factor interferes with the intrinsic phase of the coagulation process and inhibits the formation of prothrombin activator; this interferes with the rate at which thrombin is formed from prothrombin, slowing clot formation.

Clinical Manifestations

The primary presenting sign is excessive, poorly controlled bleeding. The rate of bleeding depends on the amount of factor activity and the severity of the injury that caused the bleeding. A factor activity level below 1% can cause spontaneous bleeding or severe bleeding from even minor trauma. When the factor activity level is more than 5%, bleeding is usually due to trauma and is more easily controlled. The bleeding may be superficial, may involve subcutaneous and muscle tissue, or may entail deep bleeding into joints and organ systems.

Complications

Joint and other musculoskeletal deformities, airway compression, pericardial tamponade, increased intracranial pressure, hemorrhagic shock, and death can result from uncontrolled or repeated bleeding. NOTE: Many hemophiliacs who received plasma in the early 1980s are infected with HIV. The virus was transmitted through plasma transfusions from blood banks that had contaminated blood and blood products. This occurred before reliable test measures were devised for detecting HIV in blood products and for eliminating them from the blood supply.

Diagnostic Tests

Laboratory tests reveal a normal prothrombin time, a prolonged partial thromboplastin time, and a normal bleeding time (platelet function). Assays are used to determine the factor affected and the level of factor activity. Genetic testing is performed to identify carriers.

Therapeutic Management

Surgery	None; extreme care must be exercised when these individuals need surgery for other conditions
Drugs	*Aspirin use and intramuscular injections* should be avoided because they may precipitate bleeding; inoculation against hepatitis B is important.
General	Plasma replacement of deficient factor as prophylaxis or to stop bleeding episode; use of immunosuppressives, plasmapheresis, prothrombin complexes, synthetic desmopressin (DDAVP) or aminocaproic acid (Amicar) to treat development of antibody inhibitors against a specific factor; safety precautions in activities of daily living (ADLs) to prevent injury; dental maintenance to prevent need for dental surgery or tooth pulling; education of patient and family about disease process; counseling for adaptation to chronic disease
	Experimental work is being conducted in gene transfer therapy to replace absent gene.

H

hemorrhoids (piles)

Varicosities of the veins in the rectum (internal) or on it (external) that are often inflamed and thrombosed and have a tendency to bleed

Etiology and incidence: The exact causal mechanism for hemorrhoid formation is unknown but is hypothesized to be associated with increased pressure, which causes congestion in the hemorrhoidal plexus in the anus. Increased pressure has been attributed to straining on defecation, various occupations that require prolonged standing or sitting, pregnancy, and chronic constipation. Another hypothesis suggests involvement of the vasculature of the hemorrhoidal plexus and its tendency to slide or be displaced with bowel movements in concert with a failure of the internal sphincter to relax. Hemorrhoids occur universally in children and adults and are treated as a normal finding when asymptomatic. Symptoms such as pain, bleeding, and protrusion are most often seen in adults between ages 20 and 50.

Pathophysiology: A hemorrhoid is formed when a portion of the vascular mound of the hemorrhoidal plexus weakens and prolapses after being subjected to increased vascular pressures over time. These projections from the anal lining are subject to ulceration and infection.

Clinical Manifestations

Typical symptoms include pain and bright-red blood on toilet tissue following defecation. A rectal skin tag may be present. Strangulation of a hemorrhoid may produce severe pain. Mucus production is sometimes seen.

Complications

The most common complication is strangulation of an ulcerated and edematous hemorrhoid. In rare cases, severe bleeding may occur and lead to secondary anemia.

Diagnostic Tests

Hemorrhoids are easily diagnosed by direct rectal examination or anoscopy.

Therapeutic Management

Surgery	Injection sclerotherapy to eliminate bleeding hemorrhoids; rubber band ligation for protruding, nonreducible internal hemorrhoids; photocoagulation (laser, infrared lights) to stop bleeding; hemorrhoidectomy (surgical excision) with severe intractable disease
Drugs	Topical anesthetic ointments for pain, stool softeners, analgesics
General	High-fiber diet, adequate hydration, warm sitz baths, use of wet wipes instead of toilet paper

H

hepatitis, viral

A diffuse inflammation of the cells of the liver that produces liver enlargement and jaundice

Etiology and incidence: The cause is a variety of hepatotropic viruses. To date, five viral types that cause primary hepatitis have been positively identified; these viruses are known as hepatitis A (HAV), hepatitis B (HBV), hepatitis C (HCV), hepatitis D (HDV), and hepatitis E (HEV). Viruses F and G have been discovered and may also cause primary hepatitis. Other viruses tentatively labeled as GB-A, GB-B, and GB-C are being tested to see if they differ from F and G and if they also cause hepatitis. HAV is transmitted by contaminated food and water and by the fecal-oral route; HBV and HDV are transmitted by contact with bodily fluids, HCV by percutaneous exposure to blood, and HEV by contaminated water and the fecal-oral route. NOTE: Hepatitis may also occur as a secondary infection and is associated with viruses from other primary diseases, including cytomegalovirus, Epstein-Barr, herpes simplex, varicella-zoster, coxsackie B, and rubella viruses.

Primary viral hepatitis occurs worldwide. More than 70,000 cases are reported annually in the United States, and the incidence is rising. Hepatitis A is seen most often in children and young adults, but the incidence is rising in those with HIV. Hepatitis B affects all age groups; about 10% of all transfusion-related hepatitis is this type. Hepatitis C accounts for about 20% of all cases and for most transfusion-related cases. It is seen across all age groups. Hepatitis C cases are rising rapidly. The Centers for Disease Control and Prevention estimate that 3.9 million Americans are infected and at least 12,000 of these will die annually. The annual number of deaths is expected to increase to 38,000 by the year 2010. Hepatitis D is seen in individuals who are susceptible to HBV or may be HBV carriers, such as hemophiliacs and IV drug users. The disease manifestation is severe in children. Hepatitis E is seen primarily among young adults in developing countries in Africa, Asia, or Central America. It is most severe in pregnant women.

Pathophysiology: The etiologic agent, mode of transmission, and clinical course vary according to the hepatitis type. However, the pathophysiology is the same. The causative agent invades the mononuclear cells in the liver, replicates, and sets up an inflammatory process in the parenchyma and portal ducts, causing hepatic cell necrosis, cellular collapse, and accumulation of necrotic tissue in the lobules and portal ducts. This results in interference with bilirubin excretion. Cellular regeneration and mitosis occur simultaneously with cellular necrosis, and the liver regenerates within 2 to 3 months. Continuation of the inflammatory response sets up a chronic disease process.

Risk Factors

HAV, HEV: Poor sanitary conditions, crowding, poor hygiene, recent travel to third-world countries

HBV, HCV, HDV: IV drug use with shared needles; health care workers and other occupational workers who are exposed to blood and body fluids; history of multiple sex partners; anal sex; infants or young children of infected mothers; recipients of blood products (hemophiliacs, recipients of multiple blood transfusions); recipients of hemodialysis

Clinical Manifestations

Incubation	*HAV:* 15 to 50 days; *HBV:* 45 to 180 days; *HCV:* 14 to 182 days; *HDV:* 14 to 70 days; *HEV:* 15 to 64 days
Communicability	*HAV:* last half of incubation until 1 week after onset of jaundice; *HBV:* during incubation and entire clinical course (carrier state may persist for years); *HCV:* as carrier, 1 week before clinical onset to indefinite period as carrier; *HDV:* throughout clinical disease; *HEV:* unknown
Preicteric phase	Malaise, headache, nausea and vomiting, anorexia, myalgia, chills, fever, upper quadrant abdominal pain; *HBV, HDV:* hives, itching, erythema, arthritis
Icteric phase	Appetite returns; malaise continues Jaundice with or without itching, dark urine, clay-colored stools

Complications

Complications include development of chronic hepatitis, spontaneous relapse, and cirrhosis. Severe fulminant hepatitis with rapid cellular destruction, no regeneration, and accompanying encephalopathy occur in 1% of cases and are usually fatal.

Diagnostic Tests

Serum enzymes (aspartate aminotransferase [AST, SGOT], alanine aminotransferase [ALT, SGPT]) that are eight to 20 times normal values during the prodromal and clinical phases and lactate dehydrogenase (LDH) that is 1 to 3 times normal often occur. These elevations are the hallmark of the disease. Serum bilirubin is elevated. The differential diagnosis is based on the clinical history and various laboratory tests and may be confirmed by liver biopsy. In HAV, the stool is positive for the virus 2 to 4 weeks after exposure, and the enzyme-linked immunosorbent assay (ELISA) shows a rise in HAV antibodies. Immunoglobulin M (IgM) and hepatitis B surface antigen (HbsAG) are present. In HBV, serum antigen tests detect HBeAg and HBsAg, and serum antibody tests detect a rise in anti-HBe. Serum antibody tests are used to detect HCV and HDV. HEV often diagnosed by exclusion of other etiologies of hepatitis.

Therapeutic Management

Surgery	None
Drugs	Immune globulin for prophylaxis in those exposed to HAV and HBV; vaccines (Havrix, Recombivax HB, Engerix B) for prophylaxis in individuals exposed to or at high risk of contracting HAV or HBV; HAV vaccines now routinely recommended for all children in 11 western states, where the rate of HAV is at least 20 cases per 100,000; antiemetics (chlorpromazine is contraindicated in hepatic disease) for nausea; analgesics for pain (acetaminophen is preferred); alpha-interferon for chronic HBV, HCV
General	Bed rest; diet as tolerated, with frequent, small, low-fat, high-carbohydrate meals; adequate fluid intake; appropriate infection precautions, dictated by transmission routes; monitoring by liver function tests until normal value is achieved

hernia, external

Protrusion of an internal organ (usually bowel) through an abnormal opening or weakness in the muscle wall

Etiology and incidence: Causes include congenital malformation, traumatic injury, or muscle weakening caused by factors such as pregnancy, obesity, ascites, abdominal tumors, long-term heavy lifting, surgery, or aging. Herniation may be precipitated by excessive coughing or straining during defecation. Hernias occur in all age groups and are more common in men than women. About 75% of hernias occur in the groin area.

H

Pathophysiology: External hernias may be classified as inguinal, femoral, umbilical, or incisional. Inguinal hernias involve an abdominal wall weakness where the spermatic cord in men or the round ligament in women emerges. The herniation protrudes either through the inguinal ring (indirect) or through the posterior inguinal wall (direct). With a femoral hernia, the bowel protrudes through the femoral ring into the femoral canal. Umbilical hernias occur when bowel protrudes through the inguinal ring. Incisional hernias involve protrusion through an abdominal incision that may have healed improperly.

Clinical Manifestations

The most common sign is a bulge in the inguinal, femoral, or umbilical area or at the incision site. The bulge may become larger with a shift in position or coughing. Sharp, steady pain in the affected area may also be present. Signs of hernia strangulation include increasing severity of pain and fever, tachycardia, abdominal rigidity, and absence of bowel sounds.

Complications

Incarceration or strangulation may lead to intestinal obstruction and necrosis of bowel tissue.

Diagnostic Tests

The diagnosis is made by the clinical presentation. X-ray studies may be used to confirm a suspected bowel obstruction.

Therapeutic Management

Surgery	Herniorrhaphy to repair the hernia or hernioplasty to reinforce weakened muscle with wire, fascia, or mesh; bowel resection and temporary colostomy if bowel obstruction and necrosis occur
Drugs	None
General	Manual reduction of hernia; binder or truss to prevent other herniations if individual is not a candidate for surgery

herniated disk

Rupture and extrusion of the nucleus pulposus through the external ring of an intervertebral disk, causing back pain; the usual location is the lumbosacral region of the spine

Etiology and incidence: Degenerative changes with or without accompanying trauma can lead to a weakening of the outer ring of the intravertebral disk and act as predisposing factors in the extrusion of the nucleus pulposus. The rupture is associated with severe strain or trauma. Lumbar herniation is most common and generally occurs in adults 20 to 45 years of age. Men are affected more often than women.

Pathophysiology: As the ruptured nucleus pulposus extrudes through the annulus fibrosus, the nucleus moves posteriorly and laterally into the extradural space. This often compresses or irritates the nerve root, causing sciatica and compression of the spinal cord, leading to corresponding muscle weakness and diminished sensation.

Clinical Manifestations

The predominant feature is pain in the lower back radiating down one leg or pain in the neck radiating down one arm, either of which may be sudden or insidious in onset. The pain is exacerbated by activity and jugular compression (caused by laughing, coughing, or straining at stool). Numbness and weakness may also be present in muscles innervated by the affected spinal nerve root.

Complications

Neurological deficits, particularly interference with bowel and bladder functioning, are the most common complications.

Diagnostic Tests

A clinical history, physical examination, and prolapse seen on a computed tomography or magnetic resonance imaging scan are used for diagnosis. Electromyography may define the particular root involved.

Therapeutic Management

Surgery	Microscopic laminectomy to remove a bulging disk when lesions are acutely compressing the spinal cord or pain is intractable
Drugs	Analgesics and muscle relaxants to relieve pain
General	Alternating hot and cold compresses for pain; massage; positioning to avoid strain; strict bed rest on firm surface for an acute episode, followed by structured exercise program to strengthen back and abdominal muscles; traction for cervical muscle weakness and sensory loss; back brace with lumbar origin; instruction in proper body mechanics; relaxation techniques

herpes simplex infections (fever blisters, genital herpes)

A recurrent viral infection of the skin and mucous membranes characterized by clusters of small, inflamed vesicles filled with clear fluid

Etiology and incidence: The cause is the herpes simplex virus type 1 (HSV-1) or type 2 (HSV-2). HSV-1 usually affects oral, labial, ocular, or skin tissues and is transmitted primarily by oral secretions. HSV-2 (genital herpes) affects genital structures and is transmitted by contact with genital secretions, primarily through sexual intercourse. Genital herpes is the most common sexually transmitted disease in the United States, with the highest incidence seen in men age 15 to 30. The incidence is increasing among women and neonates infected during birth by an infected mother. About 85% of the population have antibodies against HSV-1. The other 15% harbor the virus as carriers and have intermittent outbreaks, often triggered by diminished immune protection, stress, menses, sun exposure, and cold.

Pathophysiology: After initial infection the virus incubates and then forms the characteristic lesions on mucous membranes and skin. After the lesions resolve, the virus resides in the nerve ganglia and remains dormant until triggered by some stimulus or stressor that reactivates lesion formation. The disease is communicable when the lesions are present, and some transient shedding of the virus occurs even when no lesions are visible.

Risk Factors

Unprotected sexual contact (vaginal, anal, oral) with an infected partner in HSV-2
Contact with saliva or oral secretions in HSV-1
Infants of infected mothers in HSV-2

Clinical Manifestations

The classic symptoms are itching followed by the eruption of small, tense, clustered vesicles around the mouth, conjunctivae, or genitalia. These vesicles persist for a few days, then dry and crust over; they disappear in about 21 days. Atrophy and scarring may occur if lesions recur at the same site.

Complications

An initial infection of HSV-2 during pregnancy can lead to spontaneous abortion, premature labor, uterine growth retardation, and microcephaly. Blindness may result from ocular infections. Urethral strictures may develop in men, and women are at increased risk for cervical cancer. Herpes infections can be severe in individuals with AIDS, leading to esophagitis, colitis, pneumonia, and neurological syndromes.

Diagnostic Tests

A clinical examination and history lead to a tentative diagnosis, which is confirmed by culture of lesions and biopsy results.

Therapeutic Management

Surgery	None
Drugs	Analgesics for pain, topical antipruritic lotions, acyclovir to reduce symptoms in HSV-2 infections, topical and systemic antiinfective drugs for secondary infections
General	Cleansing of lesions with soap and water, lesions kept dry, mouthwashes for oral lesions, instruction about the spread and recurrent nature of the disease, use of protection during sexual activity, precautions and careful monitoring if an infected woman is considering pregnancy, emotional support to assist in coping with diagnosis

herpes zoster

See Shingles.

hiatal hernia

Protrusion of the stomach through the esophageal hiatus above the diaphragm

Etiology and incidence: The cause is unknown but is thought to be related to congenital weakness or abnormalities that often are hereditary or are due to the aging process, obesity, pregnancy, ascites, low-residue diets, and trauma. Hiatal hernias are common and occur in about 30% of the population. They are more common in women and the elderly.

Pathophysiology: Loss of muscle tone around the diaphragmatic opening predisposes a person to hernia development. The two types of hiatal hernia are sliding and rolling. Sliding hernias are more common and occur when the cardioesophageal junction and a fundic portion of the stomach are above the diaphragm, creating a weakened lower esophageal sphincter and gastroesophageal reflux. Rolling hernias involve herniation of the cardia of the stomach above the diaphragm, with possible hemorrhage, obstruction, and strangulation.

Clinical Manifestations

Sliding type	Asymptomatic or associated gastroesophageal reflux (GER) and heartburn; possible hemorrhage
Rolling type	Asymptomatic unless hemorrhage or strangulation occurs, which may cause chest pain and other manifestations imitating myocardial infarction

Complications

Esophageal laceration, perforation, or rupture with massive hemorrhage and strangulation with gangrene are the most common complications.

Diagnostic Tests

X-ray examination or esophagography is used to visualize the hernia. A Bernstein test is performed to distinguish cardiac from esophageal chest pain (a positive test result indicates esophageal pain). Cardiac conditions (e.g., acute myocardial infarction) must be ruled out if the person has acute symptoms such as chest pain.

Therapeutic Management

Surgery	Reduction of rolling hernia to prevent strangulation; fundoplication for complete mechanical incompetence of sphincter or persistent, untreatable symptoms
Drugs	GER is treated with antacids, antisecretory drugs, and gastrokinetics
General	Treatment of GER (see Therapeutic Management under Gastrointestinal Reflux Disease)

histoplasmosis

An infectious disease caused by inhaling the spores of a fungus called *Histoplasma capsulatum;* takes several forms, including acute benign respiratory, progressive disseminated, or chronic pulmonary

Etiology and incidence: Individuals located near activities where material contaminated with *H. capsulatum* is airborne can develop histoplasmosis if enough spores are inhaled. *H. capsulatum* grows in soils throughout the world. In the United States, the fungus is most prevalent along the Ohio and Mississippi River valleys and along the St. Lawrence and Rio Grande rivers. The fungus grows best in soils that are heavily rich with bat or bird droppings. Disturbances of contaminated materials cause the small *H. capsulatum* spores to become airborne or aerosolized. Once airborne, spores can easily be carried by wind currents over long distances. Histoplasmosis is not contagious; it cannot be transmitted from an infected person or animal to someone else. It can be prevented using safety practices and dust control measures to reduce worker exposure to *H. capsulatum*.

Pathophysiology: Infection occurs 3 to 14 days after inhalation of dust that contains the *H. capsulatum* spores. Once infected, the spore may be spread from the lungs through the blood to other body organs, including the liver, spleen, and lymphatic system.

The number of spores inhaled, the individuals age and overall state of health, and the susceptibility to the disease determine who becomes ill and how ill the exposed individual becomes. The number of inhaled spores needed to cause disease is unknown. Infants, young children, and older persons are at increased risks. Others at high risk are persons with weakened immune systems, those with cancer or AIDS, and persons receiving chemotherapy.

Risk Factors

Living or working in areas of high prevalence (e.g., Ohio and Mississippi river valleys and along the St. Lawrence or Rio Grande rivers)

Occupations or hobbies such as the following: bridge inspector, painter, chimney cleaner, construction worker, demolition worker, farmer; gardener, heating and air-conditioning system installer or service person, microbiology laboratory worker, pest control worker, restorer of historic or abandoned buildings, roofer, or cave explorer

Any activity that involves contact with contaminated soil or bat or bird droppings

Clinical Manifestations

Acute benign respiratory form	Dry or productive cough, malaise, infiltration pneumonia, pleural and/or substernal chest pain, low-grade fever
Progressive disseminated form	*Acute:* High fever; hepatomegaly, lymphadenopathy, splenomegaly *Chronic:* The liver lesions may lead to hepatic calcification; purpura; ulcerated lesions in larynx, mouth, nose, or pharynx
Chronic pulmonary form	Pulmonary lesions similar to tuberculosis; purulent sputum; hemoptysis; chronic, low-grade fever; cough; increasing dyspnea and eventual respiratory distress or progressive emphysema

Complications

Histoplasmosis may lead to secondary infections such as pneumonia, progressive emphysema, septic type of fever, hepatosplenomegaly, severe prostration, and death.

Diagnostic Tests

Blood test and culture	Positive serologic test for *H. capsulatum* fungal spore
Radioimmunoassay	Used to determine the level of *H. capsulatum* in the urine, serum, and other body fluids
Chest x-ray	*Acute:* To determine transient parenchymal pulmonary infiltrates

Chronic: To identify progressive
enlarged necrosis areas

Skin test   A skin test, similar to a tuberculosis
test, to determine previous infec-
tion from *H. capsulatum*

Therapeutic Management

Surgery	None
Drugs	Fungicidal and fungistatic antiinfective agents, corticosteroids, antihistamines
General	Supportive, rest
	Monitor for antifungal drug toxicity
	Teach prevention
Prevention	National Institute for Occupational Safety and Health (NIOSH) recommends that personnel use respirator protective equipment during some activities such as removal of an accumulation of bat or bird droppings from an enclosed areas such as an attic, barn, or abandoned building or when working around areas with a buildup of bat or bird droppings.

hives

See Urticaria.

Hodgkin's disease

A chronic, progressive cancer of the lymphoid tissue. (See also Cancer.)

Etiology and incidence: The cause of Hodgkin's disease is unknown. Current theory holds that it is a low-grade graft-versus-host reaction with some type of infectious agent as a cause. The incidence in the United States is low. Each year, about 7000 new cases are diagnosed in the United States, and 1600 deaths occur. Hodgkin's disease is the most common cancer in young adults. It occurs most often in two age groups, 15 to 35 and 60 to 80, and it is more common in men and boys.

Pathophysiology: The disease begins with an abnormal proliferation of histiocytes (Reed-Sternberg cells) in one lymph node, which replaces the normal cellular structure and causes tissue necrosis and fibrosis. The disease spreads through the lymphatic channels to lymph nodes throughout the body and eventually metastasizes to the liver, spleen, bronchi, and vertebrae.

Clinical Manifestations

Most individuals first notice a swelling in the cervical lymph nodes. It may be accompanied by itching, fever, night sweats, and weight loss. Later signs may include cough, dyspnea, chest and bone pain, ascites, and jaundice.

Complications

The prognosis for long-term survival is excellent with treatment. About 95% of individuals with stage I or stage II disease are cured with treatment. Untreated or advanced disease causes multiple organ failure and death.

Diagnostic Tests

The definitive diagnosis is made by lymph node biopsy, which shows the presence of Reed-Sternberg cells.

Therapeutic Management

Surgery   Excision of tumors in advanced disease, therapeutic splenectomy

Drugs   Systemic combination chemotherapy used with radiation

General   Radiation is the primary therapy, used alone or in combination with chemotherapy, particularly for stage III and stage IV disease. Colony stimulating factors (CSFs), autologous peripheral blood stem cell transplants and bone marrow transplants have also been tried with varying degrees of success.

H

hyperparathyroidism

Hyperactivity of one or more of the parathyroid glands, which is manifested as hypercalcemia

Etiology and incidence: Primary hyperparathyroidism is caused by a parathyroid adenoma, multiple endocrine neoplasia, or a genetic defect. Secondary hyperparathyroidism is caused by underlying disease such as rickets, renal failure, or osteomalacia; pregnancy; vitamin D or calcium deficiency; or an excessive intake of laxatives. Radiation exposure in the neck region may also be a precipitating factor. The disease most often occurs in adults age 30 to 70. Women are more likely than men to be diagnosed (3:2 ratio).

Pathophysiology: In primary hyperparathyroidism, one or more of the parathyroid glands hypertrophies, increasing secretion of parathyroid hormone (PTH) and elevating serum calcium levels. Increased PTH causes an increase in osteoblast formation, which increases bone turnover rate. Cysts and fibrous tissue invade the bone. Increased calcium causes renal calculi, a decrease in neuromuscular excitability, a delay in gastrointestinal motility, defects in cardiac conduction, and decreased neuronal permeability. In secondary disease the elevated PTH stems from a hypocalcemia-producing abnormality outside the gland that stimulates it to produce more calcium.

Clinical Manifestations

Manifestations include bone pain, backache, pain on weight bearing, pathological fractures, diluted urine and hematuria, fatigue, clumsiness, constipation, acute abdominal pain, mood swings, and paranoia.

Complications

Renal failure, cardiac arrhythmias, cardiac failure, central nervous system coma, and death are complications associated with untreated hyperparathyroidism.

Diagnostic Tests

Increases in total serum calcium, ionized calcium, PTH, uric acid, and chloride are the usual diagnostic findings. A thyroid scan, ultrasound, CT, or MRI may be used to locate parathyroid lesions. X-ray studies reveal bone demineralization. Intact PTH is used to distinguish primary from secondary and malignant disease.

Therapeutic Management

Surgery	Parathyroidectomy to remove adenoma or other abnormal parathyroid tissue
Drugs	Diuretics *(no thiazides, since they can lead to hypercalcemia)* to increase urinary secretion of calcium; phosphate as an antihypercalcemic
General	Treatment of the underlying disease in secondary hyperparathyroidism; increased fluid intake to at least 2 liters a day; restriction of dietary intake of calcium; monitoring of daily serum calcium, blood urea nitrogen (BUN), and potassium and magnesium levels; psychiatric evaluation and treatment for mood swings, anxiety, paranoia

H

hypertension

An intermittent or sustained elevation in systolic blood pressure (above 140 mm Hg) or diastolic blood pressure (above 90 mm Hg), or a systolic and diastolic pressure 20 mm Hg above the individual's baseline pressure

Etiology and incidence: The cause of primary (essential) hypertension is unknown. Secondary hypertension is related to an underlying disease process such as renal parenchymal disorders, renal artery disease, endocrine and metabolic disorders, central nervous system (CNS) disorders, and coarctation of the aorta. It is estimated that 60 to 85 million Americans have hypertension, and it is a major factor in cerebrovascular, cardiac, and renal disease.

Pathophysiology: Hypertension is a disease of the vascular regulatory system in which the mechanisms that usually control arterial pressure within a certain (normal) range are altered. The central nervous and renal pressor systems and extracellular volume are the predominant mechanisms that control arterial pressure. Some combination of factors affects changes in one or more of these systems, ultimately leading to both increased cardiac output and peripheral resistance. This elevates the arterial pressure, reducing cerebral perfusion and the cerebral oxygen supply, increasing the myocardial workload and oxygen consumption, and decreasing the blood flow to and oxygenation of the kidneys.

Risk Factors

Familial history of the disease
Race (blacks are at higher risk than whites and have increased incidences of mortality and morbidity from related diseases such as stroke and heart disease)
Age (occurs in 75% of women over age 75 and 64% of men over age 65)
Obesity
Sedentary lifestyle
Smoking
Stress
High-fat or high-sodium diet in genetically susceptible individuals

Clinical Manifestations

Hypertension is generally asymptomatic until complications develop. It is usually discovered on routine examination.

Complications

Complications include atherosclerotic disease, left ventricular failure, cerebrovascular insufficiency with or without stroke, retinal hemorrhage, and renal failure. When the pathological process is accelerated, malignant hypertension results; the blood pressure becomes extremely high; and nephrosclerosis, encephalopathy, and cardiac failure rapidly ensue.

Diagnostic Tests

Elevated pressures on at least two occasions from measurements taken on 3 separate days are needed to diagnose a person as hypertensive. Secondary causes are then ruled out to make a determination of primary hypertension.

Therapeutic Management

Surgery	None
Drugs	Diuretics, alpha- or beta-adrenergic blocking agents, antihypertensives, angiotensin-converting enzyme (ACE) inhibitors, calcium antagonists and/or vasodilators to reduce blood pressure (prescribed according to the stepped-care approach outlined by the 1984 Joint National Committee on Detection, Evaluation, and Treatment of High Blood Pressure)
General	Treatment of underlying disease in secondary hypertension; systematic exercise, moderate restriction of dietary sodium, decreased alcohol intake, smoking cessation, stress reduction, and weight loss, if indicated; regular monitoring of blood pressure; instruction in the importance of taking medications consistently and the potential long-term complications

hyperthyroidism (Graves' disease, thyrotoxicosis, toxic diffuse goiter, toxic nodular goiter, Plummer's disease, Basedow's disease)

A syndrome initiated by excessive production of thyroid hormones that results in multiple-system abnormalities ranging from mild to severe

Etiology and incidence: The cause of hyperthyroidism is unclear, but it is thought to be autoimmune in origin with a genetic component. The most common type of hyperthyroidism is Graves' disease, which occurs about eight times more often in women than men and is seen in about 2% of the female population in the United States.

Pathophysiology: Thyroid hormones are generally stimulatory, and excess production of these hormones produces a state of hypermetabolism in which the functions of various organ and tissue systems are increased. This is manifested by increased activity of the neuromuscular and sympathetic nervous systems. Compensatory mechanisms are called into play, and cardiac output, peripheral blood flow, body temperature, and respiratory rate increase. Other effects include increased cellular use of glucose and hyperinsulinemia, decreased supply of fats and carbohydrates, increased vitamin metabolism, increased bone mobilization and hypercalcemia, and increased secretion of adrenocorticotropic hormone and melanocyte-stimulating hormone. The organ systems eventually have trouble coping with the increased demand, and failure can result.

Clinical Manifestations

The most common signs are goiter; warm, moist skin; erythema; sweating; tremor; weakness; restlessness; insomnia; emotional lability; increased food intake; lid lag; lid retraction; proptosis; tearing; and a startled look.

Complications

Cardiac insufficiency, generalized muscle wasting, corneal ulcers, decreased libido, osteoporosis, myasthenia gravis, and impaired fertility are among the complications. The elderly are the most likely to exhibit these complications. Thyroid storm is a severe, dramatic form of hyperthyroidism with an abrupt onset and rapid progression. It is a life-threatening emergency requiring immediate treatment to prevent shock, coma, cardiovascular collapse, and death.

Diagnostic Tests

Diagnosis depends on the clinical history and examination coupled with a serum triiodothyronine and thyroxine assay and thyroid hormone binding ratio. All of the laboratory test results are elevated in hyperthyroidism.

Therapeutic Management

Surgery	Thyroidectomy in individuals who cannot receive radioactive iodine, have large goiters or toxic adenoma
Drugs	Radioactive iodine to destroy thyroid tissue (treatment of choice); thioamides to inhibit hormone synthesis; beta-adrenergic blockers to diminish clinical manifestations; iodines to reduce the size of the thyroid before surgery; corticosteroids for palliation in Graves' disease
General	Monitoring for signs of hypothyroidism, planned rest and exercise cycles, long-term follow-up, counseling for lability, instruction about medications

H

hypoglycemia

A low plasma glucose level; a plasma glucose level less than 50 mg/dl

Etiology and incidence: Three types of hypoglycemia can be considered as pathological. *Reactive hypoglycemia* occurs 2 to 4 hours after a rich carbohydrate meal. This type of hypoglycemia may be seen in individuals who have had radical gastric surgery where there may be a rapid absorption of carbohydrates, causing an early and very high plasma glucose level. This is followed by an insulin surge that reaches a peak when most of the glucose is absorbed or in individuals with early stage diabetes mellitus or alimentary hypoglycemia. *Fasting hypoglycemia* may occur when there has been inadequate food and carbohydrate ingestion. This type of hypoglycemia may be found in individuals with insulin-producing islet cell tumors (*insulinomas*), islet cell hyperplasia (*nesidioblastosis*), hormonal deficiency, liver disease, pancreatic tumors, insulin autoimmune syndromes, and renal disease. *Induced hypoglycemia* includes exogenous insulin or sulfonylurea used by persons with known diabetes, use of insulin by nondiabetics, and individuals with alcohol- or drug-induced hypoglycemia.

Pathophysiology: Regardless of cause, hypoglycemia occurs when the level of glucose in blood glucose drops. Insulin is responsible for maintaining normal blood glucose levels in conjunction with counter regulatory hormones that oppose the insulin action. Any physiology disruption resulting in an imbalance of insulin and blood glucose may lead to a state of hypoglycemia. A decrease in blood glucose results in increased secretions of epinephrine, glucagon, cortisol, and growth hormones. The release of these counter regulatory hormones result in the clinical signs that are seen in hypoglycemia. Hypoglycemia is generally episodic. Symptoms may recur and may last from a few minutes to a few hours. In most cases, the clinical signs of hypoglycemia disappear with the ingestion of food or glucose to increase the plasma glucose level.

Risk Factors

Individuals with history of radical gastric surgery, insulinoma, non-islet cell neoplasms, hormonal deficiency, liver disease, renal disease, and alcohol or drug ingestion

Clinical Manifestations

Symptoms include sweating, anxiety, tremors, tachycardia, palpitations, seizures, fatigue, dizziness, headache, behavioral changes, or visual disturbances, which are relieved by ingestion of carbohydrates.

Complications

The proven presence of hypoglycemia should be used as a sign of another underlying disorder or disease.

Diagnostic Tests

Laboratory tests	Low plasma glucose level <50 mg/dl
	Increased plasma insulin level
	Presence of insulin antibodies (may be present if the individual has had previous animal product insulin injections; will be absent if human insulin is present)
	C-peptide level (elevated fasting in nesidioblastosis)
72-hour supervised fast	Elevated insulin
	Low plasma glucose level

Therapeutic Management

Surgery	Subtotal pancreatectomy (for nesidioblastosis); insulinoma resection
Drugs	Non–life-threatening hypoglycemia: diazoxide, phenytoin, propranolol
	Life-threatening hypoglycemia: antineoplastic agents, subcutaneous glucagon, IV dextrose
General	Nutritional consultation

Diet for fasting hypoglycemia *(insulinoma or nesidioblastosis)*

Small, frequent meals with rapidly absorbable simple carbohydrates

Diet for reactive hypoglycemia

Small, freqent meals that restrict carbohydrates

hypoparathyroidism

Decreased secretion of parathyroid hormone by the parathyroid glands, manifested as hypocalcemia

Etiology and incidence: The cause is usually unintentional damage to or removal of the parathyroid glands during thyroidectomy. There is a rare idiopathic form in which the parathyroids are absent or atrophied, as well as a genetic form that is part of a polyendocrine syndrome called HAM (hypoparathyroidism, Addison's disease, and moniliasis). The idiopathic form generally occurs in childhood.

Pathophysiology: A decrease in the secretion of parathyroid hormone (PTH) leads to a reduced resorption of calcium from the renal tubules, decreased absorption of calcium in the gastrointestinal (GI) tract, and decreased resorption of calcium from bone. The serum calcium level falls, increasing neuromuscular excitability and leading to spasms and tetany.

Clinical Manifestations

Hypoparathyroidism is often asymptomatic in the early stages. The most characteristic sign is tetany with paresthesias of the lips, tongue, fingers, and feet; other signs are carpopedal and facial spasms, generalized muscle aches, and fatigue. Encephalopathy, depression, dementia, and papilledema may also be present.

Complications

Acute onset of hypocalcemia leads to laryngospasm, airway obstruction, and cardiac failure. Long-standing disease leads to bone deformities, cataract formation, reduced cardiac contractility, and heart failure. Childhood disease can lead to mental retardation and stunted growth.

Diagnostic Tests

Parathyroid deficiency is characterized by a low serum calcium level, high serum phosphorus level, and normal alkaline phosphatase level. Serum intact PTH is decreased. Chvostek's and Trousseau's signs are positive.

Therapeutic Management

Surgery	None
Drugs	Calcium supplements; vitamin D to increase calcium absorption in the GI tract
General	Calcium-rich diet; monitoring of calcium levels

H

hypothyroidism (myxedema)

A clinical state resulting from a deficiency of thyroid hormones

Etiology and incidence: The cause of some hypothyroidism is unknown but is thought to be autoimmune in origin. Other hypothyroidism is caused by destruction of thyroid or pituitary tissue by underlying disease, surgery, or radiation treatment. Hypothyroidism is a common disorder that affects all age groups. Women between ages 30 and 60 are most often affected. It also occurs in approximately 1 in every 4500 live births. The incidence is rising in the elderly population.

Pathophysiology: When the supply of thyroid hormone is inadequate, a general depression of most cellular enzyme systems and oxidative processes results, reducing the metabolic activity of the cells. This in turn reduces oxygen consumption, decreases energy production, and lessens body heat. Tissues are infiltrated by mucopolysaccharides, carotene is deposited in epidermal layers, adrenergic stimulation is decreased, protein effusion collects in the pericardial and pleural sacs, and proteinaceous ground substances are deposited in tissues.

Clinical Manifestations

Signs and symptoms are often insidious at onset. They include fatigue and lethargy; mild weight gain; cold, pale, dry, rough hands and feet; reduced attention span with memory impairment, slowed speech, and loss of initiative; swelling in extremities and around the eyes, eyelids, and face; menstrual irregularities; muscle aches and weakness; joint aches and stiffness; clumsiness; hyperstiff reflexes; decreased pulse; decreased blood pressure; agitation; depression; and paranoia.

Complications

Myxedema coma is a life-threatening complication of hypothyroidism that requires immediate treatment. Other complications include ischemic heart disease, congestive heart failure, pleural and pericardial effusion, deafness, psychosis, and anemia.

Diagnostic Tests

Serum and serum-free triiodothyronine and thyroxine (T_3, T_4) are decreased; serum thyroid-stimulating hormone (TSH) is increased in primary hypothyroidism and decreased in secondary hypothyroidism.

Therapeutic Management

Surgery	None
Drugs	Oral replacement thyroid hormone; IV form is used for myxedemic coma
General	Lifelong monitoring; instruction about lifelong thyroid hormone replacement therapy and the importance of consistent and timely use
	High-protein, high-fiber diet; early detection through thyroid screening every 1 to 3 years

H

impetigo

A superficial vesiculopustular infection of the skin found primarily on the arms, legs, and face. Ulcerative impetigo is called *ecthyma*.

Etiology and incidence: Impetigo is caused by staphylococci or streptococci transmitted by insect bites or directly from person to person through skin breaks. A secondary form of impetigo occurs with pediculosis, scabies, and fungal infections. Predisposing factors include poor hygiene, crowding, poor nutritional status, and frequent skin breaks. It is highly contagious in infants and small children, who are the most susceptible.

Pathophysiology: The bacteria colonize and incubate on the skin for as long as several weeks before initiation of the disease process. The lesions begin as small, erythematous macules beneath the stratum corneum that change to vesicles and then pustules, which rupture. In streptococcal impetigo, honey-colored crusts are formed, whereas in staphylococcal impetigo, light brown or clear crusts form. Individuals often have a mixture of both forms.

Risk Factors

Poor hygiene
Crowding
Poor nutrition
Frequent skin breaks

Clinical Manifestations

Intense itching, burning, and regional lymphadenopathy accompany the crusted skin lesions. Scratching often causes satellite lesions.

Complications

Ecthyma is a deeper form of impetigo that affects the dermis and epidermis and forms ulcers that later cause scarring. Glomerulonephritis is a severe complication that occurs in about 3% of impetigo cases.

Diagnostic Tests

The diagnosis is made by physical examination, gram stain, and culture of the lesions.

Therapeutic Management

Surgery	None
Drugs	Topical antiinfective drugs on lesions, systemic antiinfective drugs sensitive to causative agent, antipruritics for itching
General	Crusts are washed with soap and water, and cool, moist compresses are applied; isolation until lesions have healed; careful personal and family hygiene; protective devices (e.g., mittens, distractions) to reduce scratching; nails kept trimmed; nutritional therapy if needed; treatment of any underlying disease processes

influenza (flu)

An acute viral respiratory disease with clinical manifestations that often resemble a severe form of the common cold

Etiology and incidence: Influenza is caused by orthomyxovirus types A, B, and C, which are spread by direct person-to-person contact or by airborne droplet spray. Flu generally occurs in the late fall and early winter and can reach epidemic proportions when a modified form of the virus emerges for which the population has no immunity. All age groups are susceptible, but the prevalence is highest in school-age children. More than 90.4 million cases are reported annually in the United States.

Pathophysiology: After a 48-hour incubation period, the virus penetrates the surface of the upper respiratory tract mucosa, destroying the ciliated epithelium and reducing the viscosity of mucosal secretions. This facilitates the spread of virus-laden exudate to the lower respiratory tract, with resultant necrosis and desquamation of the bronchi and alveoli. The disease is generally self-limiting, with acute symptoms lasting 2 to 7 days and lingering symptoms lasting another week.

Clinical Manifestations

The onset of influenza types A and B is sudden, marked by chills, fever, generalized aches and pains, headache, and photophobia. Respiratory symptoms begin with a scratchy, sore throat; substernal burning; and nonproductive cough. Later cough becomes severe and productive, and weakness, fatigue, and sweating persist. Influenza C produces milder symptoms.

Complications

The most common complication is viral pneumonia or a secondary bacterial pneumonia. Individuals who have a compromised respiratory system and the elderly are most susceptible.

Diagnostic Tests

Tissue culture of nasal secretions or fluorescent antibody staining of secretions is positive for virus.

Therapeutic Management

Surgery	None
Drugs	Analgesics for headache, aches, and pains; nasal sprays for congestion *(no aspirin for children because Reye's syndrome may result);* antitussives for cough; flu vaccine for prevention; antiviral drugs (amantadine, rimantadine) for early intervention for influenza type A. Drugs GS4104 and zanamavir (inhaled antiviral) in clinical trials to treat type A and type B influenza should be available by year 2000.
General	Adequate hydration, rest, careful handling of items in the environment and proper handwashing to reduce the spread of the virus

I

intestinal obstruction

The contents of the intestines fail to move through the intestinal canal; intestinal obstruction may be mechanical or functional.

Etiology and incidence: Bowel obstruction occurs from one of two causes: mechanical blockage or a functional obstruction. The mechanical obstruction is caused by a blockage of the lumen of the bowel by feces, intussusception, adhesions, volvulus (twisting of the bowel), tumor, inflammation, or a foreign body. Functional obstruction, also referred to as *ileus,* occurs where there is a loss of function of the peristalsis of the intestinal tract.

Pathophysiology: If there is a blockage or lack of peristalsis within the intestinal tract, an accumulation of fluids and gas build proximal to the obstruction. The gas, high in nitrogen concentration, and the fluids accumulate and cause the bowel to swell. The edematous bowel secretes more fluids and electrolytes and causes more distention. This continued fluid and gas accumulation causes further compromise. If not treated, the distention may lead to pressure necrosis of the bowel wall. Significant abdominal distention may also cause impaired breathing, and the intraabdominal pressure may cause decreased venous blood flow to the legs.

Risk Factors

Abdominal surgery resulting in adhesions or incarcerated hernia
  or intestinal distention
Spinal fractures
Use of narcotic drugs or diphenoxylate (Lomotil)
Congenital abnormalities of the intestines

Clinical Manifestations

General	History of lack of "normal" bowel movement, early onset of cramping abdominal pain, abdominal distention
Gastrointestinal/ abdomen	Vomiting, failure to pass gas, blood in stool, localized tenderness, constant abdominal pains, guarding and rebound tenderness

| Bowel sounds | *Mechanical obstruction* peristalsis has a high-pitched, tinkling sound; *paralytic ileus* is absence of bowel sounds or low infrequent sounds |

Complications

If untreated, it may progress to necrosis and gangrene of the bowel, leading to a life-threatening situation.

Diagnostic Tests

X-ray	*Abdominal series* x-rays indicate large amounts of gas in the bowel; fluid and gas levels may be diagnostic for intestinal obstruction
	Barium enema stops at the point of obstruction
Laboratory	Serum electrolytes may indicate electrolyte loss; increased WBC count indicates strangulation of bowel

Therapeutic Management

Surgery	Surgery exploration, resection, and sometimes colostomy may be life saving.
Drugs	Antibiotics if strangulation is present
General	Nasogastric or intestinal suctioning may assist to reduce trapped fluids and gases and to reduce inflammation. Colonoscopy may assist with reduction of volvulus by releasing trapped gas and fluid.

irritable bowel syndrome (spastic colitis)

A noninflammatory motility disorder of the large bowel that alters bowel habits and causes abdominal pain and distention

Etiology and incidence: The cause of irritable bowel syndrome (IBS) is unknown, but it is associated with diet, drugs, toxins, gastrointestinal (GI) hormones, prostaglandins, and emotional factors. IBS is a common GI disorder that accounts for about half of all presenting GI complaints in the United States. Women are affected more often than men, and whites and Jews more often than other ethnic groups. All age groups are affected, although the disease is predominant in those under age 35.

Pathophysiology: The pathophysiology of IBS is still unclear. However, two patterns can be identified: one with painful constipation and diarrhea and the other with painless diarrhea. Hypermotility with high-amplitude pressure waves is present in painful IBS and hypomotility in painless IBS. Myoelectric activity is increased in both patterns, as is contractile activity after meals.

Clinical Manifestations

The primary symptoms are either painless, urgent diarrhea that occurs after meals, or alternating diarrhea and constipation accompanied by abdominal pain, bloating, flatulence, headache, and fatigue.

Complications

IBS is associated with an increased risk of diverticulitis and colon cancer.

Diagnostic Tests

A careful history of bowel habits and emotional stimuli, along with a rectal examination that elicits pain in a tender rectum, is important. Manometric studies are done to evaluate electrical response, as are tests to rule out other bowel diseases.

Therapeutic Management

Surgery	None
Drugs	Anticholinergics to reduce pain; bulk-forming agents and antidiarrheal drugs to regulate stool
General	High-fiber, low-lactose, caffeine-free, low-fat diet; counseling for emotional effects

Kaposi's sarcoma

A malignant vascular tumor of the endothelium that originates in multifocal sites

Etiology and incidence: The etiology is unknown, but cytomegalovirus (CMV) is a suspected cause. At one time the incidence of Kaposi's sarcoma (KS) was confined to a select population of older men of Jewish or Italian origin and to those who were severely immunocompromised. In late 1980, however, an alarming increase in cases occurred among sexually active, homosexual men between ages 25 and 50. KS is currently the most common AIDS-related cancer, occurring in at least one third of those diagnosed with AIDS in the United States. It is endemic in equatorial Africa and accounts for more than 10% of malignancies in Zaire and Uganda. (See also AIDS.)

Pathophysiology: KS lesions begin in the endothelial cells, which originate in the middermis, oral mucosa, lymph nodes, and gastrointestinal viscera. The lesions spread to the skin, lungs, liver, and bones. Skin lesions are typically reddish brown or purple and are various shapes and sizes.

Risk Factors for Individuals With HIV

Male gender (10:1 male:female)
Homosexuality
Multiple sex partners
History of cytomegalovirus and other sexually transmitted
    diseases
Use of inhaled nitrates

Clinical Manifestations

Individuals can have varying degrees of cutaneous and systemic involvement. The presenting signs are usually multiple skin and oral mucosal lesions that are small, round, and pink and progress to red or purple. Later symptoms indicate systemic disease and include diarrhea, weight loss, cough, dyspnea, and fever.

Complications

Associated opportunistic infections and the immunosuppression associated with AIDS complicate the course and treatment of KS.

Diagnostic Tests

The initial diagnosis is made from the presence of the characteristic lesions and a history of AIDS or Jewish or Italian heritage. The definitive diagnosis is made by biopsy of the skin lesions.

Therapeutic Management

Surgery	Excision or electrodesiccation of skin lesions
Drugs	Combination chemotherapy for progressive or widespread disease; alpha-interferon for minimal or slow-progressing disease
General	Irradiation of skin lesions; radiation as palliation

K

keratitis

Inflammation of the cornea of the eye

Etiology and incidence: Causes of keratitis include dryness, injury, irritations, infections, ischemia, and nutritional deficiencies. This often starts as a superficial inflammation of the epithelium, but if not treated, may invade subepithelial tissues or may go even deeper into the inner layer of the cornea.

Pathophysiology: The epithelium may become damaged due to injury or irritations. Inflammation, pain, blurring of vision, and other visual disturbances may result. If not treated, the inflammation of the cornea may result in damage to the cornea membrane and loss of membrane integrity. This in turn may lead to infection and/or ulceration of the cornea. Infection may result from various bacteria including *Staphylococcus, Streptococcus,* and *Pseudomonas;* fungi including *Herpes zoster;* and parasites such as *Acanthamoeba.* The *Acanthamoeba* parasite is commonly found in fresh water, soil, and airborne dust. Most individuals with this last infection are contact lens wearers who use distilled or tap water to clean or rinse their lenses. The severity of corneal destruction depends on the organism, promptness of identification and treatment, and the overall health of the individual. A large number of individuals who acquire *Acanthamoeba* keratitis must undergo a corneal transplant to regain useful vision.

Risk Factors

Overuse or exposure of eye to dryness, trauma, chemical irritation, or use of topical anesthetics
Contact lens wearer with poor lens-cleaning habits

Clinical Manifestations

Eye pain, discharge and/or increased lacrimation, blurred vision, halo vision seen when looking into light; photophobia, and purulent exudate may be noted. Opacity or irregular light refection may be noted on the corneal surface. The cornea may appear dull and uneven. Severe cases may show evidence of corneal ulceration with whitish appearance around the margin of the lesion.

Complications

Corneal ulceration, optic atrophy, or loss of sight in affected eye are all possible complications.

Diagnostic Tests

Fluorescein stain applied to cornea of eye to determine a break in epithelium (green color indicates corneal epithelium damage); culture of corneal tissue and/or ulcer scraping to determine infective organism

Therapeutic Management

Surgery	Severe cases may require corneal transplantation
Drugs	Antiinfective, antiviral, and/or anti-amoeba agents sensitive to identified organism; mucolytics for inhibiting collagenase; analgesics for pain; mydriatic-cycloplegic agents for iris inflammation and pupillary constriction
General	Pressure dressings on eye and ice compresses for 10 to 15 minutes several times per day may assist with discomfort, education about causes and use of contact lens, hospitalization for severe cases

K

kidney cancer (renal cancer)

Renal cell and clear cell adenocarcinomas account for 80% of kidney cancer. Other tumor types include transitional cell, squamous cell, and nephroblastoma.

Etiology and incidence: The cause of kidney cancer is unclear. Environmental factors have been implicated. Hereditary forms have also been identified. More than 29,000 individuals are diagnosed with kidney cancer and about 12,000 die in the United States annually. About 20% of childhood malignancies and 3% of adult malignancies occur in the kidneys. The average age of diagnosis is 55 to 60, and men are affected 1.5 times as often as women.

Pathophysiology: Tumor cells originate in the renal parenchyma and grow into a well-defined tumor, often surrounded by perinephric fat, which slows infiltration of adjacent tissues. Metastasis occurs by venous or lymphatic routes, and the most common metastatic sites are the lungs, bones, liver, and brain.

Risk Factors

Use of tobacco products (implicated in 30% of diagnosed cases)
History of acquired cystic disease, von Hippel-Lindau disease (VHL)
Familial history of hereditary papillary renal carcinoma (HPRC) or hereditary renal carcinoma (HRC)
Chronic irritation from renal calculi
Exposure to petrochemical products, asbestos, cadmium, or radiation
Obesity, particularly in females
Analgesic abuse (phenacetin containing analgesics)
History of renal dialysis, end-stage renal disease

Clinical Manifestations

Signs and symptoms develop late in the disease; hematuria is the most common presenting sign, followed by flank pain, a palpable abdominal mass, and/or fever of unknown origin.

Complications

The prognosis for metastatic lesions is poor because kidney tumors are resistant to radiation and chemotherapy. Complications include hypertension from pedicle compression.

Diagnostic Tests

Abdominal ultrasound and CT scans help detect masses that warrant further diagnostic study. Biopsy by needle aspiration or tissue sample is definitive.

Therapeutic Management

Surgery	Nephrectomy with removal of regional lymph nodes
Drugs	Hormone therapy (progesterone, testosterone) is showing some promise; interferon and autolymphocyte therapy have been used investigationally
General	None

K

labyrinthitis

An inflammation or infection of the inner ear that involves the cochlear or vestibular portion of the labyrinth

Etiology and incidence: This is a rare but potentially serious problem. The two basic types of labyrinthitis are *serous labyrinthitis*, which may occur secondary to drug or alcohol intoxication or allergies and *diffuse labyrinthitis*, which may occur when a chronic or acute otitis media gains entrance to the labyrinth through the round or oval window or through an erosion of the bony capsule. It may also occur after ear or mastoid surgery. In this second type of labyrinthitis, there may be destruction of the soft tissue structures. This in turn may cause permanent hearing loss.

Pathophysiology: In both serous and diffuse labyrinthitis, cellular infiltration of serous fluid or serofibrinous exudate occurs. If not recognized and treated, soft tissue structures are destroyed. This is what may cause total, permanent hearing loss. Chronic labyrinthitis can develop after an initial bout of labyrinthitis. The internal ear is filled with granulations that begin to change into fibrous tissue and then calcify as new bone in the labyrinth space. When this occurs, complete deafness in the affected ear occurs.

Risk Factors

Nasal or ear surgery
Viral infections
Chronic ear infections

Clinical Manifestations

Vertigo, tinnitus (ringing in the ears), and sensorineural hearing loss. Vertigo or dizziness is manifested when the vestibular structures are involved and causes problems with balance and equilibrium. Tinnitus occurs when the infection is located in the cochlea. Severe cases may also include nystagmus, which is an abnormal rhythmic, jerking movement of the eyes. This accompanies the symptoms of vertigo and occurs during labyrinth dysfunction. Other clinical signs include pain, fever, ataxia, nausea, and vomiting.

Complications

Dehydration and electrolyte imbalance from vomiting; falls secondary to dizziness and vertigo; deafness.

Diagnostic Tests

Positional maneuvers
Audiometry

Therapeutic Management

Surgery	None
Drugs	Antibiotics if the cause is thought to be bacterial; antiemetics to treat nausea and vomiting
	Vestibular suppressants and antivertigo medications to decrease severity of dizziness and vertigo
General	Bed rest to decrease head movement and turning of the head
	Safety and prevention of falls are primary concerns
	After the episode is over, the individual should have a complete audiologist evaluation to determine possibility of hearing loss

L

laryngitis

Acute: A self-limiting condition caused by a viral infection, environmental irritants, or voice overuse

Chronic: Laryngitis lasting more than 3 weeks

Etiology and incidence: Acute laryngitis may be the result of a bacterial or viral agent that affects the larynx, subglottic area, and epiglottis. Other causes of both acute and chronic laryngitis include membrane irritation and injury from irritants such as smoking, voice overuse, endotracheal intubation, acid reflux, and alcohol ingestion. Other causes of chronic laryngitis include allergies, chronic tonsillitis, and adenoiditis.

Pathophysiology: The inflammation of the mucous membranes in the lining of the larynx and vocal cords may be acute or chronic. Most prevalent is laryngitis associated with voice overuse and/or environmental irritants. When acute laryngitis is found in combination with an upper respiratory infection, a virus is generally the cause. Laryngitis may also occur in conjunction with pneumonia, influenza, tracheitis, and bronchitis.

Risk Factors

Acute

Voice overuse
Exposure to environmental irritants
Recent upper respiratory infection

Chronic

History of smoking and alcohol use
Exposure to environmental irritants

Clinical Manifestations

Acute   Sore throat, change in voice tone, hoarseness that
                 becomes worse throughout the day, aphonia
                 (complete loss of voice), fever, malaise, pain on
                 swallowing, scratchy throat, and dry cough
                 In severe cases, stridor and dyspnea may be
                 present. Indirect examination of the larynx

reveals redness and edema of the vocal cords and
swollen lymph nodes.

Chronic   Frequent clearing of throat and complaints of a
chronic dry cough

Change in voice tone; hoarseness is worse in the
morning and evening and improves during the
middle of the day

Reddened laryngeal mucosa without noted
swelling

Nodules on the cords may be present, especially in
individuals with history of smoking. Duration of
hoarseness is often over 3 weeks.

Complications

Laryngeal swelling may cause airway compromise in severe
acute cases.

Diagnostic Tests

Acute   None unless symptoms last more than 3 to 4
weeks.
Chronic   Lateral and anterior-posterior radiographs of the
neck; laryngoscopy to rule out other problems

Therapeutic Management

Surgery   Chronic laryngitis with polyps may require surgical
polyp removal
Drugs   Analgesics and/or antipyretic agents for discomfort; antibiotics if causative agent is thought to be
bacterial

Steroids may be used in severe cases to decrease
laryngeal edema.
General   Avoid talking and give the voice rest. Cool or
warm steam mist may alleviate discomfort.

Chronic laryngitis may require avoidance or
removal of irritants and correction of faulty
voice habits.

latex allergy

An immunoglobulin E–mediated reaction to proteins retained in finished natural rubber latex products

Etiology and incidence: Latex allergies have emerged in the 1990s as one of the most pervasive problems in health care; it is a serious and growing problem. Latex is the milky sap of the rubber tree *Hevea brasiliensis*. This natural rubber product contains proteins. Latex allergy is the reaction to certain proteins in the latex rubber. Health care workers are at increasingly greater risk of acquiring latex allergies. It is currently estimated that 1 in 10 health care professionals develops a latex allergy due to repeated exposure to latex protein allergens found in powdered latex gloves. It is further estimated that up to 60% of children with spina bifida and other individuals with chronic illnesses that require frequent operations are especially susceptible to developing a sensitization toward latex.

Pathophysiology: The amount of latex exposure needed to produce sensitization or an allergic reaction is unknown. Increasing exposure to latex proteins increases the risk of developing allergic symptoms. Although latex-containing products have only 2% to 3% protein, it is this protein that is thought to be the allergen in type-1 hypersensitive individuals. The precise protein responsible for causing allergic contact dermatitis latex type-1 hypersensitivity has not yet been identified and may be different for individual patients.

Risk Factors

Although all health care professionals are at risk, those at highest risk are surgical workers, emergency care workers, and obstetrics workers.

Children with spina bifida or others with conditions requiring frequent operations

Persons with congential urogenital abnormalities requiring indwelling catheters

Employees in the rubber industry

Persons with history of other IgE dependent allergies, such as rhinitis, asthma, or food allergies with a positive skin test

Clinical Manifestations

Known exposure to latex; clinical signs include local skin redness and urticaria. More severe reactions may involve respiratory symptoms such as rhinitis, sneezing, itchy eyes, scratchy throat, bronchospasm, laryngeal edema, respiratory distress and/or respiratory failure, and other typical allergic reaction signs and symptoms.

Complications

Complications include anaphylactic shock and respiratory and cardiac arrest leading to death.

Diagnostic Tests

History	Atopic history, hives under rubber or latex gloves, hand dermatitis related to gloves, allergic conjunctivitis after rubbing eye with hand that has been in contact with latex, swelling around mouth after dental procedures or blowing up a balloon, vaginal burning after pelvic examination or contact with condom
Immunological evaluation	Skin prick, intradermal, and patch contact skin tests; serologic testing (e.g., radioallergosorbent test [RAST] or enzyme-linked immunosorbent assay [ELISA]). The Food and Drug Administration (FDA) has approved a standardized latex reagent for skin testing to be used for research only. This is not yet available for public use.

Therapeutic Management

Surgery	None
Drugs	Epinephrine for reaction (may be autoinjector and carried by individual); B-agonist inhaler; prednisone; other anaphylactic life-supporting medications

General	Immediate assessment and interventions for acute reaction, including cardiac monitoring and if needed, respiratory support
	Report sensitivity to health care workers. Wear medical alert bracelet or tag. Sensitive individual should carry "hypoallergenic" latex gloves and condoms. Become aware of natural rubber-containing products.
Prevention	Use nonlatex gloves for activities that are not likely to involve contact with infectious materials.
	Use appropriate barrier protection, including powder-free gloves. These gloves reduce exposures to latex protein.
	When wearing latex gloves, do not use oil-based hand creams or lotions.

leukemia (acute lymphocytic leukemia, acute myelogenous leukemia, chronic lymphocytic leukemia, chronic myelogenous leukemia)

An acute or chronic cancer involving the blood-forming tissues in the bone marrow; may be classified as myeloid or lymphoid

Etiology and incidence: The cause of the various leukemias is unclear, although a viral association is suspected in some types. Exposure to certain toxins (e.g., benzene, ionizing radiation) has been implicated, as have genetic defects and a genetic predisposition. Leukemia accounts for 2% of all cancers diagnosed in the United States each year, and more than 20,000 deaths occur annually from some form of leukemia. Acute lymphocytic leukemia (ALL) is most common in children age 3 to 5. However, it also accounts for 20% of diagnosed adult leukemias. Acute myelogenous leukemia (AML) is an adult disease with a median age at onset of 50 years. Chronic myelogenous leukemia (CML) occurs between the ages of 20 and 60, with a peak incidence between 50 and 60 years of age. Chronic lymphocytic leukemia (CLL) is the most common leukemia in the United States, accounting for 30% of cases diagnosed each year. The median age of onset is 60 years, and it occurs twice as often in men as in women.

Pathophysiology: Whatever the etiologic agent, a transformation of leukocytes and leukocyte precursors into malignant cells occurs. Large numbers of these immature, abnormal cells proliferate rapidly, accumulating in the bone marrow, replacing the normal cells, and suppressing normal hematopoiesis. Proliferation also occurs in the lymph nodes, liver, and spleen. Eventually all body organs are involved in the leukemic process.

Clinical Manifestations

Acute forms of the disease are more rapidly progressive than chronic forms, and acute cell forms are less mature and predominantly undifferentiated.

ALL   Fatigue; dyspnea on exertion; anorexia; weight loss; headache; swollen cervical lymph nodes; swollen,

L

painful joints; splenomegaly; about 10% of cases are asymptomatic

AML   Fatigue, dyspnea on exertion, anorexia, weight loss, headache, swollen cervical lymph nodes, recurrent infections unresponsive to standard treatment, easy bruising, epistaxis, gingivitis

CML   Often asymptomatic for a period, followed by insidious onset of nonspecific symptoms (fatigue, dyspnea, anorexia, weight loss, fever, night sweats); lastly, splenomegaly, pallor, bleeding, and marked lymphadenopathy

CLL   Insidious, asymptomatic onset with lymphadenopathy, followed by fatigue, anorexia, weight loss, and dyspnea; anemia, thrombocytopenia, and bacterial, viral, and fungal infections are present in advanced disease

Complications

The prognosis is better among individuals with acute forms of leukemia and for those who experience total remission after the first course of treatment. Children have a better survival rate than adults. Persons with CLL are most likely to develop second malignancies, and people with CML have the shortest survival rates, often dying of a blast crisis. Other complications of leukemia include infection, hemorrhage, organ failure, and recurrence of the disease.

Diagnostic Tests

The leukocyte count is elevated from 15,000 to 500,000/mm^3 or higher; a large number of immature neutrophils are present; bone marrow biopsy shows a massive number of WBCs in the blast phase; and RBCs, Hgb, and Hct are decreased. Tumor markers aid in distinguishing the type of leukemia.

Therapeutic Management

Surgery	None
Drugs	Chemotherapy to induce remission and consolidation or maintenance chemotherapy after remission in acute leukemias, chemotherapy in stage III

CLL cases, chemotherapy in CML before bone
marrow transplantation, corticosteroids in
ALL and CLL, interferon in CML

General   Radiation for palliation or as a pretreatment for
bone marrow transplantation, transfusions,
reverse isolation procedures, antibiotics to treat
secondary infection

Bone marrow transplantation is the only curative
modality in CML and is used after relapse in
acute leukemias.

L

liver cancer, primary

Hepatocellular carcinomas are the most prevalent of the primary liver tumors, although cholangiocarcinomas, angiosarcomas, and hepatoblastomas also are seen.

Etiology and incidence: Chronic hepatitis B virus is a known etiologic agent. Hepatitis C virus, cirrhosis, and hemochromatosis are also associated with the development of liver cancer. The incidence of primary liver cancer in the United States is low. Most of these individuals have underlying cirrhosis. In certain areas of Africa and Southeast Asia, however, liver cancer is the leading malignancy and one of the leading causes of death. Most are associated with hepatitis B infections.

Pathophysiology: Most cancer cells originate in the parenchyma and rapidly form a tumor that extends and invades adjacent structures such as the stomach and diaphragm. Metastasis occurs to the regional nodes, lung, bone, adrenal gland, and brain.

Risk Factors

Ethanol abuse
Anabolic steroid abuse
Pesticide and herbicide exposure
Exposure to vinyl chloride
Ingestion of food contaminated with fungal aflatoxins

Clinical Manifestations

Abdominal pain, right upper quadrant mass, epigastric fullness, and weight loss are the most common presenting signs and symptoms. Systemic metabolic signs may include hypoglycemia, hypercalcemia, hyperlipidemia, and erythrocytosis.

Complications

The prognosis in liver cancer is grim; the survival rate is only about 5%. Complications include liver failure, gastrointestinal hemorrhage, and cachexia.

Diagnostic Tests

The alpha-fetoprotein blood value is elevated in 70% of cases; ultrasound and CT scans can help visualize masses. A biopsy is needed for definitive diagnosis.

Therapeutic Management

Surgery	Resection of tumor is only a potentially curative modality.
Drugs	Chemotherapy is experimental and not particularly effective to date.
General	Radiation cannot be given in sufficient doses to be effective; radiolabeled antibodies have been used, with limited success.

L

lung cancer

The major histological types of lung cancer are non–small cell cancers (squamous cell carcinoma, adenocarcinoma, and large cell undifferentiated carcinoma), which account for 90% of lung cancers, and small cell lung cancers, which make up the remaining 10%.

Etiology and incidence: Cigarette smoking is implicated in approximately 80% to 90% of all cases of lung cancer. Occupational exposure to asbestos, radon, nickel, chromium, hydrocarbons, and arsenic is linked to 10% to 15% of lung cancers. The role of air pollution and home exposure to radon gas is unclear. Lung cancer is the leading cause of cancer death for both men and women in the United States and kills more than 157,000 persons per year. More than 170,000 cases are diagnosed each year, and the incidence for women is rising rapidly.

Pathophysiology: Squamous cell carcinomas usually begin in the larger bronchi, often causing bronchial obstruction and spreading by direct extension and lymph node metastasis. Adenocarcinomas are peripheral tumors that begin in fibrotic lung tissue and spread through the bloodstream, commonly metastasizing to the brain, liver, and bone. Large cell undifferentiated carcinoma, which may arise in any area of the lung, disseminates early, spreading through the bloodstream. Small cell carcinoma is centrally located and is the fastest growing type of lung cancer, with rapid metastasis to the brain, liver, and bone.

Risk Factors

Smoking
Passive smoking (nonsmokers with chronic exposure to cigarette smoke)
Exposure to asbestos, radon, nickel, chromium, hydrocarbons, and arsenic particularly in combination with smoking
Exposure to radiation

Clinical Manifestations

A chronic cough, a change in the volume and color of sputum, chronic upper respiratory tract infections, and aching in the chest are common presenting symptoms. Wheezing, fatigue, and chest tightness may also be present.

Complications

The prognosis is poor. The long-term survival rate in individuals with localized disease is only 35%, and most people have extension and metastasis on diagnosis. Overall the survival rate for all individuals regardless of stage is 10%. Complications include superior vena cava syndrome, paraneoplastic syndromes, and cor pulmonale.

Diagnostic Tests

A history of smoking and a chest x-ray are the principal sources of diagnostic suspicion. A sputum cytology test is positive in about 75% of cases. Retrieval of cells through bronchoscopy or needle or tissue biopsy provides the definitive diagnosis.

Therapeutic Management

Surgery	Resection of tumor and surrounding tissue, lobectomy or pneumonectomy
Drugs	Systemic multidrug combination chemotherapy, biologic response modifiers
General	Radiotherapy before and after surgery and for palliation, smoking cessation, prevention through education about dangers of tobacco and environmental irritants

lupus (systemic lupus erythematosus)

A chronic, multisystem, inflammatory connective tissue disorder

Etiology and incidence: The cause of systemic lupus erythematosus (SLE) is unknown, but it is thought to be an autoimmune disease with interrelated environmental, hormonal, viral, and genetic factors. More than 500,000 individuals in the United States have diagnosed cases of SLE. Nine times as many women as men are affected, and three times as many blacks as whites.

Pathophysiology: After the etiologic agent or agents are introduced, the body forms antibodies directed against "self" tissues, cells, and serum proteins. The regulatory components of the immune system are severely compromised by these autoantibodies. The number and activity of suppressor T-cells are both diminished, allowing unrestrained proliferation of B-cells and resultant hypergammaglobulinemia. Combinations of autoantibodies and autoantigens form, circulate, and are deposited within capillary complexes, renal glomeruli, renal interstitia, serosal membranes, and the choroid plexus, as well as in the pleural vasculature. The formation of these immune complexes triggers an inflammatory response, leading to chronic destruction of host tissue.

Clinical Manifestations

Signs and symptoms vary with the acuteness of the disease and the distribution of the immune complexes in body tissues. No characteristic clinical pattern exists, but the following manifestations may be seen:

1. *Skin:* Malar or discoid rash (butterfly rash) with scaling, plugging of hair follicles and scarring, painless ulcerations of nasal and oral mucosa, photosensitivity-induced rash
2. *Joints:* Tenderness, swelling, arthritis-like pain
3. *Lungs:* Pleuritis, pleuritic pain, dyspnea, cyanosis
4. *Kidneys:* Oliguria, bladder spasms, edema, proteinuria
5. *Neurological effects:* Seizure activity, depression, psychoses
6. *Blood:* Anemia, thrombocytopenia
7. *Cardiac effects:* Pericarditis, murmurs, electrocardiographic changes

8. *General:* Fatigue, headache, fever, malaise, nausea, vomiting, anorexia, weight loss, abdominal pain

Complications

SLE is a chronic, relapsing disease often marked by long periods of remission. If acute episodes can be successfully controlled, the long-term prognosis is good. The 10-year survival rate approaches 95% in the United States. Concomitant infections and renal failure are the leading causes of death.

Diagnostic Tests

Antinuclear antibody (ANA) tests are positive in 98% of SLE cases. A positive ANA test should lead to use of a test for anti-deoxyribonucleic acid antibodies. A high titer in this test is almost specific for SLE.

Therapeutic Management

Surgery	Joint replacement for chronic synovitis, kidney transplant for renal failure
Drugs	Nonsteroidal antiinflammatory drugs for mild disease, steroids and immunosuppressives for severe disease, antiinfective drugs for secondary infections, antimalarials for skin rash
General	Plasmapheresis to reduce circulating immune complexes, renal dialysis for renal failure, aggressive management of intercurrent infection, long-term medical monitoring; balanced diet, careful monitoring if pregnant, keeping a disease-related log to trace conditions that trigger flare-ups, early treatment of flare-ups, counseling to adapt to long-term disease

L

lyme disease

A multisystem infectious disease transmitted by a tick bite and characterized by an early skin lesion

Etiology and incidence: The disease is caused by a spirochete called *Borrelia burgdorferi*. Lyme disease is the most common vector-transmitted disease in the United States. Persons of all ages are vulnerable, and the highest incidence is among individuals living in and around wooded areas. It is endemic in the northeastern, midwestern and western United States.

Pathophysiology: The spirochete enters the skin at the site of a tick bite. It incubates for 3 to 32 days and then migrates outward to the skin, forming a pinkish red rash that resembles a bull's-eye target. It may then spread to other skin sites and various organ systems via the lymphatics and bloodstream. An inflammatory cycle is set up, and cardiac, neurological, and joint abnormalities are common developments.

Clinical Manifestations

The disease first manifests itself as a red skin macule or papule at the bite site with accompanying flulike symptoms. These are often missed or ignored by the individual. In about 50% of cases, other lesions develop soon after onset.

Complications

After weeks or months, neurological abnormalities such as meningitis, meningoencephalitis, neuritis, and radiculopathies appear in about 15% of cases. Myocardial abnormalities such as atrioventricular block, myopericarditis, and cardiomegaly occur in 8% of cases. Joint inflammation, pain, and arthritis develop in 50% of cases as long as 2 years after transmission.

Diagnostic Tests

A physical examination with characteristic lesions and a positive enzyme-linked immunosorbent assay (ELISA) is indicative of the disease.

Therapeutic Management

Surgery	None
Drugs	Antiinfective drugs to combat infection
General	Bed rest, treatment of complications, prevention by wearing appropriate clothing in wooded or grassy areas and using bug repellent

L

lymphoma, non-Hodgkin's

Neoplasms of the lymphoid tissue

Etiology and incidence: The cause is unknown, but theories involving immune deficiencies and viral origins are under investigation. More than 43,000 cases are diagnosed and more than 24,000 deaths occur annually in the United States. The peak incidence occurs in preadolescence, with a drop during adolescence and then a steady increase with age in adulthood. Men and whites are at slightly higher risk than women and blacks. For unknown reasons, the incidence is on the rise in the United States.

Pathophysiology: Normal cells in the lymph nodes are replaced with immature, rapidly progressive leukocyte cells of either the T-cell or B-cell type. Rare cases involve histiocytes. Spread is via the lymphatic system to regional and distal sites, including the skin, bone marrow, brain, and gastrointestinal system.

Clinical Manifestations

A wide variety of signs and symptoms is possible, but many individuals have painless lymphadenopathy, typically of the cervical or inguinal nodes. Other symptoms are fatigue, malaise, fever, anemia, weight loss, night sweats, abdominal pain, and skin lesions.

Complications

The prognosis for individuals with low-grade tumors is good with early treatment. Rapidly progressive intermediate- and high-grade tumors have a poor prognosis. Complications include central nervous system disease, spinal cord compression, and superior vena cava syndrome.

Diagnostic Tests

A definitive diagnosis is made through lymph node biopsy.

Therapeutic Management

Surgery	Excision of tumors in advanced disease; therapeutic splenectomy
Drugs	Systemic combination chemotherapy with radiation
General	Radiation is the primary therapy, used alone or in combination with chemotherapy, particularly for stage III and stage IV cancer; bone marrow or peripheral blood stem cell transplantation is used as a salvage treatment.

L

malaria

An infectious disease transmitted by a mosquito bite and characterized by fever, sweats, and chills

Etiology and incidence: Malaria is caused by four species of protozoan parasites: *Plasmodium vivax, P. falciparum, P. malariae,* and *P. ovale.* Infection occurs through the bite of an infected mosquito or by contact with blood products from an infected individual. It is estimated that there are more than 100 million cases of malaria worldwide each year; 1 million persons die of the disease annually in Africa alone. Most endemic areas are in the tropics, and underdeveloped countries are particularly hard hit. Relatively few cases are reported in the United States annually, and most involve travelers to endemic regions.

Pathophysiology: A mosquito carrier bites a human host and injects the sporozoites, which reside and multiply in the parenchymal cells of the liver. After a maturation period averaging 2 to 4 weeks, merozoites are released and invade the erythrocytes. The infected erythrocytes rupture and release merozoites, pyrogens, and toxins, which cause hemolysis, sluggish blood flow in the capillaries, and adherence of infected erythrocytes to venous walls, obstructing blood flow, increasing the permeability of the capillaries, and causing tissue extravasation, particularly in the brain and gastrointestinal system.

Clinical Manifestations

The incubation period is followed by a 2- to 3-day prodromal period marked by low-grade fever, malaise, headache, joint aches, and chills similar to the flu and often misdiagnosed and treated as such. A paroxysmal pattern is then established, beginning with a shaking chill and followed by fever and sweats. After the fever and sweats (usually lasting 1 to 8 hours), the person feels well until the next chill begins. One cycle ranges from 20 to 72 hours, depending on the parasite involved.

Complications

Chronic malaria with accompanying parasitemia may occur in partially immune individuals in hyperendemic areas. It is characterized by recurring symptoms resembling a mild, short attack of acute malaria. Blackwater fever is a rare complication characterized by severe hemolytic anemia and renal failure. Uremia and renal failure are common complications. Cerebral malaria causes seizure, psychosis, and coma. Pulmonary edema and splenic rupture are also seen. Untreated malaria caused by *P. falciparum* has a 20% mortality rate.

Diagnostic Tests

A physical evaluation revealing the paroxysmal pattern and an enlarged spleen plus a history of exposure to an endemic area within the year are significant. A blood smear that isolates the parasite provides the definitive diagnosis.

Therapeutic Management

Surgery	None
Drugs	Antimalarial drugs for acute attacks and as prophylaxis if traveling to endemic areas; vaccines are experimental
General	Individual prophylaxis includes insect repellent, covering of skin, use of mosquito netting for bed, and avoidance of outdoors at night when in endemic areas; community prophylaxis includes control of mosquito breeding grounds and protection of the blood supply.

M

measles

See Rubella and Rubeola.

Ménière's disease

A chronic disease of the inner ear characterized by recurrent vertigo, tinnitus, and hearing loss

Etiology and incidence: The cause of Ménière's disease is unknown, although a genetic link has been suggested. Other theories have proposed trauma, infection, otosclerosis, or syphilis as inciting factors. Adults of both genders between 30 and 60 years of age are usually affected, and most cases are unilateral although 15% to 30% become bilateral 2 to 5 years after a unilateral onset.

Pathophysiology: The pathogenesis of Ménière's disease is poorly understood but is thought to center on overproduction or decreased absorption of endolymph, which causes a degeneration of the neural end organ of the labyrinth and cochlea and rupture of the labyrinth. The rupture allows endolymph into the perilymphatic space, causing a temporary paralysis of sensory structures.

Clinical Manifestations

The hallmark manifestations are an attack of prostrating vertigo with nausea and vomiting, worsening tinnitus, and sensory hearing loss with a feeling of fullness or pressure in the affected ear. The attack may last from a few hours to a day, and then it gradually subsides. Between acute attacks the person has progressive hearing loss and a persistent background humming and has an intolerance to loud noises.

Complications

Progressive hearing loss is the primary complication.

Diagnostic Tests

A history of the characteristic symptoms and a positive caloric test are indicative of Ménière's disease.

Therapeutic Management

Surgery   Decompression of the endolymphatic sac helps in about 65% of cases; labyrinthectomy or vestibular neurectomy to destroy end organs and neural connections relieves vertigo in 90% of cases, with stabilization or improvement of hearing loss in 75% of cases.

Drugs   Vestibular suppressants or anticholinergics for symptomatic relief of vertigo; antiemetics and sedatives to prevent vomiting and promote rest during acute attack; diuretics, antihistamines, and vasodilators during remission

General   Bed rest with safety precautions, avoidance of sudden head movements during acute attack; low-sodium diet to reduce fluid retention is helpful in some cases

M

meningitis, bacterial

An infection and inflammation of the meninges of the brain and spinal cord resulting in altered neurological function

Etiology and incidence: Bacterial meningitis can be caused by any number of bacteria, but 80% of cases are caused by one of three strains: *Neisseria meningitidis, Haemophilus influenzae,* and *Streptococcus pneumoniae.* The disease occurs worldwide and is both endemic and epidemic. Spread is through droplet contact, and the disease can be transmitted as long as the respiratory tract contains the causative bacteria. Children under age 5 are at greatest risk. Pneumococcal meningitis is the most common form of adult meningitis.

Pathophysiology: The bacteria invade the respiratory passages and are disseminated by the bloodstream to the cerebrospinal fluid (CSF) space and the meninges of the brain and spinal cord. A growing exudate damages cranial nerves, obliterates CSF pathways, and induces vasculitis and thrombophlebitis. The exudate also generates metabolites and cytokines, which damage cell membranes, disrupt the blood-brain barrier, and cause cerebral edema and ischemic brain damage.

Clinical Manifestations

A prodromal respiratory illness may precede symptoms of fever, severe headache, stiff neck, and vomiting. Changes in consciousness then occur, beginning with irritability, drowsiness, and confusion, followed by stupor and coma. Seizures are common.

Complications

Complications include hydrocephalus, blindness, deafness, arthritis, myocarditis, pericarditis, and cognitive deficit.

Diagnostic Tests

Cultures of CSF, respiratory secretions, and blood are positive for the causative agent.

Therapeutic Management

Surgery	None
Drugs	Antiinfective drugs specific for the causative agent, analgesics for muscle pain and headache, vaccine for prevention in at-risk populations, antiinfective drugs for those in close contact with an infected individual; corticosteroid use is under investigation
General	Adequate hydration and balancing of electrolytes, monitoring and control of intracranial pressure, hemodynamic monitoring, ventilatory support if necessary, seizure precautions, secretion precautions to prevent spread, comfort measures for photophobia, monitoring of contacts with infected individuals

migraine

M

See Headache.

mononucleosis

An acute viral infectious disease characterized by fatigue, fever, pharyngitis, and lymphadenopathy

Etiology and incidence: Mononucleosis is caused by the Epstein-Barr virus (EBV) and transmitted via prolonged contact with infected saliva or through blood transfusion. After the primary infection the virus remains in the host for life and is periodically shed in nasal secretions. At any given time, 15% to 20% of the adult population are active carriers. Mononucleosis is common in the United States, Canada, and Europe, particularly among adolescents and young adults.

Pathophysiology: EBV invades the host and incubates for 4 to 6 weeks. It then replicates in the nasopharynx and moves to the lymphatic system, where it infects B lymphocytes and stimulates the secretion of an antigen. T lymphocytes proliferate in response to the antigen, producing a generalized lymph node hyperplasia.

Clinical Manifestations

The hallmark signs are profound fatigue; a fever that peaks in the late afternoon at 101° to 105° F (38.3° to 40.6° C); severely painful and exudative pharyngitis; and symmetric lymphadenopathy. Splenomegaly is usually present in the second or third week. Mild hepatomegaly may also be present. A maculopapular rash, palatal petechiae, and periorbital edema are less common signs.

Complications

The prognosis is excellent; complications are rare but include splenic rupture, anemia, Guillain-Barré syndrome, meningitis, and encephalitis.

Diagnostic Tests

The presence of clinical manifestations plus a differential WBC count showing lymphocytes and monocytes over 50%; a heterophil agglutination antibody test with an antibody titer greater than 1:40; and an EBV-immunogobulin M test with antibodies over 1:80 are all suggestive of mononucleosis. Liver function tests (aspartate aminotransferase [AST], alamine aminotransferase [ALT], bilirubin) elevated if the liver is involved.

Therapeutic Management

Surgery	Removal of the spleen in cases of rupture
Drugs	Nonaspirin analgesics and antipyretics; steroids for treating impending airway obstruction
General	Bed rest during the acute phase, saline throat gargles, adequate hydration, avoidance of heavy lifting and contact sports for 2 months after recovery to prevent injury to spleen

M

multiple sclerosis

A chronic, progressive central nervous system disease with a disseminating demyelination of the nerve fibers of the brain and spinal cord, characterized by exacerbation and remission of varied multiple neurological symptoms

Etiology and incidence: The exact etiology of multiple sclerosis (MS) is unknown, but an immunological abnormality, allergic response, or slow-acting virus is suspected. MS is the most prevalent demyelinating disease and the third leading cause of disability in young and middle adulthood. More than 8,000 cases are diagnosed in the United States each year.

Pathophysiology: Multifocal plaques of demyelination form continuously and are distributed randomly throughout the white matter of the central nervous system, with accompanying destruction of oligodendroglia and perivascular inflammation. As myelin breakdown continues, lipid byproducts undergo phagocytosis, and the myelin sheath is destroyed. This leads to a decrease in velocity and blockage of nerve conduction and interference with or failure of impulse transmissions. Cell bodies and axons are preserved early in the disease, but eventually the axons are stripped bare. Discrete lesions extend and coalesce into larger lesions. Astrocytic processes proliferate, transforming older lesions into glial scars. The scars stop the inflammation and edema of the lesion, leading to remission early in the disease process. However, as the disease progresses, symptoms become permanent.

Clinical Manifestations

Signs and symptoms depend on the size, age, activity, and location of the lesions. Remissions may last months or years early in the disease. Later remission intervals are shorter, and eventually permanent, progressive disablement occurs.

Early	The onset is generally insidious and symptoms are transient, beginning with paresthesias in extremities, trunk, or face; clumsiness and muscle weakness; transient visual disturbances and optic pain; ataxia; bladder incontinence; and vertigo

Midcourse	Emotional lability, apathy, and shortened attention span; seizures; diplopia; dysarthria; static tremor; spasticity, gait disturbances; transient bowel incontinence
Late	Dementia, scanning speech, nystagmus, intention tremor, hemiplegia, generalized muscular weakness and atrophy, inability to stand and walk, loss of bowel and bladder control

Complications

Some individuals have frequent attacks, leading to rapid incapacitation with an unremitting, progressive course that ends in death within 1 to 2 years. Others are prone to complications related to progressive disease and disuse syndrome, such as pressure sores, contractures, pathological fractures, pneumonia, renal infection, and septicemia. Death usually is caused by complications rather than the primary disease.

Diagnostic Tests

Diagnosis is elusive and indirect and is deduced from clinical features and laboratory tests, which include elevated cerebrospinal fluid (CSF); immunoglobulin G (IgG), coupled with normal serum IgG; normal CSF protein; slowed nerve conduction in evoked potential studies; and CT and MRI scans of lesions.

Therapeutic Management

Surgery	Rhizotomy for unresponsive spasms, contracture releases
Drugs	Muscle relaxants for spasticity, corticosteroids for acute attacks; immunosuppressive therapy is in clinical trials
General	Balance of rest and activity; long-term rehabilitation (occupational, physical, and speech therapy) to maintain activities of daily living, adapt to progressive loss of function, prevent disuse syndrome, and promote bowel and bladder control; assistive devices (canes, walkers, bracing, casting, wheelchairs); counseling and psycho-

logical support of individual and family; respite home care; ventilatory assistance and communication devices in end-stage disease; care in feeding if dysphagia is present; evaluation for cognitive dysfunction; plasmapheresis and total lymphoid irradiation are under investigation

mumps (parotitis)

An acute, contagious viral disease, characterized by unilateral or bilateral edema and enlargement of the salivary glands

Etiology and incidence: The causative agent is the paramyxovirus, and the disease is spread by droplet or direct contact with infected saliva. It is most communicable immediately before and during the glandular swelling. Mumps is most often seen in children ages 5 to 15, although it may occur at any age. Adults are more likely to have a severe course of the disease. Permanent immunity occurs after infection. About 25% to 30% of cases are subclinical.

Pathophysiology: After a 2- to 3-week incubation period, the virus invades one or more salivary glands, causing tissue edema and infiltration of lymphocytes. Cells in the glandular ducts degenerate and produce necrotic debris, which plugs the ducts.

Clinical Manifestations

Onset begins with fever, headache, and malaise about 24 hours before swelling of the gland or glands (usually the parotid glands), either unilaterally or bilaterally. Pain is noted on chewing and swallowing. The glands remain swollen about 72 hours before receding.

Complications

Occasionally, particularly in adults, other glands in the testes, ovaries, breasts, and thyroid are involved, and the disease course is often more severe. Complications include meningoencephalitis, pericarditis, deafness, arthritis, nephritis, and in rare cases, sterility in men.

Diagnostic Tests

Characteristic swelling
Positive cell cultures from saliva or urine

Therapeutic Management

Surgery	None
Drugs	Analgesics, antipyretics, live mumps virus vaccine for active immunity
General	Bed rest, hydration, isolation during communicability, compresses on swelling, support of scrotum with orchitis
Prevention	MMR (measles, mumps, rubella) vaccine, given at age 1 with second dose at ages 4 to 6

muscular dystrophy

A group of inherited, progressive, degenerative muscle disorders characterized by an insidious loss of muscle strength in a variety of muscle groups. Duchenne's muscular dystrophy (DMD) is the most common of the disorders.

Etiology and incidence: DMD and Becker's muscular dystrophy (BMD), a clinical variant of DMD, are X-linked recessive disorders involving the gene that encodes dystrophin. Males are exclusively affected, and the incidence in the United States is one in every 3,000 live male births. These disorders typically manifest in boys ages 3 to 7. Females are carriers. Other dystrophies (Landouzy-Dejerine dystrophy [LDMD], Leyden-Möbius dystrophy [LMMD], Erb's dystrophy, and mitochondrial and congenital myopathies) are also inherited, but the specific genetic link is less clear. These disorders are seen in children and adults, affect males and females, and are milder.

Pathophysiology: Dystrophin, a protein product in skeletal muscle, is absent in individuals with DMD and reduced in those with BMD. The resulting pathogenesis is not clear, but lack of dystrophin is thought to impair fast muscle fiber function and to induce a number of biochemical anomalies, including intracellular accumulation of calcium. A number of systemic sequelae have also been noted. Serotonin in the platelets is reduced, and nonmuscle cells have reduced adhesiveness and generalized membrane abnormalities. Central nervous system neuropathology is noted, as is reduced gastrointestinal motility. Platelet function and the vascularity of endothelial cells are abnormal.

Clinical Manifestations

DMD	Delays in gross motor development; difficulty walking, running, climbing stairs, and riding a tricycle appears at about age 3 to 5; progressive weakness with waddling gait, lordosis, difficulty rising from a sitting or supine position; calf muscle hypertrophy; scoliosis; contractures and joint deformities; inability to ambu-

	late by about age 12; mild mental retardation; respiratory and accessory muscles involved in end stage with cardiomegaly
BMD	Onset occurs at age 5 to 25; symptoms are similar to but milder than DMD.
	Ambulation is lost about 20 years after onset.
	Contractures, scoliosis, and ventilatory failure are rare, and the life span usually is normal
LDMD	Onset from age 7 to 20; weakness of facial and shoulder girdle muscles; difficulty whistling, closing eyes, and raising arms; footdrop develops late; life span is normal
LMMD/Erb's	Adult onset with weakness of pelvic girdle (LMMD) and shoulder girdle (Erb's)

Complications

The major complications of DMD are disuse atrophy, contractures, and cardiopulmonary problems, resulting in respiratory infections. Death is usually a result of complications rather than the primary disease.

Diagnostic Tests

DMD and BMD are diagnosed through clinical evaluation and the characteristic manifestations; electromyography reveals rapidly recruited myopathic motor units without spontaneous activity; muscle biopsy shows necrosis and varied muscle fiber size; dystrophin immunoblotting is done in which dystrophin is absent (DMD) or abnormal (BMD). Other types are distinguished primarily on clinical grounds.

Therapeutic Management

Surgery	Contracture release, spinal instrumentation to correct scoliosis, tracheostomy in end-stage DMD
Drugs	Random clinical trials are being conducted with steroids; antiinfective drugs for bacterial infections in end-stage DMD

General   Long-term rehabilitation (occupational and physical therapy) to maintain activities of daily living and help adapt to progressive loss of function, prevent disuse syndrome, and promote bowel and bladder control; assistive devices (canes, walkers, bracing, casting, wheelchairs); counseling and psychological support of individual and family; respite home care; ventilatory assistance and communication devices in end-stage DMD; family genetic counseling, identification of carriers

M

myasthenia gravis

A progressive neuromuscular disease of the lower motor neurons characterized by muscle weakness and fatigue

Etiology and incidence: The cause of myasthenia gravis (MG) is unknown although evidence points to a systematic autoimmune disorder. More than 80% of individuals with MG also have thymic abnormalities, but the link is unclear. The incidence is 3 to 6 per 100,000 individuals in the United States. The age of onset is either 20 to 30 years (primarily in women) or 50 to 60 years (primarily in men).

Pathophysiology: An antigen attack on the acetylcholine receptor of the postsynaptic neuromuscular junction results in dysfunction of the receptor, which fails to act on the acetylcholine. Because of this, nerve impulses do not pass on to the skeletal muscle at the myoneural junction.

Clinical Manifestations

The most common manifestations are ptosis, diplopia, and muscle fatigue after exercise. Dysarthria, dysphagia, ocular palsy, head bobbing, and facial and proximal limb weakness are also reported. Symptoms are milder on awakening and become worse as the day progresses. Rest temporarily improves symptoms. Respiratory involvement leads to breathlessness and reduced tidal volume and vital capacity. Manifestations can be remitting, static, or progressive. Factors such as stress, menses, heat, and illness can exacerbate symptoms.

Complications

Myasthenic crisis is an acute exacerbation of symptoms; it usually involves respiratory distress and can lead to respiratory failure or aspiration and cardiopulmonary arrest.

Diagnostic Tests

A characteristic pattern of fatigue and weakness on exertion that improves with rest and a positive Tensilon test, are indicators. A CT scan may indicate the presence of thymoma;

electromyography may show muscle fiber contraction with progressive decremental response.

Therapeutic Management

Surgery	Thymectomy for treatment of thymoma and remission of adult-onset MG
Drugs	Anticholinesterases and corticosteroids to counteract muscle weakness and fatigue; immunosuppressants with autoimmune pathogenesis; influenza shots to prevent respiratory infection
General	Plasmapheresis to treat weakness and fatigue, ventilatory support in respiratory crisis, physical therapy to prevent disuse problems and occupational therapy to aid in activities of daily living, balance of exercise and rest; instruction about cholinergic crisis caused by excessive anticholinesterase medication, counseling for long-term adaptation to disease, information about the importance of preventing respiratory infection or recognizing and treating symptoms early

M

myeloma, multiple

A progressive, hematologic neoplastic disease of the plasma cells

Etiology and incidence: The etiologic factors are not clearly understood, but chromosomal abnormalities, genetic factors, viruses, and chronic antigen stimulation have been implicated as probable contributors. Multiple myeloma is a relatively rare disease that occurs primarily in those over age 40 and peaks around age 60. Men and women are equally affected, but the disease rate for blacks is 14 times that of whites. More than 13,000 cases are diagnosed in the United States each year, with 9,400 deaths.

Pathophysiology: Multiple myeloma involves an abnormal growth and proliferation of plasma cells and the development of single or multiple plasma cell tumors in the bone marrow. This leads to mass destruction of bone marrow and bone throughout the body. Plasma cells also produce an M protein immunoglobulin that coats the RBCs and inhibits the production of effective antibodies; this can lead to anemia. Metastasis is via the lymph nodes to the liver, kidneys, and spleen.

Risk Factors

Occupational exposure to petroleum products, asbestos, or radiation

Clinical Manifestations

Early symptoms are nonspecific and include fatigue, weakness, anorexia, and weight loss. These are followed by complaints of bone pain, particularly in the back and thorax, and frequent bacterial infections, particularly pneumonia and anemia. Later manifestations include thrombocytopenia and leukopenia; urinary changes; changes in cognitive, sensory, and motor functions; pathological fractures and vertebral collapse; spinal cord compression; and paraplegia.

Complications

The disease is progressive, and currently has no cure. Life expectancy is tied to the extent of disease at time of diagnosis; the median survival rate is 2 to 3 years. Complications include infection, hyperuricemia, hypercalcemia, pyelonephritis, renal failure, and GI bleeding.

Diagnostic Tests

The diagnosis is made based on one or more of the following criteria: plasma cell infiltration above 10% in bone marrow, a monoclonal spike on serum electrophoresis, presence of Bence-Jones protein in blood, radiographical visualization of osteoporosis and osteolytic lesions, soft-tissue plasma cell tumors.

Therapeutic Management

Surgery	Laminectomy and fusion for spinal cord compression
Drugs	Chemotherapy is the primary treatment, anti-infective drugs for bacterial infections, allopurinol for hyperuricemia, corticosteroids for hypercalcemia
General	Radiation in chemotherapy-resistant disease and for palliation of bone pain; bone marrow transplantation has been used with limited success; ambulation maintained as long as possible; physical therapy to maintain function; fracture precautions; adequate hydration to prevent dehydration associated with proteinuria; transfusions for anemia; monitoring for bleeding episodes; precautions against exposure to infections; emotional support for adaptation to chronic, terminal disease

M

myocardial infarction (heart attack)

Ischemic necrosis of the myocardium resulting from inadequate coronary artery blood flow

Etiology and incidence: More than 90% of all myocardial infarctions (MIs) are caused by obstruction of a plaque-lined coronary artery by an acute thrombus. MI also may be caused by arterial embolization from valvular stenosis or endocarditis and by arterial spasm after cocaine ingestion. Each year more than 1 million persons in the United States have an MI; one in four dies, and more than half of these deaths occur within 1 hour of onset. (See also Coronary Artery Disease and Angina.)

Pathophysiology: Occlusion of a coronary artery causes a persistent cellular ischemia that interferes with myocardial tissue metabolism, causing rapid, permanent cell damage and necrosis. The extent of necrosis is dictated by the size of the infarct, the vessel occluded, and the length of time it remains occluded. Damage initially occurs to the left ventricle but often extends to other cardiac chambers. Infarcts may be classified by the thickness of the myocardial tissue involved. Transmural infarcts (Q wave) involve the full thickness of the myocardium from the epicardium to endocardium and cause abnormal Q waves on the ECG. Nontransmural infarcts (non–Q wave) do not extend through the ventricular wall and cause ST segment or T wave ECG abnormalities.

Risk Factors

Familial history of heart disease
History of hypertension, diabetes mellitus
Smoking
Sedentary lifestyle
Obesity
High-fat diet
Elevated cholesterol and triglycerides
Stress
Driven, aggressive, impatient personality type

Clinical Manifestations

Most individuals have prodromal symptoms such as fatigue, shortness of breath, and crescendo angina days or weeks before the acute attack. The first symptom of the attack is usually a deep, substernal, visceral pain that may be described as aching, squeezing, or crushing, or as a heavy weight on the chest. The pain may radiate to the back, neck, jaw, teeth, or left arm, and it is not relieved by rest, nitroglycerin, or antacids. Other signs and symptoms include anxiety; restlessness; sweating; nausea; vomiting; cold, clammy skin; low-grade fever; and dyspnea. Females may have a different set of presenting symptoms than males. Their symtoms are often vague, diffuse, and less pronounced in nature, and ECG changes may be less visible. Common symptoms in women include nausea, vomiting, fatigue, dizziness, shortness of breath, and neck and shoulder pain.

Complications

Complications include arrhythmia, cardiogenic shock, heart failure, pulmonary edema, cerebral or pulmonary emboli, myocardial rupture, pericarditis, postmyocardial infarction syndrome, and sudden death. Forty-four percent of women and 27% of men die within the first year of an MI.

Diagnostic Tests

The diagnosis is made using a clinical history; ECG, which illustrates an elevation in the ST segment, T wave inversion, and deep Q waves; laboratory tests of cardiac enzymes (aspartate aminotransferase, creatine phosphokinase, lactate dehydrogenase), which are elevated for days after the event; CBC, which reveals an elevated white count and erythrocyte sedimentation rate; a thallium perfusion scan to determine the size and location of the infarct and resulting ischemia; and an echocardiogram, to detect contraction abnormalities of ventricles. ECG changes may be less visible in women.

Therapeutic Management

Surgery   Angioplasty post thrombolysis is *contraindicated*. Recent clinical trials have shown no benefit and possible harm from angioplasty performed within the first few days after an attack.

	Angioplasty may have a rescue role in cardiogenic shock that is unresponsive to other treatment.
Drugs	Thrombolytic drugs given within 6 hours of onset to interrupt MI evolution; aspirin and anticoagulants for antiplatelet, anticoagulant effects; beta-adrenergic blockers to reduce reinfarction and infarct size; angiotensin-converting enzyme inhibitors to reduce ventricular enlargement; vasodilators and narcotic analgesics for pain, antihyperlipidemics to lower chlosterol and triglyceride levels; stool softeners to avoid straining at stool; sedatives and tranquilizers to increase rest; estrogen supplements in post-menopausal women (can decrease risk of death by 40% to 50%)
General	Cardiovascular monitoring; oxygen therapy; bed rest; decreased environmental stimuli; monitoring for and treatment of depression, particularly about the third day; quitting smoking; restriction of caffeine and cholesterol; antiembolism hose; rehabilitation with stepped exercise program, sexual counseling; regular medical follow-up

oral and oropharyngeal cancer

Oropharyngeal cancer is classified anatomically rather than by cell type and includes cancers of the oral cavity, pharynx, and salivary glands. The oral cavity includes the lips, oral mucosa, gums, most of the tongue, and teeth. The oropharynx begins anteriorly where the oral cavity stops. It includes the base of the tongue, the soft palate, uvula, tonsils, and pharyngeal walls.

Etiology and incidence: The cause of oropharyngeal cancers is unknown, but the aerodigestive tract is exposed to a wide range of carcinogens, including tobacco products and alcohol. Although less than 5% of all cancers are oropharyngeal, the incidence and prevalence of oropharyngeal cancer is growing. Men have oropharyngeal cancer more often than women and blacks more than whites. For both genders and all races, the 1995 new case incidence was 19.4:100,000 population. Oral cancers, those of the lips and mouth, account for 3% of all cancers in men and 2% in women. More than 90% of all oropharyngeal cancers occur in individuals over age 45.

Pathophysiology: Most all oropharyngeal cancers are squamous cell cancers arising on the floor of the mouth, the ventrolateral aspect of the tongue, and the soft palate complex.

Risk Factors

Chronic exposure to tobacco including cigarettes, pipes, cigars and smokeless tobacco (chewing tobacco, snuff)
Poor oral hygiene
Prolonged heavy use of alcohol
Poorly fitting dentures that cause chronic lesions and/or ulcers

Clinical Manifestations

Early	Dysphagia; local pain; pain on swallowing; leukoplakia (white patch that does not rub off); reddened areas; mouth or throat ulcers that do not heal; hoarseness; localized pain
Later	Difficulty swallowing; excessive secretions; airway disturbance; enlarged lymph nodes

Complications

The overall 5-year survival rate for oral cavity tumors is 50% and for oropharyngeal cancers is about 35%. Complications include disfigurement; loss of hard or soft palate; nerve damage that may lead to impaired eating, chewing, or swallowing; paralysis; and difficulty with communication.

Diagnostic Tests

Biopsy	Scraping of leukoplakia and/or biopsy of a lesion for histopathological confirmation is diagnostic
X-ray and/or CT scan	To determine evidence of muscle, bone, or lymphatic involvement

Therapeutic Management

Surgery	The decision for surgery is determined on disease staging, location, and functional deficit or anticipated outcome for the disease. Surgery may range from simple tumor removal to radical resection of the cancer.
Drugs	Chemotherapy may be used to shrink tumors before surgery or radiation therapy.
General	Radiation therapy may be used as an early state treatment or a treatment where the functional deficit by surgery may be great or may be indicated postoperatively.

organic mental syndromes (organic brain syndrome)

A constellation of behavioral signs and symptoms associated with transient or permanent dysfunction of the brain and characterized by impaired intellectual functioning, confusion, and agitation

Etiology and incidence: Delirium and dementia are the most common categories and are discussed here. Delirium is a reversible, self-limiting condition characterized by a reduced ability to maintain attention to or appropriately shift attention among different external stimuli. Dementia is a structurally caused, permanent decline in memory, abstract thinking, and judgment.

Delirium most often occurs as a result of withdrawal from intoxication in chronic alcohol and barbiturate abusers and in acute inflammatory disorders such as meningitis and encephalitis. The most common cause of dementia is Alzheimer's disease. Other causes include vascular disease; HIV infection; central nervous system infection; severe head injury; toxic metabolic disturbances; normal pressure hydrocephalus; underlying neurological disease (Parkinson's disease, Huntington's chorea, multiple sclerosis, Pick's disease); and drug, alcohol, or nutritional abuse. More than 1 million persons in the United States have dementia, and the elderly are at greatest risk. As the incidence of AIDS increases, the incidence of dementia is expected to increase (an estimated 50% of individuals with end-stage AIDS develop dementia).

Pathophysiology: The pathophysiology of organic mental syndromes is not yet understood. Pathological changes vary by causation and in Alzheimer's-related dementia include atrophy of brain tissue with wide sulci and dilated ventricles, senile plaque formation, and neurofibrillary tangles. Vascular disease–induced dementia is characterized by multiple cerebral infarcts. In AIDS-related dementia, the neurons are infected with HIV, and in hydrocephalus, cerebrospinal fluid circulation and absorption are impeded.

Clinical Manifestations

Delirium	Rapid onset; disorientation, including loss of self-recognition in some instances; impaired

memory; inability to maintain or shift attention; irritability, agitation, restlessness, and hyperactivity; perceptual disturbance, hallucinations, and delusions; rambling, fragmented speech; impaired sleep-wake cycle; lucid intervals with symptoms worse at night; duration about 1 week on average

Dementia   Symptoms vary widely, but the overall picture is a slow, insidious disintegration of personality and intellect with impaired insight and judgment and loss of affect.

Memory impairment is often the most prominent initial symptom, and others include increasing rigidity of thought; restricted interests; easy distractibility; lack of initiation; speech disturbances; loss of impulse control; change of former traits or exaggeration of those traits (e.g., a neat person becomes slovenly or becomes obsessively preoccupied with orderliness); and depression.

Complications

Delirium may lead to dementia. Dementia (except that caused by trauma) is progressive; the individual eventually becomes totally oblivious to his or her surroundings and ultimately dies. Individuals with dementia are more susceptible to accidents and infection.

Diagnostic Tests

The diagnosis of delirium is based on the clinical presentation, particularly the fluctuation of symptoms with periods of lucidity, and a history of one or more etiologic agents. Electroencephalography shows a generalized slowing of background activity. A diagnosis of dementia is warranted with demonstrable impairment of long- and short-term memory and demonstrable disturbances in abstract thinking, judgment, personality, or other higher cortical functions that interfere with social activities and relationships. Attention and arousal tend to be normal in dementia, and manifestations are relatively stable, worsening over time. A definitive diagnosis is available only on autopsy.

Therapeutic Management

Surgery	None
Drugs	*Delirium:* Withdrawal of toxic agents (alcohol, barbiturates) and IV sedation with antianxiety agents for agitation, seizure activity, and tremors
	Dementia: Treatment of underlying disorders; antianxiety agents as disease progresses to relieve anxiety and frustration
General	*Delirium:* Adequate fluid and electrolytes; seizure precautions; safety precautions (e.g., to prevent wandering, climbing over bedrails); long-term treatment for substance abuse when it is the etiologic agent
	Dementia: Kept in familiar surroundings with minimal environmental changes; use of frequent orientation devices (clocks, calendars, schedules, memory books, name tags); encouragement to do familiar, repetitive routines; safety precautions to prevent wandering; use of adult day care, respite care, or home care to relieve caregiver; family support groups and counseling; prevention of disuse syndrome in end-stage disease

O

osteomyelitis

An infection of the bone and bone marrow

Etiology and incidence: Osteomyelitis is caused by a pathogen that is introduced directly through an open fracture, penetrating trauma, or surgical procedure, or indirectly from another infection that spreads through the bloodstream or from adjacent tissues. The most common pathogens are *Staphylococcus aureus, Streptococcus pneumoniae, Escherichia coli, Pseudomonas aeruginosa,* and *Haemophilus influenzae.* The incidence is highest in childhood and early adolescence, and the disorder occurs more often in boys. Those undergoing hemodialysis, drug abusers, and individuals with diabetes, sickle cell anemia, tuberculosis, decubitus ulcers, and peripheral arterial insufficiency are also at risk.

Pathophysiology: The long bones are most often involved. The invading pathogen travels to the metaphysis, located between the shaft and the epiphysis. The pathogen grows and multiplies in the metaphysis, producing pus, which eventually interferes with the blood supply in the bone, causing necrosis. An inflammatory response is set up, and macrophages are produced to combat the pathogens; necrosis continues, and the enlarging mass spreads through the bone cortex to contiguous tissues. New bone trabeculae are formed in an effort to keep the infection localized. The infection can spread to the bone marrow and to the skin through sinus tracts. Periodic drainage occurs until all dead bone is destroyed or excised. In adults the spine is often affected.

Clinical Manifestations

Pain, tenderness, edema, and warmth at the site are the most common manifestations. Bone pain on use or on palpation may be evident, as well as systemic symptoms such as fever, chills, sweats, malaise, weakness, headache, and nausea. Later signs include drainage from sinus tracts to the skin and fractures.

Complications

Osteomyelitis can lead to chronic infection, joint and skeletal deformities, and (in children) disturbed bone growth and limb shortening.

Diagnostic Tests

The diagnosis is made from the clinical presentation; a history of antecedent infection or open trauma in the preceding 2 to 4 weeks; an elevated WBC count and erythrocyte sedimentation rate; and a positive radionucleotide scan with technetium phosphate. X-ray examination may reveal bone destruction but only after 3 weeks or longer. Cultures of any identified mass are positive for the pathogen. If spread is via the bloodstream, serum cultures should be positive for the pathogen.

Therapeutic Management

Surgery	Surgical excision (saucerization) of infected and dead bone, sterilization of the abscess, bone grafts to affected site, amputation in some cases related to underlying diabetes
Drugs	Antiinfective drugs specific for pathogen
General	Splints to reduce joint pain; external fixation or casting for weakened bones to prevent fractures; initially bed rest, followed by progressive ambulation; dressing changes for draining wounds; hyperbaric oxygen therapy to increase circulating WBCs

O

osteoporosis

A generalized, progressive reduction of bone mass as bone resorption outstrips bone formation, causing skeletal weakness and fractures

Etiology and incidence: The causes of primary osteoporosis are unknown. Secondary osteoporosis may be caused by endocrine disorders such as hypogonadism, hyperthyroidism, hyperparathyroidism, and diabetes mellitus; prolonged use of substances (corticosteroids, barbiturates, or heparin); underlying disease (renal or liver disease, malabsorption syndrome, chronic obstructive pulmonary disease, rheumatoid arthritis, or sarcoidosis); and prolonged weightlessness or immobility. Postmenopausal women are the most susceptible to primary osteoporosis; an estimated 50% of postmenopausal women will develop osteoporosis and 33% will have an osteoporotic fracture in their lifetime.

Pathophysiology: As bone resorption outstrips bone formation, bone tissue mass progressively declines but the bone is morphologically normal. Cortical thickness also declines, as do the number and size of trabeculae with normal osteoid seams.

Risk Factors

Menopause or other loss of ovarian function
Race and gender (white women are most susceptible; Asian women are also more vulnerable)
Nulliparity
Familial history of osteoporosis
History of underlying skeletal disease
Chronic malnutrition, long-term lack of calcium intake
Diet high in red meat and/or sugar
Underweight, particularly coupled with intense exercise (women with anorexia are susceptible)
Smoking
Heavy intake of caffeine and or alcohol
Sedentary lifestyle, immobility

Clinical Manifestations

Individuals are typically asymptomatic early in the disease. The first symptom is usually a dull, aching, constant pain in the bones, particularly the back and chest. The pain may radiate down the leg, and muscle spasms may be present. As the spinal column mass diminishes, dorsal kyphosis and cervical lordosis increase, leading to multiple compression fractures of the spine and a reduction in height. Other fractures occur with minimal or no trauma.

Complications

Immobility from increased fractures and deformity from spinal crushing are common complications.

Diagnostic Tests

Clinical evaluation revealing bone pain, x-ray studies showing decreased radiodensity, photon absorptiometry, and quantitative CT scans showing decreased bone density of the spine aid in diagnosis.

Therapeutic Management

Surgery	Open reduction internal fixation of fractures of femur
Drugs	Calcium supplements and vitamin D for prevention and treatment, estrogen-progesterone combinations for postmenopausal women with uterus intact, estrogen supplements for postmenopausal women with no uterus, testosterone replacement for older at-risk males, nonsteroidal antiinflammatory drugs for pain
	The drug biphosphonate aldendronate (Fosamax) was recently approved by FDA and can be used to prevent bone resorption in women who cannot take estrogen supplements.
	Growth factors are under clinical evaluation.
General	Consistent exercise regimen, including moderate, weight-bearing hyperextension and resistance exercises to slow calcium loss and strengthen musculature; heat and massage for muscle spasm; orthopedic supports for back and neck to prevent stress fractures; cane to aid in walking; high-protein diet; monitoring of calcium levels
Prevention	Bone density surveys every 1 to 3 years after age 49 for early detection.

otitis externa

Inflammation or infection of the external canal or the auricle of the external ear

Etiology and incidence: This common external ear problem is seen in adults more often than in children. Individuals with diabetes are at highest risk. While many things such as allergy, bacteria, fungi, viruses, and trauma may cause it, the most common cause is water related to swimming (swimmer's ear). Allergy to metals in earrings such as nickel or chromium or chemicals in hair sprays, cosmetics, and hearing aids are common precipitating causes. Medications such as the sulfonamides and neomycin may also cause otitis externa. The condition is seen most often during hot, humid weather.

Pathophysiology: Dryness and/or infection of the external ear canal or the auricle of the ear. The presence of moisture often predisposes the ear to infection from fungus or water-living bacteria such as *Pseudomonas* or *Proteus*.

Risk Factors

Poor external ear hygiene and proper drying
Swimming in dirty or polluted water
Known exposure to allergic substances
Trauma to the ear

Clinical Manifestations

Pain and/or itching in the ear canal, discharge from the canal, and ear pain with manipulation of the pinna of the ear are all symptoms. Palpation may indicate pre- or post-auricular nodes. The external ear canal appears red and swollen. It may be difficult to see the ear canal.

Complications

Occlusion of the auditory canal occurs. If not treated, the condition may become chronic.

Diagnostic Tests

No test, other than direct clinical examination, is necessary. Culture may be done to determine infective organism.

Therapeutic Management

Surgery	None
Drugs	Topical antiinfective agents or analgesic for discomfort; topical corticosteroids may be required to reduce inflammation
General	Proper cleaning and drying of external ear and ear canal, avoidance of known allergic substances

O

otitis media

Inflammation of the middle ear

Etiology and incidence: Acute otitis media is usually the result of a bacterial or viral infection of the upper respiratory tract. When acute otitis goes unresolved, it leads to an effusion of the middle ear, called *secretory otitis media*. Otitis media is most commonly seen in infants and young children, typically in the winter and early spring.

Pathophysiology: Microorganisms migrate from the nasopharynx via the eustachian tube to the lining of the middle ear, where an inflammatory reaction is set up with edema and hyperemia, retraction of the tympanic membrane, and serous exudation. If a bacterial superinfection develops, the exudate becomes pus-filled, causing the tympanic membrane to bulge.

Clinical Manifestations

The first manifestation is a severe, resistant earache marked by an erythematous tympanic membrane. Fever, nausea, vomiting, and diarrhea may be present. Hearing loss and fullness in the ears are common.

Complications

Perforation of the eardrum, acute mastoiditis, petrositis, labyrinthitis, facial paralysis, epidural abscess, meningitis, brain abscess, sinus thrombosis, hydrocephalus, and subdural empyema are all possible complications.

Diagnostic Tests

Diagnosis is made by clinical evaluation. If pus is present, it may be cultured for the causative organism.

Therapeutic Management

Surgery	Myringotomy to drain pus or fluid from the middle ear if the tympanic membrane is bulging; tympanotomy ventilating tubes to create artificial eustachian tube in exudative otitis media

Drugs	Antiinfective drugs to combat pathogen and infection, analgesics and antipyretics for pain and fever, antihistamines in allergic individuals to improve eustachian tube function, bronchodilators for adults
General	Autoinflation techniques taught to children to prevent surgical placement of tubes, hearing evaluation, ear kept clean and dry after surgery, use of precautions when bathing to prevent getting water in the ear

O

ovarian cancer

Seventy-five percent of ovarian carcinomas are epithelial in origin; these include serous cystadenocarcinoma and mucinous, endometrioid, and clear cell tumors. Germ cell tumors make up fewer than 5% of all cancerous ovarian tumors, but in women under 20 years of age, they account for 65% of diagnosed ovarian cancers.

Etiology and incidence: The etiology has not been established, but an increasing incidence among nulliparous women suggests that uninterrupted ovulation and abnormal endocrine activity are predisposing factors. Ovarian cancer is the fifth most common form of cancer and the fourth leading cause of death from cancer in women. The annual mortality rate is over 14,500. Ovarian cancer is most common in Western industrialized nations among older white women of Northern European descent. Peak incidence is from age 60 to 65.

Pathophysiology: Ovarian cancer begins in the various tissues of the ovary and then spreads by direct extension and lymphatics to the regional nodes in the pelvis and paraaortic region and to the abdominal and pelvic peritoneum. Metastasis is commonly to the liver and lungs.

Risk Factors

Nulliparity (risk is decreased by 5-year or greater history of use of oral contraceptives)
Infertility
Delayed menopause
Family history of the disease (presence of BCRA1 gene mutation)
History of breast or uterine cancer
High-fat, low-fiber, vitamin A–deficient diet
Occupational exposure to asbestos and talc

Clinical Manifestations

Symptoms of early disease are often absent or mild and associated with other common problems. They include such things as vague abdominal discomfort, dyspepsia, bloating, flatulence, and digestive disturbances. Later stage signs and symptoms include ascites, abdominal and pelvic pain, abdominal and pelvic masses, persistent gastrointestinal symptoms, urinary complaints, and menstrual irregularities.

Complications

The prognosis is good with diagnosis at an early stage. However, because early ovarian cancer is typically asymptomatic, the chances of prompt diagnosis are slim. Complications include intestinal obstruction, ascites, and cachexia.

Diagnostic Tests

An enlarged ovary on manual examination is often the first diagnostic sign. A transvaginal ultrasound may be used to confirm the presence of a tumor. A definitive diagnosis is made by biopsy through laparoscopy or laparotomy. Tumor marker CA-125 is being evaluated as a diagnostic tool. It is predictive in only about 50% of early cases but may prove useful for tracking treatment progress. Human chorionic gonadotropin and alpha-fetoprotein levels will be elevated with a germ cell tumor.

Therapeutic Management

Surgery	Salpingo-oophorectomy with or without hysterectomy is the primary treatment
Drugs	Systemic chemotherapy as adjuvant to surgery; replacement estrogen therapy and calcium supplements after removal of both ovaries
General	Radiation therapy as adjuvant to surgery

O

ovarian cysts

A fluid- or semifluid-filled sac on the ovary

Etiology and incidence: While an ovarian cyst may occur at any time, they most often form from puberty to menopause. Most ovarian cysts are small and disappear within a few months. Only a few cysts require surgical removal. Infrequently, ovarian cysts may be related to a malignancy. These are most prevalent in perimenopausal and postmenopausal women.

Pathophysiology: There are five types of ovarian cysts: functional, inflammatory, endometrial, inclusion, and parovarian cysts. *Functional cysts* commonly are asymptomatic or cause symptoms of local discomfort. These most often disappear spontaneously within a couple of months from development. A small percentage may rupture and require surgery. *Inflammatory cysts* may form after an acute infection such as a sexually transmitted disease. There is pain and hypermenorrhea. *Endometrial cysts* (also called *chocolate cysts*) may occur secondarily in individuals who have endometriosis. The cysts may vary in size from very small to 3 to 4 inches in diameter. Large cysts may require surgical removal. Inclusion cysts are most often microscopic in size and are located just beneath the surface of the ovary. They occur most often after menopause and require no treatment. *Parovarian cysts* are found in young females. They are asymptomatic and are usually quite small.

Risk Factors

Pelvic infection or sexually transmitted disease
Young women

Clinical Manifestations

A pelvic mass is noted on bimanual examination. Abdominal discomfort, dull ache, local pain and tenderness, and hypermenorrhea are also symptoms.

Complications

Rupture of cyst
Resulting severe pain

Diagnostic Tests

Pelvic and rectal examination	To determine location and size of cyst
Ultrasonography	To confirm presence and size of cyst and to distinguish functional cysts from neoplastic cysts
Laparoscopy	Used infrequently to determine presence of endometriosis and to examine cyst

Therapeutic Management

Surgery	If necessary, laparoscopic or laparotomy surgery to drain and/or remove cyst
Drugs	Analgesic medications as needed for discomfort
General	Pelvic examinations to monitor cyst size and position
	Exercise and positioning to decrease discomfort

O

Paget's disease (osteitis deformans)

Chronic inflammatory disease of the bones that results in thickening, softening, and eventual bowing

Etiology and incidence: The etiology is unknown, although a familial pattern has been noted and a viral link is suspected. Paget's disease occurs worldwide but is more common in Europe, Australia, and New Zealand. About 2.5 million persons have been diagnosed in the United States. Men are more likely to be affected, as are individuals over age 40.

Pathophysiology: The disease begins with an initial phase of excessive bone resorption followed by a reactive phase of excessive and abnormal bone formation. The result is large, multinucleated osteoblasts; thickened lamellae and trabeculae; and fibrotic tissue, which produces enlarged, weakened, and heavily calcified bone.

Clinical Manifestations

Early disease is asymptomatic, with an insidious onset of aching, deep pain; stiffness; fatigability; headaches; and decreased hearing. Later signs include bowing and other bone deformities, such as an increasing skull size. Fractures occur with minor trauma.

Complications

Complications include vertebral collapse and resulting paralysis; blindness, deafness, or vertigo from impingement on cranial nerves; vascular collapse from increased cardiac demands; gout; and renal calculi.

Diagnostic Tests

The diagnosis is often incidental to examinations done for other reasons. X-ray examination shows increased bone density, abnormal architecture, cortical thickening, bowing, and bony overgrowth. The serum alkaline phosphatase level is elevated. Radionuclide bone scans show increased nuclide uptake at affected sites.

Therapeutic Management

Surgery	Hip replacement, spinal decompression
Drugs	Nonsteroidal antiinflammatory drugs for pain; chemotherapy to suppress bone cell activity before surgery or to prevent complications in poor surgical candidates; calcitonin, alendronate, or etidronate to inhibit bone resorption and manage disease
General	Orthoses for gait correction, balance of exercise and rest, referral to support groups

P

pancreatic cancer

Tumors arise from exocrine glands (95%) and endocrine glands (5%) in the pancreas. Ductal adenocarcinomas constitute 80% of all pancreatic tumors. Other histological types include squamous cell and giant cell carcinomas, sarcomas, plasmacytomas, and lymphomas.

Etiology and incidence: Cigarette smoking is strongly linked to the development of cancer of the pancreas. More than 28,000 cases of pancreatic cancer are diagnosed each year in the United States, and more than 26,000 persons die annually, making it the fourth leading cause of cancer death.

Pathophysiology: Most tumors begin in the head of the exocrine gland, obstruct the bile duct, and extend to the duodenum, intestines, and spine. Spread occurs to the regional lymph nodes, and common metastatic sites include the liver and lungs.

Risk Factors

Smoking
High-fat diet
Alcohol abuse
Occupational exposure to solvents and petrochemicals
History of chronic pancreatitis, diabetes mellitus

Clinical Manifestations

Symptoms occur late in the disease and include anorexia; weight loss; flatulence; bloating; constipation; upper abdominal pain, which radiates to the back and abates in a fetal position; jaundice; and thrombophlebitis.

Complications

The prognosis is extremely poor, with a 3% long-term survival rate. Complications include diabetes and alterations in mental status.

Diagnostic Tests

Ultrasound, CT scans, and endoscopic retrograde pancreatography are used to locate masses and to assist in staging of the tumor. The definitive diagnosis is made by needle or tissue biopsy.

Therapeutic Management

Surgery	Pancreatectomy or Whipple procedure; bypass of obstructions for palliation
Drugs	Chemotherapy has not been effective to date, although several combination drugs are under study; insulin after removal or resection of pancreas; analgesics for pain
General	Radiation limits tumor progression but does little for survival rate.

P

pancreatitis

Acute or chronic inflammation of the pancreas

Etiology and incidence: The most common cause of acute pancreatitis is heavy alcohol consumption and biliary tract disease. Other causes include infections (e.g., mumps, hepatitis); drugs (thiazides, steroids, azathioprine, pentamidine); vasculitis; and surgery on pancreas, stomach, or biliary tract. The most common cause of chronic pancreatitis is alcoholism. Other causes are hyperparathyroidism, stenosis of the pancreatic duct, and carcinoma. The incidence varies with location and is high where the incidence of alcoholism is high. In tropical countries such as India, Indonesia, and Nigeria, a form of idiopathic pancreatitis occurs in children and young adults.

Pathophysiology: Acute pancreatitis is a result of autodigestion in which normally excreted pancreatic enzymes digest pancreatic tissue. Bile and phospholipase A combine to cause severe tissue necrosis. Elastase dissolves elastic fibers in the blood vessels and causes hemorrhage. Release of kinins causes vasodilation, vascular permeability, and pulmonary edema. Hypercalcemia and transient hyperglycemia develop. Chronic pancreatitis results from repeated acute episodes or from a slow sclerosing process, resulting in fibrosis and obstruction of the pancreatic ducts.

Clinical Manifestations

Acute	Severe abdominal pain radiating to the back; fever, sweating, rapid pulse, shallow respirations, and decreased breath sounds; decreased blood pressure; blunted sensorium
Chronic	Intermittent or chronic dull, boring abdominal pain relieved somewhat by sitting and leaning forward; weight loss, steatorrhea, diarrhea, nausea, vomiting

Complications

Adult respiratory distress syndrome; disseminated intravascular coagulation; cardiac, renal, or pulmonary failure; infected necrosis of the pancreas; and pancreatic pseudocyst, leading to hemorrhage and rupture of the pancreas, are all possible complications that often lead to death.

Diagnostic Tests

Acute	Elevated amylase 2 to 12 hours after onset, dropping to normal within 72 hours; elevated lipase, WBCs, glucose, and serum bilirubin levels
Chronic	Pancreatic calcification, enlarged ducts, or abnormal size and consistency of pancreas on CT scan or ultrasound; secretin test with normal volume and low bicarbonate

Therapeutic Management

Surgery	*Acute:* Débridement of tissue in necrotizing pancreatitis, drainage of pancreatic pseudocyst or abscesses, removal of stones obstructing the common bile duct
	Chronic: Pancreaticojejunostomy, pancreatectomy, Whipple procedure, autotransplantation for severe intractable pain and complications
Drugs	*Acute:* Narcotic analgesics for pain, antacids by nasogastric tube, histamine receptor antagonists for gastrointestinal bleeding, antiinfective drugs for abscesses, adrenergics for hypotension
	Chronic: Analgesics for pain, pancreatic enzyme supplements, antacids, histamine receptor antagonists to improve effects of enzyme supplements, insulin or oral hypoglycemic therapy if indicated
General	*Acute:* Endoscopic sphincterotomy for biliary pancreatitis; hemodynamic monitoring; central venous pressure catheter; nasogastric tube; peritoneal lavage; correction of electrolyte imbalances; total parenteral nutrition; discontinue alcohol or drug use; NPO to rest gastrointestinal tract and diminish pancreatic activity, then low-fat, high-carbohydrate diet
	Chronic: Enteral nutritional support if indicated; discontinue use of alcohol with alcohol rehabilitation program

P

Parkinson's disease

A slowly progressive, degenerative neurological disorder, characterized by slow, impoverished movement; muscle rigidity; resting tremor; and postural instability

Etiology and incidence: Parkinsonism has been linked to a genetic defect for the alpha-synuclein protein. Individuals with this form of Parkinson's comprise less than 10% of known cases, and onset is generally early (before age 50). The disease can also be caused by drugs (neuroleptics, reserpine, metoclopramide, tetrabenazine, N-MPTP [a byproduct of heroin synthesis]); toxins (carbon monoxide, carbon disulfide, manganese); structural lesions of the midbrain or basal ganglia; vascular lesions of the striatum from repeated head trauma; and in rare cases encephalitis. Other causes are yet unidentified. Parkinsonism is the fourth most common neurodegenerative disease of the elderly. It affects about 1% of those over age 65 in the United States, and an estimated 40,000 cases are diagnosed each year. Men and women are equally affected; the mean age of onset is 57 years, and peak onset is in the seventh decade.

Pathophysiology: Some agent or event triggers a degeneration and loss of pigmented neurons in the substantia nigra, locus ceruleus, and other brainstem dopaminergic cell groups. The loss of these neurons leads to a depletion in neurotransmitter dopamine and interferes with the motor production of the basal ganglia. Interneuronal inclusion bodies (Lewy bodies) are left in surviving pigmented neurons and serve as biological markers of the disease. Clinical manifestations emerge only after 75% to 80% of the dopamine innervation has been destroyed.

Clinical Manifestations

Early	Infrequent blinking; lack of facial expression; deliberateness of speech; impaired postural reflexes, particularly in the arm; resting pill-rolling tremor of one hand that is absent during sleep
Midcourse	Progressive rigidity, slowness and poverty of movement, and difficulty initiating movement; muscle aches and fatigue; masklike, open-

mouthed facial expression; stooped posture; gait begins slow and shuffling and quickens to a run with a forward lean; hypophonic speech with stuttering dysarthria; drooling; dysphagia; forgetfulness; resting tremors of lips, jaw, tongue, and limbs; depression

Late
Severe postural instability, urinary retention, orthostatic hypotension, paranoia with visual hallucinations, delirium, dementia

Complications

Injury from falls is a common threat. Other complications include aspiration pneumonia, drug reactions, and disuse syndrome.

Diagnostic Tests

The diagnosis is based primarily on the pattern of clinical manifestations and must be distinguished from individuals with essential tremor in which the tremor is action related and without facial or gait involvement.

Therapeutic Management

Surgery
Stereotactic thalamotomy to alleviate tremors and rigidity in drug-resistant individuals

Drugs
Antiparkinsonian agents such as levodopa, carbidopa/levodopa (Sinemet), trihexyphenidyl (Artane), benztropine mesylate (Cogentin), ethopropazine (Parsidol), and bromocriptine (Parlodel) to reduce tremor and rigidity; antihistamines and anticholinergics to extend the effects of levodopa; antidepressants for depression; anticholinergics with neuroleptics to prevent parkinsonism

General
Long-term physical therapy to maintain muscle tone, function, and range of motion, as well as gait and transfer training; occupational therapy to maintain activities of daily living and teach safety skills; speech therapy to evaluate and improve swallowing abilities, reduce dysarthria,

and strengthen facial muscles; warm baths and massage to relax muscles; consistent exercise program; assistive devices (canes, walkers, wheelchairs, electric lift chairs, grab bars, raised toilet seats, bath seats, eating and hygiene devices); counseling for depression and long-term adaptation; measures to prevent skin breakdown, urinary tract infections, falls, and corneal abrasions; deep breathing to maintain vital capacity; balanced, low-protein diet; bowel and bladder programs; treatment of underlying cause in non–gene-linked parkinsonism

pediculosis (lice)

Infestation by lice of the head, body, or pubic areas

Etiology and incidence: Two species of lice cause pediculosis. *Pediculus humanus* affects the head and body, and *Phthirius pubis* infects the pubic area, eyebrows, eyelashes, and axillae. In pediculosis capitis (head lice), the lice on the scalp are transmitted by personal contact and through objects such as combs and brushes. In pediculosis corporis (body lice), the lice live in unclean underclothing and periodically feed on the skin. In pediculosis pubis (pubic lice), the lice live at the base of curly hairs, chiefly in the genital region, and are transmitted primarily by sexual contact or very close personal contact. Infestation is widespread in areas with crowded, unsanitary living conditions. Head lice are common in day care centers, schools, and other places with large numbers of children who share personal items.

Pathophysiology: The lice bite the skin and inject saliva during feeding, causing severe pruritus. Scratching causes excoriation and secondary infection. Each day, female lice lay eggs (nits), which cement themselves to the base of the hair shaft in the head and pubic area. These eggs hatch in 8 days.

Clinical Manifestations

Itching, excoriation, and secondary infection of bite lesions are common signs. Grayish-white nits may also be observed at the base of hair shafts, as can the lice themselves.

Complications

Furunculosis is an occasional complication. The lice also serve as vectors for organisms that cause typhus, trench fever, and relapsing fever.

Diagnostic Tests

A physical examination revealing nits or lice. The examination may be enhanced using fluorescent light and microscopic examination of hair shafts.

Therapeutic Management

Surgery	None
Drugs	Antiinfective shampoos, creams, lotions, and ophthalmic solutions to kill lice and nits; must be used again about 8 to 10 days after initial treatment to kill remaining hatching nits
General	Nit combs to comb out nits; elimination of body lice from clothing and bedding by washing, boiling, and steaming; elimination of lice from combs and brushes by boiling; vacuuming of carpets and upholstered furniture; cutting fingernails short and using gloves to prevent damage by scratching; prevention by instituting sanitary conditions, encouraging children not to share combs, brushes, caps, scarves, and other articles of clothing; school and community prevention and early detection programs

pelvic inflammatory disease

Infection of the fallopian tubes, which may extend to the ovaries, pelvic peritoneum, or uterine connective tissue

Etiology and incidence: Pelvic inflammatory disease (PID) is caused by a pathogen, the most common of which is *Chlamydia trachomatis*. The pathogen is usually transmitted during intercourse but may also be introduced during abortion and childbirth. Women with intrauterine devices (IUDs) are at greater risk, as are sexually active women with multiple partners. Adolescent and young adult women are most often affected. As many as 1 million women are suspected of being infected annually.

Pathophysiology: The infection typically begins intravaginally and spreads upward through the entire genital tract to the fallopian tubes. The infection, which may be unilateral or bilateral, produces a profuse exudate in the tubes that leads to agglutination of the mucosal folds, adhesions, and tubal occlusion. Peritonitis from spreading exudate is common, and the ovaries may also be invaded.

Risk Factors

Unprotected sex
Multiple sex partners
Sexual contact with urethritis or gonorrhea
Previous history of PID
Frequent vaginal douching
Infection after abortion, childbirth, insertion of IUD, uterine biopsy or pelvic surgery
History of immunological or renal disorders

Clinical Manifestations

PID may be either acute or chronic.

Acute	Onset typically occurs after onset of menses
	Progressive lower abdominal pain with guarding and rebound tenderness, fever, copious purulent cervical discharge, nausea and vomiting, malaise; urinary urgency and frequency, vaginal itching and maceration

Chronic	Chronic pain, menstrual irregularities, recurrence and exacerbation of acute symptoms

Complications

Common complications include generalized peritonitis, sterility, and ectopic pregnancy.

Diagnostic Tests

Clinical manifestations, coupled with elevated WBCs and erythrocyte sedimentation rate plus a positive culture of secretions, are diagnostic. On pelvic examination, moving of the cervix causes severe pain and rebound tenderness is present in abdomen. Laparoscopy may be used as a differential diagnostic tool.

Therapeutic Management

Surgery	Salpingolysis to remove adhesions; salpingostomy to reopen blocked fallopian tube; salpingo-oophorectomy for ruptured tube or ectopic pregnancy; in vitro fertilization for sterility
Drugs	Antiinfective drugs, usually in combinations to control and alleviate infection
General	Bed rest in semi-Fowler's position, adequate hydration, removal of IUDs, tracking and treatment of sexual partners, sexual abstinence and avoidance of tampons and douching during treatment, instruction about sexually transmitted diseases and safer sexual practices

pericarditis

A chronic or acute inflammation of the parietal and visceral layers of the pericardium and outer myocardium

Etiology and incidence: Pericarditis is most commonly idiopathic in origin but may result from viral, bacterial, fungal or parasitic pathogens from infective diseases (AIDS, tuberculosis, influenza, histoplasmosis); underlying connective tissue disorders (systemic lupus erythematosus, rheumatoid arthritis, rheumatic fever, scleroderma, periarteritis); neoplastic disease (breast cancer, lymphoma, bronchogenic cancer); metabolic disease (renal failure, myxedema); postmyocardial infarction; trauma to the chest cavity; chest surgery or hemodialysis; drugs (procainamide or phenytoin); and irradiation. Any individual with one of the above causative agents is at risk. All age groups and races and both genders are vulnerable. Pericarditis is the most common manifestation in those with AIDS.

Pathophysiology: Inflammation of the pericardium occurs by irritation or by direct extension of another disease state. The normally clear fluid in the pericardial sac is filled with an exudate of fibrin, WBCs, and endothelial cells, which coat the parietal and visceral layers of the pericardium. Friction occurs between the layers, setting up an inflammatory process in the surrounding tissues. This process may remain localized or become widespread. Pericarditis may be fibrinous or may create a pleural effusion that is serous, sanguineous, hemorrhagic, or purulent. Chronic pericarditis leads to pericardial thickening, adhesions, and scarring, which may in time calcify, rendering the pericardium useless. This impedes the diastolic filling of the heart, reduces stroke volume, and decreases cardiac output.

Clinical Manifestations

Acute	Retrosternal or precordial chest pain radiating to the neck and back; pleuritic pain that increases on inspiration and in a horizontal position; shallow, rapid breathing; dyspnea; dysphagia; restlessness; anxiety; fever, chills, and weakness

Chronic	Asymptomatic unless constriction is present, then symptoms appear with exertional dyspnea; paroxysmal nocturnal dyspnea; fatigue; peripheral edema; orthopnea; cough

Complications

Rapidly forming effusion interferes with cardiovascular dynamics and leads to cardiac tamponade, shock, and cardiovascular collapse if not treated immediately. Chronic disease leads to cardiac and liver failure.

Diagnostic Tests

Acute	History of pain; elevated WBCs, erythrocyte sedimentation rate; blood or urine culture to identify organism if infectious process is involved; electrocardiography (ECG); early ST-T segment elevation, PR interval depression, QRS voltage decrease; precordial friction rub; enlarging cardiac silhouette on serial chest x-ray studies; echocardiogram to detect pleural effusion
Chronic	Pericardial knock on auscultation; calcification on x-ray study; enlarged cardiac silhouette *ECG:* Widened P wave in leads I, II, and V6; deep Q waves; flattened or inverted T waves MRI shows thickened pericardium; echocardiogram shows presence of effusion

Therapeutic Management

Surgery	Pericardiocentesis to remove fluid, pus, or blood from pericardium in acute effusive disease or tamponade; pericardiectomy to remove visceral and parietal pericardium in chronic constrictive disease
Drugs	Antiinfective drugs to treat underlying infection; antiinflammatory drugs for effusion, fever, and pain; analgesics for pain; diuretics for chronic congestion *Anticoagulants are contraindicated, because they can cause intrapericardial bleeding and contribute to tamponade.*

General   Treatment of underlying disease
Acute: Cardiac monitoring for complications, bed
  rest, adequate hydration, comfort measures
Chronic: Restricted activity, instruction about
  surgery

P

peripheral atherosclerotic disease

Acute or chronic occlusion of the blood supply to the extremities by atherosclerotic plaques

Etiology and incidence: The most common cause is underlying atherosclerosis, and individuals with atherosclerosis are vulnerable.

Pathophysiology: The pathological processes involved in atherosclerosis are detailed under coronary artery disease. In peripheral disease, an artery in an extremity is either suddenly occluded (acute), resulting in rapid tissue ischemia, or occluded after a long-term buildup of plaque in the vessel (chronic), leading to insidious development of tissue ischemia.

Clinical Manifestations

Acute	Sudden onset of severe pain, coldness, numbness, and pallor of affected extremity; absent pulses distal to occlusion
Chronic	Intermittent claudication progressing to pain at rest; decreased pulses; pallor after elevation; dry, scaly skin with sparse hair and nail growth on affected extremity; numbness and tingling; slow healing of wounds

Complications

Necrosis and gangrene, with resultant limb loss, is the most common complication.

Diagnostic Tests

Clinical evaluation and Doppler ultrasound to locate the obstruction are used for diagnosis.

Therapeutic Management

Surgery	Thromboendarterectomy or resection with or without graft to remove obstruction and make vessel patent; amputation for uncontrolled infection, necrosis, or gangrene

Drugs   Antiinfective drugs for infection; vasodilators,
              calcium antagonists, and thromboxane inhibitors
              for chronic disease

General   *Acute:* Percutaneous transluminal angioplasty
              instead of surgery to remove obstruction; lasers,
              mechanical cutters, stents, and rotational
              sanders are also being tried to clear the blockage

              Chronic: Progressive exercise to develop collateral
              circulation; prophylactic nail and foot care to
              prevent secondary infection; careful monitoring of
              wounds, cuts, and ulcers; avoidance of all tobacco
              products and any other known vasoconstrictors

peripheral vascular disorders

A complex of vascular diseases affecting the extremities and involving the arteries, veins, and lymphatics. (See specific diseases, such as Peripheral Atherosclerotic Disease, Raynaud's Disease, Thrombosis, and Varicose Veins.)

P

peritonitis

Inflammation of the abdominal peritoneum

Etiology and incidence: Peritonitis is caused by the contamination of the peritoneal cavity by bacteria or chemicals. The condition may be either primary or secondary. Primary peritonitis is caused by acute or subacute bacterial infection of the peritoneum not associated with any underlying bowel disorder. Secondary peritonitis is the result of contamination of the peritoneum from perforation of the gastrointestinal tract. Secondary peritonitis generally occurs secondary to a perforation or rupture of one of the organs of digestion. A life-threatening irritation/infection of the peritoneum results. If not promptly recognized and treated, death may result. Perforated peptic ulcer, ruptured appendix, trauma, ischemic bowel disease, intestinal instruction, pancreatitis, and perforated colon are common causes of generalized peritonitis.

Pathophysiology: Fecal contamination and resulting infection within the peritoneal cavity is the most common cause of secondary peritonitis. The peritoneum is a semipermeable saclike closure within the abdominal cavity, enclosing the abdominal viscera and mesentery. The peritoneum also lines the abdominal wall, the undersurface of the diaphragm, and the pelvic floor. If there is a rupture of the intestinal wall, the peritoneum attempts to wall off the contamination, and a large number of polymorphonuclear leukocytes pour into the area and through phagocytosis, remove bacteria and foreign matter. The body's generalized health and systemic tissue perfusion often determine how the body fights off the potential infection. Often, the contamination body insult is significant and the body is unable to cope. Vascular dilation, hyperemia, and fluid shifts occur. The rate of fluid shift is proportional to the degree of peritoneal insult and the success of the body's peritoneal defense mechanism.

Risk Factors

Peptic ulcer
Ruptured appendix
Abdominal trauma, either blunt or penetrating
Ischemic bowel disease
Intestinal obstruction

Pancreatitis
Decreased tissue perfusion
Elderly

Clinical Manifestations

History	Sudden onset of severe abdominal pain that worsens with movement or coughing; nausea and vomiting
Clinical examination	Guarding and report of generalized and rebound tenderness during abdominal palpation; abdominal distention
Bowel sounds	Decreased or absent bowel sounds
Systemic	Rapid, weak, thready pulse; decreased blood pressure; tachypnea; decreased urinary output; fever; appears ill

Complications

Complications are more likely in the elderly, those with poor tissue perfusion, and those with abdominal cavity contamination. Complications include abscess, hypotension, acidosis, hypokalemia, and respiratory difficulties. Untreated peritonitis leads to death.

Diagnostic Tests

Laboratory tests	CBC with differential shows increased leukocytes; hemoconcentration; metabolic acidosis; respiratory alkalosis
X-rays	Abdominal x-ray to determine gas and fluid collection in large and small bowel; free gas in the abdominal cavity; bowel walls may appear thick
Peritoneal aspiration	To determine organism; aspirate appears cloudy, blood-tinged, may contain fecal material

Therapeutic Management

Surgery	Indicated to treat the primary cause of the peritonitis and to prevent further peritoneal infection
Drugs	Antibiotics to treat multiple bacterial flora contaminating the peritoneal cavity; analgesics to control pain; aggressive intervention with IV fluids, electrolytes, and colloid solutions to correct hypovolemia
General	Hospitalization immediately on diagnosis; nasogastric suctioning; NPO; cardiopulmonary monitoring with assistance if needed; blood, urine, and peritoneal cultures to determine appropriate anti-infective agents

pertussis (whooping cough)

An acute, highly communicable bacterial infection of the mucous membranes of the bronchus characterized by a spasmodic cough

Etiology and incidence: Whooping cough is caused by *Bordetella pertussis,* a nonmotile, gram-negative coccobacillus. It is usually transmitted through aspiration of droplet spray produced by an infected individual during paroxysms. Pertussis is endemic throughout the world and becomes epidemic in 2- to 4-year cycles. It occurs in all age groups, but infants and toddlers are the most susceptible. The incidence had been greatly reduced in the United States since the 1940s, when a pertussis vaccine was introduced, but an upsurge in reported cases began in the late 1980s and continues currently.

Pathophysiology: When inhaled, *B. pertussis* attaches itself to the cilia of the respiratory epithelial cells and incubates for about 7 to 10 days before producing symptoms. The pertussis toxin is absorbed from the respiratory tract into the lymph system, causing a lymphocytosis. The pathogenesis of the paroxysmal cough is unknown.

Clinical Manifestations

Pertussis has three stages, each lasting about 2 weeks. The individual is contagious from the onset of the first symptom until the end of the second stage or until the patient is treated with antibiotics.

Catarrhal	Drippy nose, sneezing, tearing, and low-grade fever; listlessness; hacking nocturnal cough
Paroxysmal	Exhausting paroxysms of prolonged coughing two to three times an hour that often end with an inspiratory whooping sound or choking and vomiting accompanied by production of copious, viscid, tenacious mucus with cyanosis and apnea
Convalescent	Diminished coughing and production of mucus

Complications

Complications most commonly occur in infants and very young children; they include bronchopneumonia, asphyxiation, convulsions, and cerebral hemorrhage, with resultant spastic paralysis and mental retardation.

Diagnostic Tests

The diagnosis is often missed in the catarrhal phase, since the disease mimics influenza or bronchitis at this point. Lymphocytosis in an afebrile individual is suggestive and should lead to culture of nasal secretions. A definitive diagnosis is made by a positive culture of nasal secretions in the catarrhal or early paroxysmal stage. Direct fluorescent antibody staining of secretions may also isolate the pathogen but is less sensitive than a culture.

Therapeutic Management

Surgery	Tracheostomy if needed
Drugs	Antiinfective drugs to treat bronchopneumonia or otitis media, erythromycin in incubation or catarrhal stage to arrest pathogen, prevention through immunization, prophylactic treatment of contacts with antiinfective drugs
General	Hospitalization of infants with IV fluids, oxygen, possible ventilatory support, and suctioning; close monitoring of fluids, electrolytes, and nutritional needs; respiratory isolation during catarrhal and paroxysmal stages; home treatment for older children and adults with bed rest; minimal stimulation; small, frequent feedings; adequate hydration; and respiratory isolation

pharyngitis

An acute or chronic inflammation of the pharynx, including the pharyngeal walls, tonsils, uvula, and palate

Etiology and incidence: A sore throat is most often the result of viral pharyngitis. There are three types of pharyngitis: viral, streptococcal, and gonococcal. Of all sore throats, fewer than 10% of adults and 30% of children have streptococcal pharyngitis. Even fewer individuals providing a history of orogenital sexual activity will have gonoccal pharyngitis.

Pathophysiology: The most common of all throat disorders. It is often preceded by a common cold and is characterized by a mild sore throat, difficulty and pain in swallowing, and a low-grade fever.

Risk Factors

Upper respiratory infection
Children are more likely to acquire streptococcal infections
Winter months
Orogenital unprotected sex with infected partner

Clinical Manifestations

General	*Viral or streptococcal:* History of sore throat; cold or upper respiratory infection, fever, especially for streptococcal pharyngitis; headache; cough; fatigue; malaise
	Gonococcal: History of orogenital sexual activity, may have no other symptoms
Throat and cervical examination	*Viral:* Red and swollen pharynx, no tonsillar or pharyngeal exudate.
	Streptococcal: Tonsillar exudate, anterior cervical adenopathy
	Gonococcal: Pharyngeal exudate, cervical lymphadenopathy

P

Complications

Pharyngeal abscess or ulcer are common complications.

Diagnostic Tests

Rapid strep screen and throat culture may be used to diagnose streptococcal pharyngitis.

Therapeutic Management

Surgery	None
Drugs	Antiinfective agents if streptococcal organism is identified
	Analgesic and antipyretics for comfort
General	Rest, humidified air, warm saline throat gargles, adequate fluid intake

phlebitis

See Thrombosis.

pleurisy

An inflammation of the visceral and parietal pleurae that envelop the lungs

Etiology and incidence: Pleurisy arises from a pleural injury, which may be caused by an underlying lung disease (e.g., pneumonia, asbestosis, or infarction); an infectious agent, neoplastic cells, or irritants that invade the pleural space (e.g., amebic empyema, tuberculosis, pleural effusion, systemic lupus erythematosus, pleural carcinomatosis, rheumatoid disease); or pleural trauma (e.g., rib fracture).

Pathophysiology: The pleura becomes edematous and congested, cellular infiltration ensues, and fibrinous exudate forms on the pleural surface as plasma proteins leak from damaged vessels. This causes the visceral and parietal pleural surfaces to rub together rather than slide over each other during respiration. The pleura becomes increasingly inflamed and stretched, causing pain on each breath.

Clinical Manifestations

The primary symptom is sudden onset of pain in the chest or abdominal wall that may vary from vague to an intense stabbing sensation. The pain is aggravated by breathing and coughing. Respirations are rapid and shallow, with guarding and decreased motion on the affected side.

Complications

Permanent adhesions that restrict lung expansion may develop.

Diagnostic Tests

Auscultation reveals a friction rub, along with the characteristic presentation of pain. A chest x-ray may reveal pleural effusion.

Therapeutic Management

Surgery	None
Drugs	Narcotic analgesic to relieve pain during deep-breathing and coughing exercises, analgesics and antipyretics
General	Treatment of underlying disease, positioning and splinting of chest, coughing and deep breathing to prevent atelectasis and infection

Pneumocystis carinii pneumonia

A fungally induced pneumonia most commonly seen as an opportunistic infection secondary to AIDS. (See also Pneumonia and AIDS.)

Etiology and incidence: *Pneumocystis carinii,* the cause of this type of pneumonia (PCP), is a fungus. PCP, or pneumocystosis, was relatively rare, seen in only a handful of severely immunosuppressed patients, until the advent of AIDS. PCP is now seen in about 80% of individuals with AIDS and is the initial AIDS-defining condition in more than 60% of HIV-positive individuals. More than 50% of all AIDS deaths are attributable to PCP infections.

Pathophysiology: The fungus lies dormant in the person's lung until the body's defenses are compromised. At that time a usually benign resident becomes an aggressive pathogen. The organisms proliferate in the alveolar spaces, facilitated by diminished cell-mediated and humoral host defenses. The organisms attach to alveolar epithelial cells, impairing replication and inducing degeneration and increased membrane permeability. This causes formation of exudate in the alveolar space, reduces surfactant levels, and results in intrapulmonary shunting of blood, decreased lung compliance, and hypoxemia.

Clinical Manifestations

Fever, dyspnea, and a dry, nonproductive cough that evolves over several days or weeks are the first symptoms. Increasing shortness of breath usually prompts the individual to seek treatment. The onset tends to be more acute in individuals who do not have AIDS.

Complications

Pulmonary insufficiency, pulmonary failure, and death can occur. The overall mortality rate with treatment is about 20%.

Diagnostic Tests

The definitive diagnosis is established through a histopathological examination, preferably of induced sputum. A chest x-ray examination may show fluffy infiltrates. A gallium scan may show increased lung uptake even if the x-ray is negative.

Therapeutic Management

Surgery	None
Drugs	Antiinfective drugs to combat the pathogen (trimethoprim/sulfamethoxazole [TMP/SMX] is the drug combination of choice); adjunctive corticosteroid therapy; prophylaxis with TMP/SMX and aerosol pentamidine for patients with AIDS who already have had one bout of PCP and in those with a CD4 cell count below 200/mm^3
General	Oxygen therapy, adequate hydration, adequate ventilation or ventilatory support, adequate nutrition; education of HIV-positive individuals about early signs and symptoms of PCP

pneumonia, bacterial/nonbacterial

An acute infection and inflammation of the bronchioles, alveolar spaces, and interstitial tissue of the lung parenchyma

Etiology and incidence: Pneumonia is caused by bacteria, viruses, fungi, or parasites. Each year in the United States, more than 4.2 million persons are diagnosed with pneumonia, and 82,000 of those individuals die, making pneumonia the sixth leading cause of death in the United States. In developing countries pneumonia is either the first or second leading cause of death. The most common types, which are bacterial, are *Pneumococcus, Staphylococcus, Streptococcus, Klebsiella,* and *Haemophilus* pneumonia.

Pathophysiology: Organisms reach the lung through aspiration, aerosolization, or hematogenous spread. This usually occurs through droplet inhalation or by aspiration of fluids in the oropharynx. Pneumonia results if a series of host defense mechanisms fails to keep the respiratory tree free of infection. Upper airway mechanisms such as nasal filtration may be bypassed, the normal flora altered, immunoglobulin A (IgA) secretion impaired, or the glottis depressed. Lower airway mechanisms such as coughing, cilia mucus, and mucociliary transport may be altered or impaired. Macrophages or cell-mediated immunity may be impaired, and immunoglobins, complement, or surfactant may be deficient in the alveoli.

The pathophysiology varies by etiologic agent. Bacterial pneumonia is marked by an intraalveolar suppurative exudate with consolidation. Mycoplasmal and viral pneumonias produce interstitial inflammation with infiltrate in the alveolar walls; there is no accompanying exudate or consolidation. Pneumococcal and streptococcal pneumonia have four distinct stages: (1) *congestion,* characterized by serous exudate, vascular engorgement, and rapid proliferation of the pathogen; (2) *red hepatization,* when RBCs, fibrin, and polymorphonuclear cells fill the alveoli; (3) *gray hepatization,* when leukocytes and fibrin pack the alveoli; and (4) *resolution,* marked by lysis and resorption of exudate by macrophages.

Viral pneumonia begins with an inflammatory response in the bronchi, which damages the ciliated epithelium. The lungs become congested and may be hemorrhagic. Intracellular viral

P

inclusions form with many viruses. In aspiration pneumonia, the bacteria is aspirated with food or liquid. If the pH of the aspirated substance is below 2.5, atelectasis, pulmonary edema, and hemorrhage occur, followed by tissue necrosis and the formation of exudate.

Risk Factors

History of viral respiratory infection
Alcoholism
Smoking
Age extremes (very young and very old at greater risk)
History of debility, dysphagia, altered consciousness
Use of therapies that depress the immune system
Underlying disease states such as diabetes mellitus, heart failure, chronic obstructive pulmonary disease, asthma or immunosuppressive disorders
Hospitalized individuals, particularly those postoperative from chest or abdominal surgery

Clinical Manifestations

Bacterial	Abrupt onset with shaking chills, cough, dyspnea, sputum production (often rust or salmon colored), pleurisy; nausea, vomiting, malaise, and myalgia also may be present
Viral	Headache, fever, myalgia, cough with mucopurulent sputum
Mycoplasmal	Malaise, sore throat, dry cough with rapid progression to productive cough with mucoid, purulent, and blood-streaked sputum
Fungal	(See *Pneumocystis carinii* Pneumonia.)
Aspiration	Dyspnea, cyanosis, hypotension, tachycardia

Complications

Septic shock, lung abscess, respiratory failure, bacteremia, endocarditis, pericarditis, and meningitis are possible complications.

Diagnostic Tests

Sputum examination	Must be obtained from lower respiratory tract; positive for pathogen
WBC count	Leukocytosis; neutrophilia in mycoplasmal or viral infection
Radiology	Consolidation in bacterial infection, bronchopneumatic type infiltrate in viral infection, clear in early mycoplasmal infection, atelectasis in aspiration pneumonia
Pulmonary function	Decreased lung volumes and compliance, increased airway resistance

Therapeutic Management

Surgery	Thoracentesis with chest tube if empyema or collapse occurs; tracheostomy if needed for patent airway
Drugs	Antiinfective drugs (broad spectrum or specific to pathogen), analgesics for pain, prophylaxis with influenza vaccine and pneumococcal pneumonia vaccine in high-risk individuals
General	Rest, humidification with nebulizer to loosen secretions, oxygen if Pao_2 is below 60 mm Hg, coughing and deep-breathing exercises, adequate hydration to liquefy secretions, suctioning with copious secretions or compromised consciousness, mechanical ventilation for respiratory failure, adequate nutritional support with supplemental feedings or total parenteral nutrition if needed, monitoring of blood gases and general respiratory status

P

poliomyelitis

An acute, communicable viral infection that affects the central nervous system, producing a range of manifestations from a subclinical or mild nonfebrile illness to aseptic meningitis, muscle weakness, and paralysis

Etiology and incidence: Polio is caused by three distinct polio enteroviruses belonging to the Picornaviridae family and labeled types 1, 2, and 3. Type 1 is the most paralytogenic and the most likely to cause an epidemic. Polio has been all but eradicated in most developed countries because of widespread vaccination. In developing countries, however, the once rare disease has reached an incidence as high as that in the United States before a vaccine was developed. The mortality rate ranges from 1% to 10%, depending on the severity and type of disease.

Pathophysiology: The polio virus enters the mouth after contact with infected feces or oral or respiratory secretions. It multiplies in the lymphoid tissue of the throat and ileum, producing a follicular necrosis. The incubation period ranges from 5 to 35 days, averaging 7 to 14 days. A transient viremia of 3 to 5 days' duration occurs when the virus is transported via the bloodstream and autonomic nerve fiber endings to the central nervous system. The viremia disappears at the onset of disease symptoms. Paralysis results when extensive damage is inflicted on the motor neurons, resulting in atrophy of associated skeletal muscle fiber groups.

Clinical Manifestations

Most cases are subclinical and produce no signs or symptoms. Clinical disease may be either minor (abortive) or major. Major illness may or may not lead to paralysis. The person is infectious from the time of infection up to 6 weeks after infection.

Minor   Develops 3 to 5 days after exposure, accounts for 85% of clinical cases, occurs primarily in young children, no central nervous system involvement; slight fever, malaise, sore throat, headache, vomiting, anorexia, and abdominal pain lasting 24 to 72 hours

Major	Develops 7 to 14 days after exposure, primarily in older children and adults; fever, severe headache, stiff neck and back, deep muscle pain, paresthesias, or hyperesthesias
	This may be followed by a loss of tendon reflexes and asymmetric weakness or paralysis, or it may involve lower extremity, respiratory, facial, palatal, pharyngeal, or bladder muscles.

Complications

Complications, which arise primarily from major paralytic disease, include respiratory failure, hypertension, cor pulmonale, soft tissue and skeletal deformities, and paralytic ileus. In paralytic polio, 50% of affected individuals recover with no residual effects, 25% have mild disability, and 25% have severe permanent residual disability. Recovery of muscle function takes 6 months to 2 years. A postpoliomyelitis syndrome has been identified, which occurs several years after the initial attack of polio. The syndrome is characterized by profound fatigue, muscle weakness, fasciculations, and muscle atrophy.

Diagnostic Tests

The definitive diagnosis is made through culture of throat washings or fecal material or from convalescent serum antibody titers, which are four times higher than acute antibody titers.

Therapeutic Management

Surgery	Tracheostomy if needed in respiratory paralysis
Drugs	Sabin (OPV) vaccine is recommended for all infants and children as prophylaxis; Salk (IPV) vaccine is recommended for individuals with underlying immunodeficiency disease; Salk vaccine is recommended for unvaccinated adults who are traveling to endemic or epidemic areas
General	*Mild:* Bed rest
	Major: Strict bed rest in acute phase; hot, moist packs for muscle spasm and pain; intermittent catheterization for urinary retention; assisted ventilation for respiratory paralysis; suctioning for

pooling secretions; physical therapy for weakened or paralyzed extremities; IVs, tube feedings for those unable to swallow; monitoring for aspiration of secretions; long-term rehabilitation for those with permanent residual disability

polycythemia

An increase in the number of circulating erythrocytes and hemoglobin concentration that is manifested in three forms: polycythemia vera, secondary polycythemia, and relative polycythemia

Etiology and incidence: The cause of polycythemia vera is unknown, and the disorder is usually seen in older Jewish men. It occurs in one in 200,000 persons in the United States. Secondary polycythemia is a compensatory response to tissue hypoxia associated with underlying chronic obstructive pulmonary disease; hemoglobin abnormalities such as carboxyhemoglobinemia, which is seen in heavy smokers; congestive heart failure; congenital heart disease; or prolonged exposure to altitudes above 10,000 feet. The incidence is about two in 100,000 persons in the United States. Relative polycythemia is caused by fluid loss and dehydration and disappears when fluids are replaced.

Pathophysiology: Polycythemia vera involves rapid, uncontrolled cellular reproduction and maturation, which causes hyperplasia of all bone marrow cells and replaces bone marrow fat. Increased megakaryocytes may be present and form clumping patterns. Bone marrow iron is absent in about 90% of affected individuals. The cellular overproduction increases blood viscosity and blood volume, and organs and tissues become engorged with blood.

P

Clinical Manifestations

Polycythemia vera	Weakness and fatigue; a feeling of fullness in the head, with headache, lightheadedness, and dizziness; visual disturbances (scotoma, double or blurred vision); dyspnea; nosebleeds; night sweats; and epigastric and joint pain; later signs include pruritus, clubbing of digits, a reddened face with engorged retinal veins, and hepatosplenomegaly

Secondary polycythemia	Above manifestations plus hypoxemia in the absence of hepatosplenomegaly and hypertension
Relative polycythemia	Often individual has no complaints or vague complaints (e.g., headache, fatigue) with ruddy complexion and slight hypertension when recumbent

Complications

Thrombosis, cerebrovascular accident, peptic ulcers, myeloid metaplasia, leukemia, and hemorrhage are common complications in polycythemia vera and result in the death of about 50% of untreated individuals within 18 months of the appearance of symptoms. The median survival rate in treated individuals is 7 to 15 years. Hemorrhage is the most common complication of secondary polycythemia. Hypercholesterolemia, hyperlipidemia, and hyperuricemia may complicate relative polycythemia.

Diagnostic Tests

Polycythemia vera	Increased RBC mass and normal arterial oxygen saturation associated with splenomegaly or two of the following: thrombocytosis, leukocytosis, elevated leukocyte alkaline phosphatase, or elevated serum B_{12}; bone marrow reveals panmyelosis
Secondary polycythemia	Elevated erythrocytes, Hct, Hgb, mean corpuscular volume; absence of leukocytosis and thrombocytosis; erythroid hyperplasia of bone marrow
Relative polycythemia	Normal or decreased RBC mass, elevated Hct, no leukocytosis, normal plasma volume; normal bone marrow studies

Therapeutic Management

Surgery	Splenectomy to treat resistant splenomegaly
Drugs	Chemotherapeutic agents to induce myelosuppression in some polycythemia vera cases; allopurinol to treat hyperuricemia; antihistamines for pruritus; analgesics for joint pain

General   *Polycythemia vera:* Phlebotomy to reduce RBC
mass; pheresis for removal of WBCs, RBCs,
and platelets; exercise to promote circulation;
monitoring for thrombus formation, hemorrhage,
and ulcer formation

Secondary polycythemia: Treatment of underlying
causes

Relative polycythemia: Fluid and electrolyte replacement, measures to prevent further fluid loss

P

polyps

Common benign grapelike growths arising or protruding from mucous membrane tissue. The masses may be sessile or pedunculated and vary considerably in size. Polyps may appear as single growths or in clusters.

Etiology and incidence: Polyps may be idiopathic or may be associated with an autosomal dominant trait (familial polyposis, Gardner's syndrome) or an underlying disease. Incidence reports are highest in North America and Europe, and polyps have been noted in as much as 50% of the population in the United States on autopsy. The likelihood of acquiring polyps increases with age.

Polyps are commonly found on the cervix, within the colon, in the nose, or on the vocal cords. The cause of each polyp type differs depending on location. For example, *vocal cord* polyps often occur secondary to chronic voice abuse, inhalation of toxic irritants, smoking, and/or allergies. *Nasal polyps* are often the result of irritation of the mucous membrane from allergy or sinusitis. *Cervical polyps* are most often seen in women who use oral contraceptives and those approaching menopause. *Colon polyps* are often an autosomal dominant trait that is often transmitted by an affected parent. The child of an affected parent has a 50% chance of acquiring colon polyps.

Pathophysiology: Normal cell proliferation and differentiation processes are altered, causing a proliferation of immature epithelial cells that accumulate to form a polyp tissue mass. Polyps are soft, pliable growths and may appear as single growths or in clusters. *Nasal polyps* are soft, pliable, nontender masses growing from the sinuses or nasal mucosa. *Vocal cord polyps* generally have a broad-base attachment to the vocal cords. This may interfere with voice tone. *Colon polyps* are often found as discrete mass lesions on the mucosal membrane of the colon. The lesions of familial polyposis may be considered precancerous adenomatous polyps. These polyps may increase in size and number until the entire colon is studded with hundreds of polyps. *Cervical polyps* generally arise from the endocervical tissue and are often bright red and vascular.

Risk Factors

Nasal: Chronic maxillary sinusitis, allergies, cystic fibrosis
Vocal cord: Chronic overuse of voice, smoking, allergies
Cervical: Oral contraceptives, menopause
Colon: Family history

Clinical Manifestations

Vocal cord polyps	Raspy voice
Nasal polyps	May be asymptomatic or may have decreased air flow on the side of the polyp
Colon polyps	May be asymptomatic; often rectal bleeding is the first sign
	Other signs include diarrhea, increased mucus in the stools, and crampy abdominal pain
Cervical polyps	Often are asymptomatic; may have some intermittent spotting or bleeding

Complications

It is dependent on location; nasal polyps may occlude airway, vocal polyps may affect voice, and colon polyps may become malignant.

P

Diagnostic Tests

Direct observation of the polyp is diagnostic. Methods of observation vary based on polyp location. Rectal examination, endoscopy, and/or barium enema are used to visualize rectal or colon polyps.

Therapeutic Management

Surgery	Most often polyps are surgically removed and sent for tissue evaluation; prophylactic proctocolectomy with ileostomy for inherited multiple polyposis syndrome
Drugs	No routine medications
General	Periodic clinical reevaluation for individuals with history of polyps

posttraumatic stress disorder

A syndrome of symptoms that occur in response to perceived severe physical or emotional trauma

Etiology and incidence: The exact prevalence of posttraumatic stress disorder (PTSD) is unknown. Some community-based studies have indicated a prevalence rate in the United States ranging from 1% to 14% of the general population. It is thought that PTSD is underreported, since many individuals with PTSD fail to seek help and therefore go undiagnosed and uncounted. The group of individuals who have been most widely identified and studied are combat veterans of the Vietnam War. Veterans who were more involved in combat or who were prisoners of war are more likely to experience PTSD than other veterans. PTSD occurs in all age groups and may follow traumatic events such as rape, physical abuse, unintentional injuries, catastrophic illnesses, major losses, community violence, and all types of natural and human origin disasters.

Pathophysiology: There is no single explanation for PTSD. Theories and research demonstrate a causative interrelationship of biological and behavioral factors. Long-standing alterations in the biological response to stress may contribute to a number of complaints commonly expressed by individuals with PTSD. The most common biological studies on PTSD focus on hormone and neurotransmitter deregulation in PTSD: neurobiological response to danger, norepinephrine, hypothalamic-pituitary adrenal axis (HPA), and opiates. Behavioral responses and experiences are also an integral component of the potential development of PTSD. Distorted perceptions of an event, inadequate coping skills, fear, and feelings of helplessness may all contribute to PTSD. The individual's interpretation of an event is a subjective process that may or may not reflect the actual reality of a situation. A distorted appraisal of a current event and a remembrance of the historic traumatic experience may interfere with the individual's ability to attach a healthy meaning to any single event. The individual has been fear conditioned, and this in turn prevents different and perhaps healthier interpretation of a similar yet nontraumatic event.

Risk factors

Past traumatic event such as combat exposure, prisoner of war;
   rape, or sexual or physical assault
Contributing factors such as unstable or problematic family
   members, domestic violence, early separation from family,
   family history of anxiety or antisocial behavior, physical
   and/or sexual abuse as a child, depression, substance abuse,
   emotional or behavioral problems, psychiatric instability

Clinical Manifestations

Hypervigilance and physiological arousal	A feeling of continued danger or fear even though the individual is in a safe environment
Guilt	A feeling of survival or self-blame guilt because the individual survived
Dissociation	A feeling of being disconnected or separated from one's own feelings. This usually occurs because the feelings are very painful or negative
Depersonalization	A feeling of detachment from oneself and from one's interaction with others
Psychogenic amnesia	Selective memory loss of a specific period related to the traumatic event or circumstance
Psychogenic fugue	Sudden, unexpected travel from the individual's home local area to another geographical location
Flashbacks	Having a vivid image of the traumatic event or circumstance
Avoidance of triggers	Avoidance of any triggers such as places, persons, or things that may trigger a PTSD episode
Comorbidity	The coexistence of other disorders such substance abuse, generalized anxiety, depression, and antisocial or borderline personality

P

Complications

Isolation and secondary psychological responses are common complications.

Diagnostic Tests

Historical presence of trauma or assault; clinical evaluation and structured interviews; repeated responses to similar triggers. Objective testing using such tools as *The Mississippi Scale Post-Traumatic Stress Disorder* and *The Clinician-Administered Post-Traumatic Stress Disorder* test.

Therapeutic Management

Surgery	None
Drugs	No specific drugs; may treat secondary psychiatric signs and symptoms such as anxiety, depression, and/or impulsive activities or thoughts
General	Counseling
	Facilitate individual and family support
	Provide milieu therapy of the individuals social environment
	Teach self-care and empowerment

preeclampsia and eclampsia (pregnancy-induced hypertension)

Preeclampsia is a disorder occurring between the twentieth week of pregnancy and the first week postpartum characterized by hypertension, proteinuria, and edema. Eclampsia is diagnosed when a woman with preeclampsia develops convulsions or becomes comatose in the absence of any other underlying neurological disorder.

Etiology and incidence: The cause of preeclampsia and eclampsia is unknown. Preeclampsia occurs in 5% of pregnant women. About one in 200 of those individuals diagnosed with preeclampsia develops eclampsia.

Pathophysiology: An increased sensitivity to angiotensin II develops, followed by vasospasms, which cause increased resistance to vascular flow and increased aterial pressure, with accompanying hemoconcentration.

Risk Factors

Primigravidas (85% of cases)
Age (less than 18 or over 35)
Grand multigravidas
Large fetus or multiple fetuses
Evidence of major uterine anomalies
Morbid obesity (over 100 pounds above normal weight range)
History of preeclampsia with previous pregnancies
History of preexisting cardiovascular conditions, diabetes mellitus, collagen vascular or renal disease

Clinical Manifestations

The primary signs of preeclampsia are a blood pressure of 140/90 or an increase of 15 mm Hg diastolic or 30 mm Hg systolic over the woman's baseline pressure, and proteinuria and nondependent edema of the hands and face. These signs may be accompanied by a sudden weight gain. Seizure activity or coma (or both) in a woman with preeclampsia is indicative of eclampsia.

Complications

A major complication of preeclampsia is abruptio placentae. Untreated preeclampsia leads to eclampsia, and untreated eclampsia is generally fatal.

Diagnostic Tests

Evaluation is based on the presenting symptoms.

Therapeutic Management

Surgery	Delivery for women with severe or unresponsive preeclampsia—vaginal delivery if cervix is ripe; cesarean section if vaginal delivery is unlikely
Drugs	*Severe preeclampsia:* IV magnesium sulfate to reduce blood pressure, addition of hydralazine if no response occurs; calcium gluconate as an antidote for excess magnesium sulfate; *diuretics are contraindicated because they reduce uteroplacental perfusion*
General	*Mild preeclampsia:* Bed rest, positioned on the left side to increase urinary output and lessen intravascular dehydration and hemoconcentration; increased fluid intake and normal salt intake; close monitoring of blood pressure daily or every other day
	Severe preeclampsia and eclampsia: Immediate hospitalization, IV with balanced salt solution and administration of drugs in preparation for delivery; vital signs and fetal heart tone every 15 minutes; intake and output measurements hourly; monitoring for signs of abruptio placentae, seizure, decrease in consciousness, HELLP syndrome (*h*emolysis, *e*levated *l*iver enzymes, *l*ow *p*latelet count)

premenstrual syndrome

A combination of affective and physical symptoms starting 7 to 10 days before menstruation and disappearing within a few hours to days after the onset of menstrual flow

Etiology and incidence: The etiology of premenstrual syndrome (PMS) is unclear, but the disorder seems to be related to fluctuations in estrogen and progesterone. Excessive aldosterone, hypoglycemia, hyperprolactinemia, allergy to progesterone, changes in carbohydrate metabolism, and psychogenic factors have also been implicated. An estimated 50% of all women experience PMS sometime before menopause. Those over age 30 are at higher risk, and the severity often increases as a woman ages.

Pathophysiology: A fall in estrogen and progesterone is accompanied by an increase in aldosterone, ovarian steroids, and antidiuretic hormone. This promotes sodium and fluid retention and results in edema. Decreased estrogen levels may also reduce brain levels of monoamine oxidase, catecholamine, and serotonin, resulting in irritability, depression, and mood swings.

Clinical Manifestations

PMS is marked by a broad manifestation of signs and symptoms that may range from mild to severe.

Physical	Fatigue, edema, weight gain, oliguria, breast fullness, headache, vertigo, syncope, paresthesias, easy bruising, palpitations, abdominal bloating, constipation, nausea, vomiting, pelvic heaviness and cramping, backache, acne, neurodermatitis, cystitis, enuresis, aggravation of allergy, and asthma
Affective	Mood swings, depression, irritability, anxiety, outbursts of anger, lethargy, insomnia, decreased attention span, forgetfulness, crying, loss of motivation, confusion, change in sexual arousal

Complications

Extreme antisocial behavior that is potentially harmful to the woman or others is a complication of PMS.

Diagnostic Tests

Evaluation is based on the symptom pattern, which appears and disappears with the menstrual cycle. Conditions such as endometriosis, an ovarian cyst, pelvic infection, underlying thyroid disease, or a psychiatric disorder must be ruled out.

Therapeutic Management

Surgery	Endometrial ablation for severe, untreatable pain; oophorectomy for severe, unresponsive symptoms
Drugs	Long-acting progestin to regulate cycles, gonadotropin-releasing hormone agonists or oral contraceptives to suppress ovulation, progesterone replacement, antiprostaglandins to reduce cramping, diuretics for edema, mild tranquilizers for agitation, antidepressants for depression, vitamin supplements
General	Restriction of sodium, caffeine, tobacco, alcohol, and refined sugar; increased intake of complex carbohydrates, protein, and fiber; consistent exercise program to release endorphins; stress reduction program; counseling with partner involvement to better understand and cope with symptoms

pressure sore (decubitus ulcer, bedsore)

Ischemic necrosis and ulceration of tissues that overlie a bony prominence and that have been subjected to prolonged external pressure from a supporting surface such as a bed or wheelchair

Etiology and incidence: Pressure sores are caused by prolonged pressure on tissues compressed between an internal body structure such as bone and an external surface. The force and duration of the pressure directly determine the size of the ulcer.

Pathophysiology: Pressure exerted over an area interferes with the blood supply to the tissue, producing ischemia and increasing capillary pressure. This leads to edema and multiple small-vessel thromboses and sets up an inflammatory reaction. If the pressure is not relieved, the ischemic tissue necroses and ulcerates.

Risk Factors

Immobilization
Sensory and motor deficits
Reduced circulation
Malnutrition
Anemia
Edema
Infection
Friction
Moisture
Incontinence
Shearing forces
Decreased tissue integrity or viability
Aging

Clinical Manifestations

Four grades or stages of ulcer formation are defined by the National Pressure Ulcer Advisory Panel Consensus Conference. These stages are classified by the degree of tissue damage observed and possess the following characteristic signs and symptoms:

Stage 1   Nonblanchable erythema of intact skin; in dark-
             skinned individuals, presenting symptoms include

skin discoloration with accompanying heat, edema, or hardness

Stage 2   Partial thickness skin loss involving the epidermis or the dermis, including blisters, abrasions, and shallow craters

Stage 3   Full thickness skin loss with damage or necrosis to subcutaneous tissue that may extend down to underlying fascia and presents as a deep crater

Stage 4   Full thickness skin loss accompanied by extensive destruction, tissue necrosis and damage to muscle, bone, or supporting structures (e.g., tendons, joint capsules)

Complications

Bacteremia and septicemia are common complications. Osteomyelitis, septic arthritis, and pathological fractures also can occur.

Diagnostic Tests

Clinical evaluation revealing the characteristic picture described under Clinical Manifestations

History of one or more predisposing and contributing factors

Therapeutic Management

Surgery   Sharp débridement to remove eschar and dead tissue in large ulcers

Stage 3 or 4 ulcers that do not respond to conservative treatment: direct closure, skin grafting, skin flaps, muscle flaps, and free flaps

Joint disarticulation with large stage 4 ulcers

Drugs   Topical applications (e.g., enzymatic ointments) to débride necrotic tissue, hydrophilic gels for reepithelialization, topical antibiotics to suppress infection, platelet-derived epidermal growth factors for tissue healing

Do not use topical antiseptic agents (e.g., povidone iodine, iodophor, hydrogen peroxide, sodium hypochlorite, acetic acid) to clean ulcers because they are cytotoxic.

General   Elimination of pressure through frequent
           turning, special beds, mattress overlays, wheel-
           chair pads filled with gels, air, water, sand,
           or other pressure-relieving ingredients; use of
           lifting devices to prevent shearing; débride-
           ment with wet dressings; irrigation with whirl-
           pool baths; electrical stimulation to promote
           antibacterial effects and stimulate muscle
           protein synthesis; balanced nutrition; control
           of incontinence and careful cleansing

Prevention Instruction in ulcer prevention (e.g., frequent
           use of pressure relief measures such as turning,
           raising off buttocks, shifting weight when
           seated); daily skin inspections; use of pressure
           relief mattress overlays and wheelchair
           cushions; clean, dry clothing and bed linens
           free of wrinkles and treated with fabric
           softener; lotion on all skin surfaces, especially
           over bony prominences, to reduce friction

P

prostate cancer

Adenocarcinomas account for most prostate cancers. The rest are transitional cell, squamous cell, endometrioid, or sarcomatous cancers. (See also Cancer.)

Etiology and incidence: The cause is unknown but appears to be related to endogenous hormones. A genetic component may also play a role. Prostate cancer is the most commonly diagnosed cancer in men in the United States, with more than 244,000 cases reported annually. It is the second leading cause of cancer deaths in men, with more than 40,000 deaths reported annually. It strikes those over age 50 most frequently (more than 85% are over age 65) and the incidence and mortality rates are higher in black men.

Pathophysiology: Adenocarcinomas usually begin in the lower posterior prostate and grow slowly to encompass the entire gland. The tumor spreads directly to the bladder and levator ani muscles and, via the lymphatic system, throughout the pelvis. Metastasis occurs through the bloodstream to the bones, liver, lungs, and kidneys.

Risk Factors

Age (70% of men over age 80 have evidence of disease)
Race (blacks, particularly young blacks, have higher rates)
Familial history in first-degree relative
Diet with high fat-intake (particularly saturated fats)

Clinical Manifestations

Early signs mimic benign prostatic hypertrophy; they include difficulty initiating and stopping the urinary stream, frequency and pain on urination, and a weak urinary stream.

Complications

The prognosis is good with tumors that have not metastasized more than 70%, and even with metastasized disease, treatment may achieve long-term palliation. Complications of advanced disease include thrombosis, pulmonary emboli, retrograde ejaculation, and impotence.

Diagnostic Tests

Palpable nodules on digital rectal examination and an elevated prostate-specific antigen offer suspicions of tumor. A needle biopsy is the definitive follow-up. Transrectal ultrasonography is used to assess size and shape of tumor.

Therapeutic Management

Surgery	Prostatectomy for localized tumor, transurethral resection when the bladder is involved, bilateral orchiectomy for metastatic disease
Drugs	Hormone therapy or chemotherapy for palliation
General	Radiation (external beam and/or interstitial implant) as a primary treatment alternative to surgery and for palliation; counseling for changes in sexual functioning; cryosurgical ablation

P

prostatic hypertrophy, benign

A progressive enlargement of the periurethral prostate gland

Etiology and incidence: The etiology of benign prostatic hypertrophy (BPH) is unknown but is thought to be related to hormonal changes as a man ages. It is most commonly seen in men over age 50 and can be expected to affect at least 50% of the male population. The incidence of BPH continues to rise as longevity increases.

Pathophysiology: Multiple fibroadenomatous nodules grow in the periurethral glands of the prostate, displacing the fibromuscular prostate. The lumen of the prostatic urethra becomes progressively compromised, and outflow of urine is obstructed.

Clinical Manifestations

A man may be asymptomatic for years before signs of progressive urinary frequency, urgency, nocturia, dribbling, and hesitancy occur. This is accompanied by a diminution in the size and force of the stream and a feeling of fullness in the bladder region after urination. Recurring urinary tract infections may be common.

Complications

Renal complications arise from prolonged obstruction; they can include hydronephrosis, renal infection, azotemia, renal calculi, uremia, and renal failure.

Diagnostic Tests

A clinical evaluation revealing an enlarged, indurated, and tender prostate in conjunction with typical manifestations is suggestive of BPH. An elevated prostate-specific antigen, postvoid residual, and decreased peak and mean flows on a uroflow test aid in diagnosis. Cystoscopy and cystometrography allow visualization and assessment of the degree of urethral obstruction.

Therapeutic Management

Surgery	Transurethral resection of the prostate is the definitive treatment of choice; alternatives include intraurethral stent, balloon dilation, microwave therapy, cryotherapy, incisional resection laser ablation, and ultrasonic aspiration.
Drugs	Alpha-antagonists or hormonal agents to reduce prostate's size (these may cause erectile dysfunction, loss of libido, feminization, and thromboembolism)
General	Intermittent catheterization

P

prostatitis

An inflamation of the prostate gland

Etiology and incidence: Prostatitis may be acute or chronic, bacterial, or nonbacterial. Nonbacterial prostatitis (also called *prostatosis*) is the most common type of prostatitis. Acute and chronic bacterial prostatitis is less commonly seen. *Acute prostatitis* is found in two of 10,000 outpatient visits. There is increased risk associated with men ages 20 to 35 who have multiple sexual partners and those who engage in high-risk sexual behaviors (e.g., lack of condom use or anal intercourse). *Chronic prostatitis* is more prevalent than acute prostatitis. It is estimated that as many as 35% of men over age 50 may have chronic prostatitis. Factors that may predispose a person to develop chronic prostatitis include excessive alcohol intake, perineal injury, and sexual practices. *Nonbacterial prostatitis* is the most common of all the types of prostatitis. It may be associated with or follow a urinary tract infection, urethritis, or epididymitis.

Pathophysiology: Acute and chronic prostatitis are both caused by a bacterial infection of the prostate. Bacteria often enter through the urethra following urethral instrumentation (e.g., catheterization or cystoscope), trauma, bladder outlet obstruction, or infection elsewhere in the body. Common causative agents include *E. coli, Proteus, Klebsiella, Pseudomonas,* and *Enterobacter.* Although the causative agent of nonbacterial prostatitis has not been identified, *Chlamydia* has been implicated as a possible pathogen.

Risk Factors

Urethral instrumentation
High-risk sexual behaviors (lack of condom use and/or anal intercourse)
Recurrent urinary tract infections, urethritis or epididymitis
Excessive alcohol intake
Age (20 to 35 for acute; over age 50 for chronic)

Clinical Manifestations

Acute prostatitis	Sudden onset of fever, chills, myalgia, arthralgia, and general malaise; localized discomfort or pain in the perineal area or low back and prostate; associated urinary symptoms include urgency, frequency, nocturia, diminished urine stream, dysuria, and a burning sensation in the urethra; pain in the testicles and with ejaculation *Examination findings:* Firm, swollen prostate that is tender and warm to the touch; enlarged and tender inguinal lymph nodes; urethral discharge
Chronic prostatitis	Recurrent urinary tract infections; low back pain; perineal or pelvic floor pain; testicular pain; pain or burning with urination; pain with ejaculation and with bowel movements; incontinence of urine; and abnormal urine color In some cases, no symptoms *Examination findings* include an enlarged tender prostate, swollen scrotum, tender and enlarged inguinal lymph nodes, and urethral discharge.
Nonbacterial prostatitis	Frequent urination; pain and/or burning with urination; low back pain; pain in testes and with ejaculation; pain with bowel movements *Clinical examination* reveals firm, tender, and swollen prostate. There may be urethral discharge and scrotal swelling or tenderness.

Complications

Sterility may result from prostatitis.

Diagnostic Tests

Urinalysis and urine culture

Blood test to examine for systemic infection

Diagnosis of nonbacterial prostatitis is made by demonstrating the presence of inflammatory cells in the expressed prostatic secretions in the presence of negative prostatic secretion and bladder cultures. Intravenous pyelogram (IVP) may be done to ensure bladder neck patency.

Therapeutic Management

Surgery	Infrequent; however, transurethral resection of the prostate may be performed for chronic prostatitis if antibiotic therapy is not successful
Drugs	Antiinfective agents (often intravenous for acute prostatitis) specific to cultured organism; stool softener for bowel movement discomfort
General	Acute and chronic may require urinary catheterization or suprapubic caterer, warm tub or sitz baths, and increased fluid intake
	Education about cleanliness of the genitals, safe sex, and alcohol intake

psoriasis

A recurrent chronic disease of the skin, characterized by dry, scaly plaques and papules of varying size

Etiology and incidence: The cause is unknown but is thought to be related to genetic and environmental factors that trigger an overproduction of epidermal cells. The onset typically occurs between ages 10 and 40, and the disorder affects 2% to 4% of the U.S. population. Whites are at greater risk than blacks, as are those with a family history of psoriasis.

Pathophysiology: Three main pathological components are at work in psoriasis, to varying degrees. An increased miotic rate causes rapid epidermal cell turnover and shortened transit time of the cell from the basal layer to the epidermis. Faulty keratinization of the horny layer causes easy desquamation and diminished protection for underlying tissue. Dilation of dermal vessels and intermittent discharge of leukocytes into the dermis cause hot, red skin.

Clinical Manifestations

The onset is gradual, and the disorder is characterized by chronic exacerbation and remission. The scalp, elbows, knees, back, and buttocks are the most common sites. The nails, eyebrows, axillae, and anal and genital regions may also be affected. The lesions are well-defined, dry, nonpruritic papules or plaques overlaid with shiny silver scales, and they heal without scarring. The skin may be reddened and hot to touch. Affected nails are pitted, discolored, thickened, and crumbly.

Complications

Common complications include psoriatic arthritis and exfoliative psoriatic dermatitis, which can lead to crippling and general debility.

Diagnostic Tests

The diagnosis is based on examination of characteristic lesions.

Therapeutic Management

Surgery	None
Drugs	Topical corticosteroids, keratolytics used in lotion, cream, ointment, or shampoo form to treat lesions; antineoplastic agents for severe recalcitrant disease
General	Shortwave or longwave ultraviolet light therapy; lubricants to soften skin; exposure to sunlight but avoiding sunburn; stress- reduction programs; prevention of mechanical injury to skin; instruction that lesions are not communicable; counseling if body image is affected and to adapt to chronic nature of disease

pulmonary embolism

Sudden blockage of a pulmonary artery by foreign matter, which impedes the blood flow to the lung tissue

Etiology and incidence: The most common cause is a thrombus, which typically forms in the leg or pelvic vein but may be seen in other locations. Other causes include fat, amniotic fluid, air, and gas. Pulmonary embolism is the third most common cardiovascular disease in the United States. It is estimated that up to 5% of hospital deaths are attributable to pulmonary emboli.

Pathophysiology: Emboli in any form travel through the bloodstream and lodge in one or more pulmonary arteries. The area of the lung supplied by the affected artery becomes underperfused but is still ventilated. This results in physiological dead space or wasted ventilation and contributes to hyperventilation. Histamine release from the embolus produces reflex bronchoconstriction, leading to further hyperventilation. Depletion of alveolar surfactant results in diminished lung volume and compliance. If the clot is large enough and interferes greatly with pulmonary perfusion, it may result in pulmonary hypertension.

Risk Factors

History of thrombophlebitis, myocardial infarction, severe
    burns, congestive heart failure, venous insufficiency,
    polycythemia vera, chronic pulmonary disease, autoimmune
    hemolytic anemia, or cancer
Major surgery or fractures of lower extremities
Pregnancy and childbirth
Prolonged immobility
History of chronic illness
Obesity
Use of oral contraceptives or estrogen supplements

Clinical Manifestations

The manifestations of a pulmonary embolus (PE) are nonspecific and vary in degree and intensity, depending on the size of the embolus, the extent of occlusion, the amount of collateral circulation, and preexisting cardiopulmonary function. Small emboli may be asymptomatic. The chief manifestation is breathlessness. Other symptoms include anxiety, restlessness, tachypnea, sweating, cough, hemoptysis, chest pain, fever, and rales. Cyanosis may be present with a massive embolus.

Complications

Cardiac arrhythmias, cor pulmonale, atelectasis, shock, hepatic congestion, and necrosis are complications. Pulmonary infarction is an uncommon complication of PE that results in hemorrhagic consolidation and tissue necrosis distal to the occlusion. Death following a PE usually occurs within 1 to 2 hours of the initial event. Those with underlying cardiovascular or pulmonary disease and those with a large embolus are at greater risk of dying. Untreated individuals risk recurrent emboli and about a 50% chance of death.

Diagnostic Tests

The diagnosis is suggested by the presenting clinical picture and confirmed by the following procedures:

Pulmonary angiogram	Visualization of intraarterial filling defects
Lung perfusion scan	To detect perfusion defects
Ventilation scan	To detect altered ventilation patterns
Blood gases	Arterial hypoxemia (decreased Pao_2 and $Paco_2$)
Electrocardiography	To rule out myocardial infarction; a PE is characterized by tall, peaked P waves, depressed ST segments, T-wave inversions, and supraventricular tachyarrhythmias
Chest x-ray	Unilateral elevation of the diaphragm, enlarged pulmonary artery, and pleural effusion 2 hours or longer after the event

Therapeutic Management

Surgery	Embolectomy for large emboli unresponsive to treatment; umbrella filter in inferior vena cava to trap multiple emboli before they reach the lung; interruption of blood flow through the inferior vena cava by ligation for multiple emboli

Drugs   Anticoagulants to halt clot propagation (heparin is used in the acute phase and is replaced by coumadin, which may be administered for 6 months to life; medications should overlap for 5 to 7 days to achieve effective blood levels of coumadin); fibrinolytic enzymes may be used in place of anticoagulants for clot lysis, particularly of large clots; analgesics for pain; vasopressors, dopamine to treat hypotension

General   Oxygen therapy; bed rest in acute phase, followed by progressive mobilization; hemodynamic and cardiac monitoring; facilitation of breathing; intake and output measurements to monitor renal function; observation for bleeding as a side effect of anticoagulants, and safety measures to prevent bleeding; information about long-term anticoagulant therapy; antiembolism hose and instruction in preventing pooled blood in the lower extremities

P

pyelonephritis

An acute or chronic infection and inflammation of the kidney or renal pelvis (See also Urinary Tract Infection.)

Etiology and incidence: Acute pyelonephritis is caused by a bacterial invasion that moves from the urethra to the bladder to the ureters to the kidney. The infecting bacteria are commonly normal intestinal and fecal flora that grow readily in urine. The annual incidence of pyelonephritis in the United States is 16 in 100,000; the annual nosocomial incidence rises to 73 in 100,000. Chronic pyelonephritis most typically occurs as a result of repeated acute episodes but may also be caused by metastatic disease.

Pathophysiology: Bacteria ascend the urinary tract and colonize one or both kidneys. The kidney enlarges as the inflammatory process is activated, and parenchymal tissue is destroyed. Chronic inflammatory cells appear within a few days, and medullary abscesses and papillary tissue necrosis occur. Patchy spots of infection develop and spread to the pelvic and calyceal epithelia and the cortex. If the process becomes chronic, atrophy, calyceal deformity, and parenchymal scarring occur.

Risk Factors

Individuals with a condition that interferes with the dynamics of normal urine flow are at greater risk. This includes those with underlying obstructions (strictures, calculi, tumors, prostatic hypertrophy), neurogenic bladder, vesicourethral reflux, diabetes, or renal disease; those who are sexually active or pregnant; and those undergoing medical or surgical procedures such as catheterization or cystoscopy. Women are more susceptible than men because of the anatomical construction of the female urinary system.

Clinical Manifestations

The onset is fairly rapid and is characterized by dull, constant flank pain, chills, and fever. Concomitant signs of a lower urinary tract infection (e.g., urinary frequency, dysuria) occur in about one third of individuals.

Complications

The most common complication of acute disease is septic shock or chronic pyelonephritis (or both). With chronic disease there is a 2% to 3% chance of developing end-stage renal failure.

Diagnostic Tests

Presenting clinical symptoms are confirmed by urinalysis, which reveals antibody-coated bacteria, bacteriuria, WBC casts, and pyuria; a CBC shows an increase in WBCs. Renal function studies may assist in the diagnosis of chronic disease.

Therapeutic Management

Surgery	Correction of underlying obstructions
Drugs	Oral or parenteral antiinfective drugs to combat infection; continuous suppression antiinfective therapy may be used to treat recurrent or chronic infection; antipyretics for fever
General	Increased fluid intake; urine cultures to track effectiveness of antiinfective drugs; instruction in preventing infection (cleansing perineum, proper wiping technique, adequate fluid intake, cleansing after sexual activity)

P

rabies

An acute, viral, infectious, communicable disease of the central nervous system (CNS) characterized by CNS irritation, paralysis, and death

Etiology and incidence: The causative agent is a neurotropic rhabdovirus that is often present in the saliva of infected animals and is usually transmitted to humans through the bite of a rabid animal. Dogs are the most common source of infection, but bats, raccoons, skunks, foxes, cats, and cattle are all known to carry rabies. Rabies is fairly rare in the United States, where vaccination has largely eliminated canine rabies. Rabid dogs are prevalent in Latin America, Africa, and Asia, where they are a health risk to humans.

Pathophysiology: The virus travels from the site of entry via the peripheral nerves to the spinal cord and brain, where it incubates for 10 days to 1 year. It then multiplies and travels from the CNS through the efferent nerves to many body tissues, including the salivary glands, saliva, urine, cerebrospinal fluid, corneal cells, and skin. It causes vessel engorgement, edema, and punctate hemorrhages in the meninges and the brain, and diffuse degenerative changes occur in the neurons of the brain and spinal cord. Negri bodies may be formed in the hippocampus or neurons in the cerebellum, cortex, and spinal cord.

Clinical Manifestations

Signs and symptoms manifest in three stages: a prodrome (lasts 1 to 10 days), acute neurological or furious rabies (lasts 2 to 7 days), and paralytic or dumb rabies.

Incubation	Itching, hyperesthesia, and pain radiating from the bite wound
Prodrome	Headache, nausea, fever, chills, apathy, malaise, anxiety, irritability, restlessness, depression
Acute	Agitation, excessive salivation, marked motor activity followed by laryngeal and pharyngeal spasms, dysphagia, and hydrophobia; 1- to 5-minute periods of thrashing, hallucination, biting, seizures, and disorientation, followed by calmness and lucidity; autonomic

	hyperactivity with supraventricular arrhythmias, deregulated blood pressure, and tachypnea
Paralytic	Progressive paralysis in an ascending fashion, with ensuing coma and death, usually within 12 days of symptom onset

Complications

Death is almost certain without prompt treatment. It is usually caused by fluid depletion and cardiovascular or respiratory collapse and may occur during the acute or paralytic stage.

Diagnostic Tests

Diagnosis is difficult in humans before the onset of symptoms, and virus isolation and antibody testing, although effective, may not prove positive until after the individual dies. An animal bite in humans should trigger immediate action. If the bite is from an apparently healthy domestic animal, the animal should be held for 10 days for observation in case of rabies symptoms. If the animal is rabid or suspected of being rabid, it should be killed immediately and its brain subjected to a fluorescent antibody test and viral isolation. If the bite is from a wild animal such as a skunk, raccoon, bat, fox, or other carnivore, the animal should be considered rabid unless it is available for testing and tests negative, or the geographic area is free of rabies.

Therapeutic Management

Surgery	None
Drugs	Rabies vaccine (active immunity) and rabies immune globulin (passive immunity) administered prophylactically after a bite from an animal suspected of being or tested as rabid; preexposure vaccination should be considered for individuals at high risk for exposure to rabid animals (e.g., veterinarians, spelunkers, animal handlers, and laboratory workers who handle infected tissues)

R

General   Immediate cleansing of the wound with soap and water, flushing of deep puncture wounds as prophylaxis; once symptoms develop, treatment is supportive only to control respiratory, circulatory, and CNS damage; individual should be placed in isolation, and staff should use precautions in handling body secretions

Raynaud's disease

Episodic vasospasm of the small cutaneous arteries, usually in the fingers but occasionally in the toes, nose, or tongue, that results in intermittent pallor or cyanosis of the skin

Etiology and incidence: Raynaud's disease may be idiopathic, or it may occur secondary to other underlying conditions such as connective tissue disorders, obstructive arterial disease, neurogenic lesions, trauma, or drug intoxication. Attacks are often triggered by stress or cold or are seen in conjunction with migraines and angina. Raynaud's disease is a rare occurrence. The idiopathic type accounts for somewhere between 70% and 90% of reported cases and is most often seen in young women.

Pathophysiology: The pathophysiology is not fully clear but involves a severe constriction of cutaneous vessels followed by vessel dilation and then a reactive hyperemia. Catecholamine release and prostaglandin metabolism are thought to play a role in the process. Vessels may thicken with advanced disease.

Clinical Manifestations

Intermittent attacks lasting from a few minutes to hours cause the fingers to blanch, then become cyanotic, and finally turn red and throb with pain. In long-standing disease, the skin becomes smooth, shiny, and tight with a loss of subcutaneous tissue. Small, painful ulcers may appear on the tips of the fingers.

Complications

Recurring infection and gangrene are rare complications of severe Raynaud's disease.

Diagnostic Tests

The diagnosis is made from the clinical pattern and by abnormal perfusion patterns on digital plethysmography or peripheral arteriography.

Therapeutic Management

Surgery	Sympathectomy for individuals with progressive symptoms
Drugs	Reserpine to reduce vasoconstriction; alpha-adrenergic blocking agents and calcium antagonists to dilate peripheral vessels; use of prostaglandins is under study
General	Avoidance of exposure to cold and mechanical and chemical irritants; quitting smoking; stress-reduction programs, such as biofeedback; treatment of underlying causes in secondary disease

renal calculi (kidney stones)

The precipitation of normally occurring crystalline substances into irregularly shaped stones, which are deposited in the urinary tract, most commonly in the renal pelvis or calyces

Etiology and incidence: The precise etiology of renal calculi formation is unknown. Renal calculi are common, and about one in 1000 adults in the United States are hospitalized with them. Four of five individuals who develop calculi are men, and the peak onset is ages 20 to 30.

Pathophysiology: Certain conditions increase the supersaturation of urine with stone-forming salts, induce preformed salt nuclei, or reduce the production of crystal growth inhibitors. This allows the precipitation process to occur and stones to form, ranging in size from microscopic to several centimeters in diameter.

Risk Factors

Obstruction and stasis of urine
Urinary tract infection
Dehydration and concentration of urine
Prolonged immobility
Vitamin A deficiency; dietary excess of vitamin D, calcium, vitamin C, protein, tea, or fruit juice
Underlying disease of the small bowel; an underlying metabolic disorder (e.g., hypercalcemia or hyperparathyroidism); and hereditary disease (e.g., cystinuria)
Anatomical abnormalities of the kidney or ureters

Clinical Manifestations

Many calculi are asymptomatic. If they obstruct the calyx, pelvis, or ureter, they cause severe pain that is typically described as traveling from the costovertebral angle to the flank and then to the suprapubic region and external genitalia. Back- or abdominal pain, or both, may also be present. Chills, fever, nausea, vomiting, abdominal extension, and hematuria are also common.

Complications

Large stones can remain in the renal pelvis or calyx or hang up in the ureter and cause infection, necrosis, or obstruction, with subsequent hydronephrosis.

Diagnostic Tests

The diagnosis is based on clinical features plus an x-ray of the kidneys, ureter, and bladder, which demonstrates calculi, and a urinalysis, which may show hematuria, pyuria, and crystalline sludge in the sediment. Intravenous pyelography and CT scans are also used to locate and visualize stones.

Therapeutic Management

Surgery	Pyelolithotomy or nephrolithotomy to remove large stones in kidney or ureterolithotomy to remove stones in the ureter that are not amenable to other treatment; nephrectomy when the kidney has been irreparably damaged
Drugs	Percutaneous stone dissolution with chemical solvents to shrink large uric stones in preparation for other retrieval methods; antiinfective drugs to treat infection; narcotic analgesics for pain; diuretics to prevent urinary stasis; cholestyramine for prophylaxis; for hypercalcinuria, allopurinol to reduce uric acid
General	Small, solitary calculi without infection or obstruction may be treated by increasing fluid intake to encourage passage; extracorporeal shock wave lithotripsy (ESWL) is the treatment of choice for stones less than 2 cm in diameter; percutaneous nephrolithotomy is used in conjunction with ESWL to remove stones larger than 2 cm; cystoscopy with basket extraction can be used to remove calculi less than 1 cm in diameter that are lodged in the ureter
Prevention	Increased fluid intake; treatment of underlying conditions; reduction of excess calcium, phosphorus, purine, and oxalates in diet

renal failure, acute

Sudden impairment of renal function marked by rapid, steadily increasing azotemia with or without oliguria

Etiology and incidence: Acute renal failure (ARF) may be caused by (1) prerenal factors that interfere with renal perfusion (e.g., fluid and electrolyte depletion, hemorrhage, septicemia, cardiac or liver failure, heat stroke, burn-induced fluid depletion, myoglobinuria); (2) postrenal factors that cause obstruction (e.g., prostatism, calculi, tumors of the bladder or pelvis); or (3) renal factors that directly impair renal function (e.g., acute tubular injury, acute glomerulonephritis, disseminated intravascular coagulation, arterial or venous obstruction, tubulointerstitial nephritis, intrarenal precipitation). About 1% of all hospital admissions in the United States are for ARF, and the mortality rate is about 50%. ARF caused by prerenal or postrenal factors is more treatable than ARF caused by renal factors.

Pathophysiology: Prerenal azotemia results from inadequate renal perfusion. As the glomerular filtration rate is reduced, sodium and water resorption is enhanced, causing oliguria. Urinary osmolarity is high, and urine sodium concentrations are low. Four mechanisms may be at work, either independently or in concert, in ARF caused by renal factors: (1) a decrease in renal blood flow; (2) a reduction in glomerular permeability; (3) tubular obstruction; and (4) diffusion of glomerular filtrate across injured tubular epithelium. Other mechanisms are unclear at present. Postrenal azotemia results from obstruction and subsequent glomerular or tubular dysfunction and mimics renally caused ARF in manifestation.

R

Risk Factors

Age (the very young and very old)
Dehydration
Underlying renal disease, diabetes mellitus
Hypotension
Sepsis, burns, jaundice
Recent surgery
Multiple organ system failure

Drug therapy (multiple drugs, aminoglycosides, angiotensins, angiotensin converting enzyme [ACE]-inhibitors, cyclosporin, cisplatin)

Exposure to heavy metals, radiographic contrast media

Clinical Manifestations

Prerenal	Nausea, vomiting, diarrhea, decreased tissue turgor, dry mucous membranes, bad taste in the mouth, oliguria, somnolence, fatigue, hypotension, tachycardia
Renal	Nocturia, fatigue, decreased mental acuity, fever, skin rash, edema, headache, anorexia, nausea, vomiting, oliguria or anuria, weight gain, rales, hypertension
Postrenal	Renal signs plus difficulty voiding, changes in urine flow, possibly flank pain

Complications

ARF can lead to renal shutdown, which affects all other body systems and if left untreated leads to death. Even with treatment, pulmonary edema, hypertensive crisis, acidosis, hyperkalemia, and infection are common, and death occurs in as many as 50% of all diagnosed cases.

Diagnostic Tests

Diagnosis is directed to classification of the condition as prerenal, renal, or postrenal.

Urine	*Prerenal:* Decreased pH, urine sodium, and oliguria; increased specific gravity; normal creatinine and sediment
	Renal: Decreased specific gravity, increased urine sodium and creatinine, oliguria or normal volume, sediment contains casts, pyuria
	Postrenal: Normal specific gravity, urine sodium, and creatinine; sediment normal or hematuria possible
Serum	Decreased pH, calcium, and bicarbonate; increased potassium, chloride, phosphate,

blood urea nitrogen, creatinine, and osmolality; sodium normal or decreased; Hgb
and Hct elevated with dehydration and
decreased with hypervolemia; decreased
adhesiveness of platelets

Ultrasound/ Kidneys may be enlarged
CT scan

Renal scan/ To visualize obstructions, tumors, and
IV urogram masses

Therapeutic Management

Surgery	Renal transplantation when cause is renal and unre-sponsive to other treatment
Drugs	Alkalinizing agents for acidosis; potassium-removing resins for hyperkalemia; vasodila-tors, angiotension antagonists, or calcium antagonists to treat hypertension; diuretics in pre-renal disease to increase perfusion unless oli-guria is present; dopamine if vasopressor is needed; antiinfective drugs for associated infec-tions (only antibiotics excreted primarily by the liver are used)
General	Limitation of all drugs that require renal excretion; balance of fluid intake and output (I&O), avoid-ing fluid overload; high-carbohydrate, low-protein feedings, essential amino acid replacement by IV and at least 100 g glucose per day; decreased potassium and sodium intake if levels are elevated; vitamin supplements; careful management of skin care to reduce dryness and prevent injury or infection; careful monitor-ing of I&O, weight, electrolytes, vital signs, cardiac status, and mental status; peritoneal or hemodialysis the treatment of choice when milder measures fail; information about dietary and fluid restrictions, medications, and dialysis

R

renal failure, chronic

Slow, insidious, and irreversible impairment of renal excretory and regulatory function

Etiology and incidence: The causes of chronic renal failure (CRF) include chronic glomerular disease (e.g., glomerulonephritis); chronic infection (e.g., pyelonephritis or tuberculosis); congenital anomalies (e.g., polycystic kidneys); vascular disease (e.g., hypertension); endocrine disease (e.g., diabetes); collagen disease (e.g., systemic lupus erythematosus); obstructive processes (e.g., calculi); and nephrotoxins.

Pathophysiology: In CRF, the renal system experiences ischemia, inflammation, necrosis, fibrosis, sclerosis, and scarring. Nephrons are permanently destroyed, and the kidneys become unable to respond to excessive or decreased salt and fluid intake. Synthesis of erythropoietin diminishes, and the kidneys are unable to excrete end products of metabolism. CRF occurs in three stages: diminished renal reserve, then renal insufficiency, and finally renal failure and uremia. As failure is occurring, a number of substances that are normally excreted accumulate in the body, including nitrogenous waste, electrolytes, and uremic toxins. Eventually all organ systems are affected.

Clinical Manifestations

Individuals with diminished renal reserve are asymptomatic. Those with moderate renal insufficiency may have only vague symptoms such as nocturia or fatigue. Lassitude and decreased mental acuity are often the first signs of CRF. These may be followed by neuromuscular twitching, cramps, and seizure activity. Anorexia, nausea, vomiting, stomatitis, and a metallic taste in the mouth are uniformly present. Advanced disease symptoms include tissue wasting; itching, uremic frost, and yellow-brown discoloration of the skin; gastrointestinal (GI) bleeding; hypertension; and coma.

Complications

All organ systems are affected by end-stage renal disease, and death is imminent without renal transplantation although life may be prolonged with dialysis.

Diagnostic Tests

Urine	Acidic pH, low osmolality, fixed specific gravity, proteinuria, casts; WBCs and RBCs may be present in sediment
Serum	Decreased pH, bicarbonate, magnesium; increased potassium, sodium, hydrogen, phosphate, calcium ions; increased uric acid, blood urea nitrogen, osmolality; decreased iron and iron-binding capacity; decreased creatinine clearance
CBC	Decreased Hgb, Hct, and RBC survival time; reduced platelets and decreased adhesiveness
X-ray of kidneys, ureter, and bladder/ultrasound	Small, contracted kidneys

Therapeutic Management

Surgery	Renal transplantation; insertion of Tenckhoff catheter for peritoneal dialysis; insertion of internal arteriovenous fistula for hemodialysis
Drugs	Alkalinizing agents for acidosis; potassium-removing resins for hyperkalemia; antihypertensives for hypertension; diuretics for edema and hypertension; phosphate binders for hyperphosphatemia; antiinfective drugs for infection; anticonvulsants for seizures; antiemetics for nausea; H_2-receptor antagonists for GI irritation; antipruritics for itching; laxatives and stool softeners for constipation; calcium, iron, and vitamin replacements
General	Diet low in protein, sodium, potassium, and phosphate, high in calories and calcium, and supplemented with essential amino acids; balanced fluid intake and output; monitoring of intake and output, weight changes, vital signs, electrolytes, and cardiac and mental status; careful skin

R

care; energy conservation with activities of daily living; peritoneal dialysis or hemodialysis to treat end-stage disease; long-term emotional support, counseling for adaptation to chronic, potentially fatal disease

retinal detachment

Separation of the sensory layers of the retina from the pigmented epithelium

Etiology and incidence: The most common cause is a hole or tear in the retina. Other causes may be seepage of vitreous fluid into the subretinal space as a result of inflammation, choroidal tumors, or systemic disease. Detachment may also occur as a result of vitreous traction placed on the inner lining of the retina from the contraction of fibrous band formations associated with diabetic retinopathy, sickle cell disease, or other retinal degeneration. Retinal detachment is most common after age 40 unless it is associated with trauma.

Pathophysiology: As vitreous fluid fills the subretinal space, the sensory layers of the retina progressively pull away from the pigmented epithelium. Separation may occur suddenly or may develop slowly over years.

Risk Factors

Degenerative changes associated with aging
Myopia
Cataract surgery
Trauma
Gender (twice as common in males)
History of retinopathy of prematurity, diabetic retinopathy

Clinical Manifestations

R

Retinal detachment may be totally asymptomatic until the macular area is invaded, reducing central vision and often fracturing images. Lightning flashes or floaters also may be present, particularly if separation is fairly rapid.

Complications

Untreated detachments may lead to severe vision impairment or blindness.

Diagnostic Tests

The diagnosis is made by indirect ophthalmoscopy, which reveals tears, breaks, and detachment.

Therapeutic Management

Surgery	Photocoagulation, diathermy, or cryothermy to burn or freeze tear margins and promote inflammation and scarring to seal the hole or tear
	Scleral buckle: An implant is used to encircle the eyeball, indent the sclera, and draw it flat against the retina in cases of large or multiple holes or tears.
Drugs	Mydriatics to dilate the pupil before and after surgery, prophylactic antiinfective drugs to prevent uveitis, steroids to control inflammation, antacids to prevent gastric irritation from steroids, narcotic analgesics to aid in maintaining sustained positions with scleral buckle, stool softeners for 4 to 6 weeks to prevent constipation
General	Eye patches 1 to 2 days after surgery to promote rest of the eyes; with scleral buckle, strict bed rest and specific head positioning to promote adhesion (position is maintained with foam wedges for 4 to 5 days); orientation measures if eyes are bilaterally patched; avoidance of heavy lifting, vigorous exercise and head jarring

rheumatic fever

A nonsuppurative, acute inflammatory complication from a group A streptococcal infection characterized by lesions in the connective tissues of the joints, heart, central nervous system (CNS), and subcutaneous tissues.

Etiology and incidence: The causative agent of rheumatic fever (RF) is a group A streptococcus, and the disease usually is a delayed complication of an upper respiratory infection. The role of predisposing host and environmental factors is unclear. Malnutrition and overcrowding seem to be factors. However, recent outbreaks in the United States tend to be among white middle-class children and young adults. An autoimmune theory and genetic predisposition have also been hypothesized. More than 2.1 million cases are reported annually in the United States, and more than 5000 deaths occur from the disease. Children are most susceptible, and the disease is twice as common among females.

Pathophysiology: A week to a month after a streptococcal throat infection, the streptococcal agent begins to damage the cardiac connective tissue by forming lesions that fragment the collagen fibers, infiltrate cellular lymphocytes, and leave fibrin deposits. Aschoff nodules (bullous hemorrhagic lesions) then develop, surrounded by large mononuclear and polymorphonuclear leukocytes, and the result is pericarditis, myocarditis, and left-sided endocarditis. The leaflets and chordae of the heart valves are infiltrated and thicken, resulting in stenosis and insufficiency. Joint tissue is infiltrated by lesions and Aschoff's nodules, causing a polyarthritis that is reversible and migratory, favors large joints, and lasts 1 to 2 days in the affected joint before moving on. Subcutaneous nodules may form under the skin over bony prominences, and a transient nonpruritic rash (erythema marginatum) may form on the trunk and proximal regions of the extremities. The CNS may also become involved, since streptococcal antigens cause cross-reactive antibodies to bind to the nerve tissue, where damage is caused by lymphocytes. After the damage occurs, as long as 6 months may lapse before the onset of chorea, which causes involuntary, purposeless, nonrepetitive movements that subside without neurological deficit in 3 to 6 months.

R

Clinical Manifestations

The five major manifestations of RF (carditis, polyarthritis, subcutaneous nodules, erythema marginatum, and chorea) can appear alone or in combination, producing a number of clinical disease patterns. Signs and symptoms of each of the major manifestations are given below.

General	Low-grade fever, anorexia, malaise, pallor, weight loss, abdominal pain that mimics appendicitis
Carditis	Tachycardia, gallop rhythm, effusion, diastolic murmurs, cardiac enlargement, pericardial friction rubs, congestive heart failure, high-pitched apical murmur of mitral regurgitation, low-pitched apical middiastolic flow murmur, diastolic murmur from aortic regurgitation, mitral and aortic stenotic murmurs with chronic valvular disease
Polyarthritis	Heat, swelling, redness, and severe tenderness of major joints, with migration from joint to joint, lasting 1 to 2 days and then moving on, for about 1 month
Subcutaneous nodules	Firm, painless nodules 0.5 to 1 cm in diameter that are found in crops over bony prominences and that persist 1 to 2 weeks before resolving gradually
Erythema arginatum	Nonpruritic macular eruptions on the trunk and proximal extremities; individual lesions clear within hours, but the rash may persist for months
Chorea	Involuntary, purposeless, rapid movements of the extremities, facial grimaces, speech disturbances, muscle weakness, and emotional lability
	These conditions develop up to 6 months after other symptoms and last about 2 weeks before gradually subsiding.

Complications

Rheumatic heart disease caused by damage to mitral and aortic valves is the most common complication and may eventually lead to death. Individuals who have RF are susceptible to recurrent bouts of the disorder.

Diagnostic Tests

The diagnosis is made using the guidelines of the American Heart Association; these include evidence of a previous streptococcal A infection, the presence of two of the five major manifestations or one major and two general manifestations, and a positive C-reactive protein serum test or an elevated erythrocyte sedimentation rate.

Therapeutic Management

Surgery	None
Drugs	Antiinfective drugs specific for group A streptococci during RF and afterward for prophylaxis; antipyretics for fever; nonsteroidal antiinflammatory agents for polyarthritis; corticosteroids for carditis; diuretics and digitalis for signs of congestive failure; sedation for chorea
General	Bed rest, then limited activity for carditis; nonstimulating environment for chorea; oxygen and restriction of sodium for cardiac failure; information about the recurrent nature of RF and the importance of (1) long-term prophylactic treatment and (2) notifying health care personnel (dentists, physicians, nurses) about rheumatic history before treatment for other conditions

R

Rocky Mountain spotted fever

An acute, febrile, infectious, rash-producing disease

Etiology and incidence: The cause is the *Rickettsia rickettsii* organism, which is transmitted through the bite of an adult *Ixodes* tick. The disease is seen most often from May to September, when adult ticks are active and humans are likely to be outdoors in tick-infested areas. The incidence is highest in children under age 15 and in those who frequent tick-infected areas for work or recreation.

Pathophysiology: The organism enters humans through a prolonged bite (4 to 6 hours) by an adult tick. *R. rickettsii* then localizes and proliferates in the vascular endothelium of small and medium blood vessels, producing widespread swelling and degeneration that result in thrombi and vasculitis and affect the skin, subcutaneous tissues, heart, lungs, kidneys, liver, spleen, and central nervous system.

Clinical Manifestations

The incubation time between bite and symptoms ranges from 3 to 12 days. The shorter the incubation period, the more severe the manifestations. The onset is abrupt and is marked by a severe headache; intermittent fever; chills; pain and aching in the back, bones, muscles, and joints; anorexia; nausea; vomiting; a thick, white covering on the tongue; and a nonproductive cough. Skin eruptions develop on the wrists, ankles, and forehead within 2 to 5 days of symptom onset, and the rash spreads to the entire body, including the palms, soles, and scalp, within 2 days. The lesions become petechial and coalesce into hemorrhagic areas that ulcerate and peel; restlessness, insomnia, delirium, and coma may ensue.

Complications

Untreated cases lead to complications such as pneumonia; tissue necrosis, with gangrene of the digits; disseminated intravascular coagulation; circulatory failure; renal failure; and cardiac arrest with sudden death.

Diagnostic Tests

The diagnosis is made through a history of a tick bite, a pattern of symptoms, and blood cultures that isolate the causative agent. Immunofluorescent tests that detect the organism in a punch biopsy of affected cutaneous tissue are also used.

Therapeutic Management

Surgery	None
Drugs	Antiinfective, rickettsiostatic drugs until individual is afebrile; antiinfective drugs in combination with corticosteroids if treatment is started later in the disease process; analgesics for pain; antipyretics for fever; *aspirin is avoided because it can cause hemorrhage*
General	Rest; fluid and electrolyte replacement; meticulous mouth and skin care; monitoring for complications

R

rubella (German measles)

A mild, febrile, highly communicable viral disease characterized by a diffuse, punctate, macular rash

Etiology and incidence: Rubella is caused by a ribonucleic acid (RNA) virus that is spread by airborne droplets or direct contact with nasopharyngeal secretions. The disease is communicable from a week before the rash appears to 5 days after the rash disappears. Rubella is common in childhood, but it also affects adults who were not infected during childhood. Infection confers lifelong immunity. Epidemics are seen during the spring of each year, and major epidemics occur in 6- to 9-year cycles. The incidence declined dramatically after the advent and widespread use of a vaccine in the 1960s, and less than 250 cases are reported annually in the United States.

Pathophysiology: The virus invades the nasopharynx and travels to the lymph glands, causing lymphadenopathy. After 5 to 7 days, it enters the bloodstream, causing a viremia and stimulating an immune response that results in a skin rash. The rash lasts about 3 days. Subclinical infection may remain for as long as 5 days after the rash disappears.

Clinical Manifestations

Prodrome	Swollen suboccipital, postauricular, and postcervical glands; fever, sore throat, cough, fatigue
Rash	Tiny reddish spots on the soft palate on the last day of prodrome or the first day of the rash; light pink to red, discrete, maculopapular rash that starts on the face and trunk and spreads to the upper and lower extremities
Post rash	Headache, mild conjunctivitis

Complications

Complications include transitory arthritis, encephalitis, purpura, and congenital rubella syndrome. Congenital rubella syndrome occurs in an infant born to a woman who contracts rubella during the first trimester of pregnancy. The result can be abortion, stillbirth, or congenital rubella. About 25% of exposed infants develop the syndrome and have such defects as cataracts, deafness, microcephaly, mental retardation, heart defects, hepato-splenomegaly, jaundice, and bone defects. Many die within 6 months of birth.

Diagnostic Tests

The diagnosis is made on the appearance of the rash plus a positive culture of pharyngeal secretions and a fourfold increase in specific antibodies.

Therapeutic Management

Surgery	None
Drugs	Antipyretics for fever; active immunization in all persons over age 12 months with no evidence of immunity, except those who have a compromised immune system or are pregnant
General	Isolation from pregnant women

R

rubeola (red measles)

A highly contagious, acute viral disease characterized by Koplik's spots and a spreading maculopapular rash

Etiology and incidence: Rubeola is caused by a paramyxovirus and is spread by airborne droplets or direct contact with nasopharyngeal secretions. The disease is communicable from 4 days before the rash appears until the rash disappears. Before the advent of a vaccine in the 1960s, epidemics were seen every 2 or 3 years among small and school-age children in the United States. Now outbreaks occur primarily in previously immunized adolescents and adults and in unimmunized children. Slightly more than 500 cases are reported annually in the United States. Infection confers lifelong immunity.

Pathophysiology: The virus invades the nasopharynx and the respiratory epithelium, incubates, and multiplies there for about 7 to 14 days. It spreads via the lymphatics, producing hyperplasia and viremia, which spreads by means of the leukocytes to the reticuloendothelial system. The reticuloendothelial cells necrose and set up a secondary viremia, which infects the respiratory mucosa and produces edema. Two to 4 days after the respiratory invasion, the virus travels to and invades the cells of the epidermis and oral epithelium, stimulating a cell-mediated response and producing Koplik's spots, followed in 1 to 2 days by a skin rash. The rash lasts 4 to 7 days before fading.

Clinical Manifestations

Prodrome	Fever, coryza, hacking cough, conjunctivitis, photophobia, lymphadenopathy
Rash	Koplik's spots on the buccal mucosa 2 to 4 days after prodrome onset; irregular maculopapular rash starts on face and neck and spreads to trunk and extremities
Post rash	Brownish desquamation

Complications

Complications include secondary bacterial infections (e.g., otitis media or pneumonia); viral pneumonia; and encephalitis and delayed, subacute, sclerosing panencephalitis.

Diagnostic Tests

The diagnosis is made on the basis of the symptom pattern plus a positive culture of pharyngeal or conjunctival secretions or of blood or urine, plus a fourfold increase in specific antibodies.

Therapeutic Management

Surgery	None
Drugs	Antipyretics for fever; active immunization for persons over age 15 months except those with compromised immune systems; passive immunization (immune globulin) for high-risk contacts; prophylactic antiinfective drugs in high-risk children; vitamin A supplementation is under study
General	Bed rest in a quiet, darkened room during prodrome; isolation during prodrome and rash; skin care; tepid baths; monitoring for complications

R

scabies

A transmissible parasitic infestation of the skin characterized by burrows, intense itching, and excoriations

Etiology and incidence: Scabies is caused by the *Sarcoptes scabiei* mite and is easily transmitted by skin-to-skin contact. The mite cannot live long off the human body and is rarely transmitted in any other fashion. Incidence is worldwide and flourishes in areas where overcrowding and poor sanitation are common.

Pathophysiology: The impregnated female mite burrows under a superficial layer of skin, forming a tiny tunnel. She extends the tunnel daily as she deposits feces and two or three eggs to incubate and hatch. After 20 days, she dies. The eggs hatch and form adult mites within 10 days.

Clinical Manifestations

The individual is asymptomatic for 30 to 60 days after initial contact unless he or she has been previously sensitized. In those cases, symptoms appear within 48 hours. The first symptom is severe itching that is most intense at night. The burrows are seen as very fine, wavy dark lines that range from a few millimeters to 1 cm in length. They are seen primarily in finger webs, on the palms, on flexor wrist and elbow surfaces, in the axillary folds, around the areolae in girls and women and on the genitals in boys and men, on the buttocks, and around restrictive clothing lines. In infants, they may be seen on the face. Scratching causes excoriation, papules, pustules, crusting, and secondary superimposed bacterial infections.

Complications

The individual may have a postscabies pruritus that is self-limiting.

Diagnostic Tests

The diagnosis is made from visualization of the lesions and scrapings that show the mite on microscopic examination.

Therapeutic Management

Surgery	None
Drugs	Permethrin cream applied to entire body for 24 hours as a scabicide; corticosteroid cream for itching, which may take 1 or 2 weeks to subside; systemic antiinfective drugs for persistent secondary infections
General	Examination of all close contacts for infestation; treatment of all members in the household, including pets; cool soaks or compresses to reduce itching

S

scarlet fever

An acute, contagious bacterial disease characterized by a skin rash and a strawberry tongue

Etiology and incidence: The cause of scarlet fever is a circulating erythrotoxin that is produced by a group A beta-hemolytic streptococcus. It is spread by airborne droplets, contact with nasopharyngeal secretions, or ingestion of contaminated milk or other food. It is communicable from the point of infection through the active disease phase and postdisease in individuals with sinusitis or otitis media. The disease is seen predominantly in children.

Pathophysiology: The invading streptococcus releases an erythrogenic toxin that stimulates a sensitivity reaction in the individual. The result is widespread dilation of small capillaries and toxic injury to the vascular epithelium, particularly in the kidneys, liver, and heart.

Clinical Manifestations

Signs and symptoms appear 1 to 3 days after exposure to the agent, starting with a prodromal period.

Prodrome	Abrupt high fever, chills, tachycardia, nausea, vomiting, headache, abdominal pain, malaise, sore throat
Enanthema	Enlarged, reddened tonsils covered with patchy exudate; red, edematous pharynx; after the first day, the tongue is coated and white with red, swollen papillae (white strawberry tongue) until the white coat sloughs off on the fourth day, leaving a red strawberry tongue; red punctate lesions on the palate
Exanthema	Rash appears 12 hours after prodromal symptoms; rash is pinhead-size red lesions that rapidly cover the body except for the face; the rash concentrates in the axial folds, on the neck, and in the groin and lasts 4 to 10 days; the face is flushed on the cheeks with a circumoral pallor; after a week, desquamation and peeling begin on the palms and soles

Complications

Complications include otitis media, sinusitis, peritonsillar abscess, and severe, disseminated toxic or septic disease (fulminating scarlet fever), which may cause septicemia and hepatic damage.

Diagnostic Tests

The diagnosis is made from clinical signs and a positive Schultz-Charlton reaction skin test or a positive throat culture.

Therapeutic Management

Surgery	None
Drugs	Antiinfective drugs to combat the streptococcal agent, antipyretics for fever, analgesics for pain
General	Bed rest while febrile, isolation with secretion precautions for 24 hours after initiation of antibiotics, adequate fluids, gargles and throat washes for throat, room humidification for comfort

seborrhea

See Dermatitis.

S

seizures (convulsions, epilepsy)

Paroxysmal episodes of sudden, involuntary muscle contractions and alterations in consciousness, behavior. sensation, and autonomic functioning. The episodes may be partial (simple, complex), generalized (absence, myoclonic, tonic, clonic, tonic-clonic) or are unclassified. Seizures are labeled epilepsy if they are recurrent.

Etiology and incidence: The etiology of seizures may be idiopathic or symptomatic. Identified causes include pathological processes in the brain (e.g., vascular anomalies or lesions, space-occupying lesions, trauma, acute cerebral edema, infection, degeneration, and neuronal injury); endogenous or exogenous toxic substances (e.g., uremia, lead ingestion, alcohol intoxication, or phenothiazides); metabolic disturbances; febrile states; developmental abnormalities; or birth defects. Seizures affect about 2% of the U.S. population, and nearly 1.4 million of those individuals have chronically recurring seizures (epilepsy).

Pathophysiology: Seizures result from a generalized disturbance in cerebral function. An internal or external stimulus causes abnormal hypersynchronous discharges in a focal area in the cerebrum that spread throughout the cerebrum. During the seizure, neuropeptides and neurotransmitters are released and blood flow is increased. Extracellular concentrations of potassium are increased, and concentrations of calcium are decreased. Changes occur in pH and utilization of glucose increases. It is hypothesized that the seizure ceases when the neuronal cell membrane hyperpolarizes and causes the neuronal cells to cease firing, suppressing the surface potentials of the cerebrum. Partial seizures begin locally with a specific aberration of sensory, motor, or psychic origin, reflecting the cerebellar origin of the seizure. A complex partial seizure progresses to impairment of consciousness. A generalized seizure affects both consciousness and motor function from the onset. Absence seizures last 10 to 30 seconds and involve twitching and loss of contact. Myoclonic seizures involve intermittent contraction of muscles without loss of consciousness. Tonic seizures are marked by prolonged involuntary muscle contraction with a 30- to 60-second loss of consciousness. Clonic seizures involve intermittent muscle contractions and loss of consciousness for several minutes. Tonic-clonic seizures involve loss of consciousness with sustained muscle contractions, followed by intermittent muscle contractions and then a limp body state.

Clinical Manifestations

Simple partial	*Motor:* Recurrent involuntary muscle contractions of one body part (e.g., face, finger, hand, or arm) that may spread to other, same-side body parts
	Sensory: Auditory or visual hallucinations, paresthesias, vertigo
	Psychic: Sensation of déjà vu, complex hallucinations or illusions, unwarranted anger or fear, pupillary dilation, sweating
Complex partial	*Onset:* May have aura before onset
	Motor: Automatisms (patting body parts, smacking lips, aimless walking, picking at clothes), unintelligible muttering, staggering gait
	Sensory: 1 to 2 minutes of loss of contact with surroundings, hallucinations
Generalized	*Absence:* Transient loss of consciousness, flickering of eyelids or intermittent jerking of hands
	Myoclonic: Rapid, jerky movements in extremities or over entire body, which may cause a fall
	Tonic: Sudden abnormal dystonic posture, deviation of eyes and head to one side
	Clonic: Symmetric jerking of extremities for several minutes with loss of consciousness
	Tonic-clonic: Aura of epigastric discomfort, outcry, loss of consciousness, cyanosis, fall; tonic then clonic contractions, then limpness, sleep, headache, muscle soreness, confusion, and lethargy; loss of bowel and bladder control

S

Complications

Complications may occur as a result of the onset of seizure activity and can include injury from a fall or from jerking, as well as airway occlusion and aspiration. A condition known as *status epilepticus,* in which motor sensory or psychic seizures follow one another with no intervening periods of consciousness, is a medical emergency. Failure to get immediate treatment can lead to hypoxia, hyperthermia, hypoglycemia, acidosis, and death.

Diagnostic Tests

The presence of seizures is diagnosed by clinical history and examination. The diagnostic priority is to distinguish idiopathic seizure activity from symptomatic activity.

CT/MRI/positron emission tomography	Structural changes
Skull x-ray	Evidence of fractures, shift in calcified pineal gland, bony erosion, separated sutures
Cerebral angiography	Vascular abnormalities, subdural hematoma
Echoencephalography	Midline shifts in brain structures
Urine	To detect medication toxicity
Serum	Hypoglycemia, electrolyte imbalance, increased blood urea nitrogen, increased blood alcohol levels
Electroencephalography	*Tonic-clonic:* High, fast voltage spiked in all leads
	Absence: 3/s, rounded, spiked wave complexes in all leads
	Complex partial: Square-topped, 4-6/s spike wave complexes over involved lobe
	Inherited pattern: 2.5 to 3/s spike and wave pattern; presence of delta waves indicates destroyed brain tissue

Therapeutic Management

Surgery	Resection of epileptic focus or stereotactic lesions in the brain
Drugs	Anticonvulsants to prevent or control seizure activity
General	*During seizure:* Safety precautions to prevent injury (e.g, loosen restrictive clothing, roll on side to prevent aspiration, place a small pillow under the head, ease from a standing or sitting position to the floor)

Do not place a finger or other object into the person's mouth to protect or straighten the tongue—it is unnecessary and dangerous; do not try to hold the person still because you may injure the individual or yourself.

Maintain a patent airway; note frequency, type, time, involved body parts, and length of seizure; monitor vital signs and neurological status; reorient individual as seizure ceases.

Other: Eliminate causative or precipitating factors; encourage normal lifestyle, moderate exercise, and participation in sports with proper safeguards.

A driver's license is permitted in most states if the person is seizure-free for 1 year.

Alcohol is contraindicated, and medical and laboratory monitoring of anticonvulsant blood levels and possible side effects should be conducted.

Provide information about the importance of taking medications as directed and not deleting doses, as well as individual and family support to adapt to seizure disorder.

Instruct to wear a medical identification tag.

S

shingles (herpes zoster)

An acute, central nervous system infection involving the dorsal root ganglia that is characterized by vesicular eruption and neuralgic pain in various areas of the skin

Etiology and incidence: Shingles is caused by the varicella-zoster virus, the same virus that causes chickenpox. It is theorized that the virus lies dormant in the dorsal root ganglia after a chickenpox outbreak and is reactivated by local trauma, acute illness, emotional stress, systemic disease (particularly Hodgkin's disease), immune system compromise, or immuno-suppressive therapy. About 3% of the U.S. population has shingles. Individuals over age 50 persons with HIV are more likely to develop the disease.

Pathophysiology: The reactivated virus travels from the dorsal root ganglia down the sensory nerve and inflames and infects the skin of the affected ganglion.

Clinical Manifestations

Prodrome	Chills, fever, malaise, gastrointestinal upset 3 to 4 days before eruption
Eruptive phase	Crops of vesicles on an erythematous base appear on the skin above the affected dermatome with hyperesthesia, severe pain, burning, and itching; after day 5 the lesions dry out and crust over and may scar as they heal
Postherpetic phase	Neuralgia that may persist for months or years

Complications

Herpes zoster ophthalmicus may result in vision loss. A generalized outbreak of shingles may lead to acute urinary retention and unilateral paralysis of the diaphragm. In rare cases, shingles may be complicated by central nervous system infection, muscle atrophy, transient paralysis, and ascending myelitis.

Diagnostic Tests

Physical examination	Characteristic lesions
Cytologic smear	Direct identification of multinucleated cells
Culture	Varicella virus in vesicular fluid

Therapeutic Management

Surgery	None
Drugs	Analgesics for pain, antipruritics for itching, antiviral agents for immunocompromised individuals and the elderly during eruptive phase to accelerate healing and reduce neuralgia, tranquilizers for severe neuralgia
General	Wet compresses on lesions, avoidance of scratching and spread to other body regions, cryotherapy or transcutaneous electrical nerve stimulation for neuralgia

sickle cell anemia

A chronic hemolytic anemia characterized by sickle-shaped red blood cells

Etiology and incidence: Sickle cell anemia results from a genetic mutation in a hemoglobin molecule that is transmitted from parent to child. The disease is most prevalent in tropical Africa and in those of African descent. People from the Mediterranean region, Puerto Rico, Turkey, India, and the Middle East may also have the disorder. Between 45,000 and 75,000 black persons in the United States have the disease, and 2.5 million more carry the trait. If two persons carrying the trait have children, the child has a 1 in 4 chance of developing the disease and a 1 in 2 chance of being a carrier.

Pathophysiology: The erythrocytes of individuals with sickle cell anemia contain more hemoglobin (Hgb) S than Hgb A. Consequently, the erythrocytes become rigid, rough, elongated, and crescent shaped when oxygen tension decreases. A decrease in oxygen tension is caused by hypoxic conditions or elevated blood viscosity. These "sickled" cells are easily destroyed as they enter the smaller blood vessels in the body. They accumulate in the capillaries, impairing circulation and causing pain, tissue and organ infarction, and hypoxia, which, in turn, causes more sickling.

Clinical Manifestations

Signs and symptoms are seldom seen before age 6 months. When they do occur, manifestations are the result of anemia, chronic disease, and vasoocclusive events known as sickle cell crises.

General	Characteristically, the individual has a history of chronic fatigue, dyspnea, joint swelling and aching, chest pain, ischemic leg ulcers, and multiple infections. Jaundice or pallor, tachycardia, hepatomegaly, and cardiomegaly also may be present. Children tend to be small for their age, and growth or puberty may be delayed. Adults tend to have narrow

	shoulders and hips, long extremities, a curved spine, and a barrel chest.
Sickle cell crisis	Sleepiness, difficulty staying awake; severe abdominal, thoracic, muscular, or bone pain; dark urine, hematuria; pale lips, tongue, palms, and nail beds; lethargy; listlessness; irritability; fever (these conditions last days to weeks)

Complications

Sickle cell anemia causes system-wide, long-term complications that include multiple infections, hemolytic anemia, chronic obstructive pulmonary disease, congestive heart failure, retinopathy, neuropathy, myocardial infarction, cerebrovascular accident, pulmonary emboli, splenic failure, and renal failure. These complications eventually lead to death. The average life span for an individual with sickle cell anemia is currently about age 40.

Diagnostic Tests

Stained blood smear	Visualization of sickled cells
Sickle cell blood prep	Sickling noted after deoxygenation
Turbidity tube test	A mix of blood and Sickledex in a turbid solution indicates presence of Hgb S
Hgb electrophoresis	Presence of Hgb S and Hgb A indicates sickle cell trait; presence of only Hgb S indicates sickle cell anemia
Blood	Decreased erythrocyte life span

S

Therapeutic Management

Surgery	None
Drugs	Analgesics for pain, antiinfective drugs starting at age 4 months for prophylaxis against infection, pneumococcal and influenza vaccines for prophylaxis against influenza and pneumonia, hydroxyurea to reduce pain crisis and provide an increment in Hgb content, iron supplements for low folic acid level

General   Blood transfusions in aplastic crisis or before
           general anesthesia and surgery; chronic transfu-
           sion therapy for those under age 18 who have had
           a stroke, individuals with recalcitrant leg ulcers,
           and pregnant individuals

           Crisis: Rest, hydration; oxygen; monitoring of vital
           signs; cardiovascular, fluid and electrolyte, and
           blood gas monitoring; monitoring for signs
           of renal involvement, pulmonary embolism,
           and vessel occlusion

           Other: Measures to prevent infection; early, aggres-
           sive treatment of infection, dehydration, vomit-
           ing, and diarrhea; avoidance of dehydration,
           strenuous exercise, exercise in high altitudes,
           and smoking; protecting extremities from cold;
           adequate hydration and balanced diet; balance
           of rest and exercise; genetic screening and
           counseling for high-risk individuals and carriers;
           support groups and counseling for long-term
           adaptation to chronic disease

sinusitis

An acute or chronic inflammatory process affecting the paranasal sinuses

Etiology and incidence: Sinusitis is caused by bacteria (streptococci, staphylococci, pneumococci, *Haemophilus influenzae*); viruses (rhinovirus, influenza virus, parainfluenza virus); and fungi (aspergilli, Dematiaceae, Mucoraceae, *Penicillium* sp.). Onset often occurs after an acute respiratory infection but may also be triggered by a dental procedure or gum infection, allergic rhinitis, diving or swimming episode, or sudden drop in temperature. Sinusitis may also be associated with anatomical abnormalities of the nose. Fungally induced sinusitis most often is seen in immunosuppressed individuals such as those with AIDS, leukemia, lymphoma, or multiple myeloma or in persons with poorly controlled diabetes. More than 35 million cases are reported in the United States annually, and the rates are higher among women and those living in the southern United States.

Pathophysiology: Some factor precipitates a swollen nasal mucous membrane, which obstructs the ostium of the paranasal sinus. The oxygen in the sinus is absorbed into the blood vessels in the mucous membrane and sets up a negative pressure (vacuum) in the sinus, inducing pain. If the vacuum is maintained, a transudate is formed from the mucous membrane and fills the sinus, serving as a medium for transient bacteria, viruses, or fungi. Serum and leukocytes then rush to combat the resulting infection, causing a painful positive pressure in the obstructed sinus. The mucous membrane becomes hyperemic and edematous.

S

Clinical Manifestations

Signs and symptoms include tender, swollen areas over the involved sinus; malaise and slight fever with rhinorrhea; and seropurulent or mucopurulent drainage. Pain is specific to the sinus. Maxillary sinusitis causes pain in the maxillary area, toothache, and frontal headache. Frontal sinusitis causes frontal pain and headache. Ethmoid sinusitis causes pain behind the eyes and a splitting frontal headache. Pain from sphenoid sinusitis occurs in the occipital region.

Complications

Repeated sinus attacks may lead to permanent damage to the mucosal lining and a condition known as chronic suppurative sinusitis. Frontal sinusitis may lead to severe intracranial complications, including brain abscesses, which may prove fatal. Fungal sinusitis, particularly in severely immunosuppressed individuals, can be fatal.

Diagnostic Tests

Culture	Causative organism in sinus discharge
Transillumination	Involved sinus produces a dark shadow (a normal sinus is light)
Sinus x-rays/CT scans	To determine extent of sinus involvement

Therapeutic Management

Surgery	Endoscopy to create nasal window in acute maxillary sinusitis; Caldwell-Luc procedure for chronic maxillary sinusitis; ethmoidectomy for ethmoid or sphenoid sinusitis; creation of an osteoplastic flap to drain frontal sinus; débridement of tissue in fungally induced sinusitis
Drugs	Antiinfective drugs specific to causative agent, analgesics for pain and headache, antihistamines to reduce secretions, nasal spray vasoconstrictors to open nasal passages, adrenergics for chronic sinusitis
General	Irrigation and drainage of affected sinus; steam inhalation to promote drainage; hot, moist compresses to nose to relieve pain and congestion; avoidance of smoking and other nasal irritants and allergens

skin cancer

Skin cancers can be divided into two groups: melanomas and non-melanomas. Three distinct types of nevi (moles) give rise to melanomas: common acquired, dysplastic, and congenital melanocytic; they produce four types of melanoma: superficial spreading (70%), nodular (15%), lentigomaligna (less than 10%), and acrolentiginous (less than 5%). Non-melanomas are typically either basal cell or squamous cell in origin.

Etiology and incidence: Environmental factors such as ultraviolet radiation and chronic sun exposure in direct interaction with skin type are directly linked to the development of non-melanoma skin cancer. The precise cause of melanoma is unknown though ultraviolet radiation in interplay with hereditary (chromosomal abnormalities) and immune incompetence is strongly suspected.

Skin cancer is the most common of all malignancies. An estimated 800,000 cases are diagnosed annually in the United States alone. More than 34,000 of these are melanomas, and the incidence of melanoma is increasing by approximately 4% a year. More than 7500 deaths are attributed to skin cancer each year, and 5500 of these are from malignant melanomas.

Pathophysiology: Basal cell carcinomas vary considerably in appearance but usually begin as a small, shiny, flesh-colored nodule on the skin. The carcinoma enlarges slowly and develops a pearly border with telangiectases on the surface. It often bleeds, crusts, and then bleeds again in a chronic cycle. It rarely metastasizes but does invade adjacent tissue structures. Squamous cell carcinomas are usually scaly and crusty or nodular, warty, and raised and often develop in keratotic tissue or old scars. They eventually ulcerate and invade the underlying tissue. They rarely metastasize, but when they do, the lungs are the most common site. Malignant melanomas arise from a mole that begins to show changes in size, color, shape, and consistency. They begin by growing on the epidermis and then invade the dermis and subcutaneous tissues. Once this occurs, the tumor metastasizes fairly rapidly through the vascular and lymphatic systems. Common metastatic sites include the bones, brain, liver, and lungs.

S

Risk Factors

Non-melanoma

Fair complexion, light hair, blue eyes (i.e., skin that burns easily
  and is difficult to tan)
Occupations that require prolonged sun exposure
Albino
Long-term x-ray exposure
Occupational exposure to radium, arsenic, coal tar, and creosote
Family history of the disease
History of chronic irritation or inflammatory diseases of the
  skin (e.g., leprosy, lupus, granulomas, ulcers, burn scars)
Immunodeficiencies
Genetically inherited syndromes (e.g., xeroderma pig-
  mentosum, familial dysplastic nevus syndrome, Bazex's
  syndrome)

Melanoma

Large number of moles greater than 2 mm (more than 120
  moles between 1 and 5 mm; more than 5 moles greater
  than 5 mm)
Large number of moles on buttocks or raised moles on arms
Moles that are atypical (e.g., asymmetrical or with no clear
  border)
Tendency to freckle
History of one or more blistering sunburns
Extensive exposure to sunlight in early childhood
History of non-melanoma skin cancer, acne, or dysplastic nevus

Clinical Manifestations

A skin lesion that does not go away and that grows larger over
time or a mole that changes appearance is a possible sign, as are
itchiness, scaling, oozing, bleeding from a mole or lesion, and
changes in sensation. For melanomas, four manifestations are key
in early detection and are known as the ABCD rule. Melanomas
tend to be *asymmetrical,* with a notched or indistinct *border,*
variegated in *color,* and a *diameter* of greater than 6 mm.

Complications

The prognosis for non-melanoma carcinomas is excellent with
intervention because metastasis is rare. The long-term prognosis
for melanomas is tied to the thickness of the tumor at the time of

diagnosis. Tumors over 3 mm deep carry a survival rate of less than 50%. Metastasized disease reduces the survival rate dramatically. Common complications include scarring and disfigurement at the site of tumor removal.

Diagnostic Tests

Tissue biopsy and a histological examination form the base for definitive diagnosis.

Therapeutic Management

Surgery	Excision is the treatment of choice for melanoma; excision, cryosurgery, electrodesiccation and curettage, and Mohs chemosurgery are used for non-melanomas
Drugs	Topical chemotherapeutic agents to treat premalignant actinic keratosis; interferon to treat recurrent or advanced basal cell carcinoma; hyperthermic regional perfusions in combination with surgery to treat melanomas
General	Radiation in combination with surgery for extensive nonmelanomas; radiation may be used instead of surgery in elderly patients or to treat non-melanomatous lesions of the nose, eyelids, or lips (melanomas are radioresistant); prevention education about sun exposure and use of sunscreens and protective clothing when in the sun

S

spina bifida

A developmental malformation of the spine in which the posterior vertebral laminae fail to close, leaving the meninges and spinal cord exposed. The three common types are (1) spina bifida occulta, in which the only defect is vertebral and the meninges and spinal cord are normal; (2) spina bifida with meningocele, in which the meninges protrude through the vertebral opening, forming a cyst filled with cerebrospinal fluid and covered with skin; and (3) spina bifida with myelomeningocele, in which the protruding cyst also contains a portion of the spinal cord and spinal nerves and is covered by a thin membrane.

Etiology and incidence: The etiology is unclear, but the most recent hypothesis suggests a genetic predisposition involving a polygenic interaction with environmental factors such as maternal malnutrition, alcohol, organic solvents, drugs, toxins, or potato blight. This interaction precipitates a faulty closure of the neural groove on day 28 of gestation. The geographic distribution and incidence of spina bifida vary widely, but it is the most common developmental defect of the central nervous system. It occurs in approximately 0.6 of every 1000 live births in the United States and the incidence has been steadily declining in recent decades. It is more common in infants of European descent, females, and those in poverty.

Pathophysiology: During the normal formative stages of the nervous system, a decided depression known as a neural groove appears on the dorsal ectoderm of the embryo at approximately 20 days of gestation. The groove deepens rapidly, spreads laterally, and then fuses dorsally to form the neural tube. Neural tube formation begins in the cervical region and advances caudally and cephalically until day 28 of gestation, when both ends of the tube seal themselves off. Spina bifida occurs when the neural tube fails to close or when a closed tube splits as a result of abnormal cerebrospinal fluid pressure.

Clinical Manifestations

Manifestations vary widely, depending on the degree and location of the spinal defect. Sensory and motor disturbances parallel one another.

Occulta	Typically asymptomatic; dimple or hair growth on the skin over the malformed vertebra; weakness in feet, bowel, or bladder sphincter possible as child grows if defect goes undetected and uncorrected
Meningocele	External cystic sac seen on spinal cord at birth; hydrocephalus possible; weakness in legs or bowel and bladder sphincters is rare if defect is surgically corrected
Myelomeningocele	*At birth:* Round, raised, poorly epithelialized sac on spinal cord that may be bluish and may be leaking or ruptured; hydrocephalus; loss of partial or total motor and sensory control below the level of the lesion; poor anal sphincter and detrusor tone; possible rectal prolapse; constant urine dribbling or urinary retention; possible joint deformities and kyphosis formed in utero
	Developing in childhood: Clubfeet, contractures in ankles, knees, and hips; hip dislocations; scoliosis; decreasing ability to ambulate; incontinence; urinary tract infections (UTIs); constipation; skin breakdown; obesity

Complications

An immediate complication often seen after birth with a leaking or ruptured sac is meningitis. Other immediate complications include hypoxia and hemorrhage. Other congenital abnormalities such as cardiac or gastrointestinal malformations may also be present. Long-term complications are associated with motor and sensory disability and include respiratory infection and failure, renal infection and failure, permanent skeletal deformities, and decubiti. In the 1950s, most individuals with myelomeningocele died in infancy. Now, most have a near normal life expectancy with careful and consistent health care.

Diagnostic Tests

Clinical evaluation	Pigmented spots, hairy patches, and spinal sinuses seen at birth may indicate spina bifida occulta; motor and sensory function tests determine level of injury in myelomeningocele; palpation of fontanelles and increasing head circumference indicate hydrocephalus
Ultrasound/CT/MRI	Abnormalities of head or spine or both
Myelography	Spinal defects
Intravenous pyelography	Abnormalities in renal system
Urodynamics	To assess detrusor and sphincter function
Fetal ultrasonography	May detect major myelomeningocele defects
Alpha-fetoprotein	Elevated at 16 to 18 weeks' gestation

Therapeutic Management

Surgery	Repair and closure of defect within 24 to 72 hours after birth; ventriculoperitoneal shunt to treat hydrocephalus; shunt revisions as child ages or if shunt is not patent or functional; corrective orthopedic procedures for contractures, clubfeet, scoliosis (spinal instrumentation), hip dislocations; vesicostomy for vesicourethral reflux; augmentation enterocystoplasty to increase bladder capacity and reduce bladder pressure; placement of artificial urinary sphincter or ureteral sling to aid bladder emptying; urinary diversion to control chronic urine leakage and retention
Drugs	Collagen injection in sphincter submucosa to control bladder incontinence; stool softeners and laxatives for constipation; antispasmodics

to treat bladder spasms; antiinfective drugs for UTI

General *Initial care:* Monitoring for associated defects and complications; measures to prevent infections; monitoring of patency and functioning of ventriculoperitoneal shunt; adequate hydration and nutrition; normal infant stimulation; meticulous skin care; proper positioning and body alignment; monitoring of intake and output; emotional support of family; teaching parents to hold, feed, and stimulate infant and any special techniques needed for care; physical therapy and range-of-motion (ROM) exercises; safety measures for decreased sensation

Long term: Consistent medical monitoring by neurologists/neurosurgeons for shunt function and revision and spinal cord tethering; orthopedic surgeons for treatment of contractures, gait analysis, and bracing; urologists for bladder and kidney function; pediatricians for minor infections, bowel program and coordination; physical therapists for maintenance of ROM, prevention of contractures, gait training, strengthening, and endurance; occupational therapists for activities of daily living; intermittent catheterization for bladder control; weight-maintenance diet to prevent obesity and maintain ambulation; counseling for long-term adaptation; case management for long-term support and education of individual, family, and school and coordination of ongoing care

Prevention American Academy of Pediatrics recommends that all women of childbearing age take a 0.4 mg supplement of folic acid a day and that women contemplating pregnancy take 4.0 mg daily one month before conception through the first trimester of pregnancy. This can reduce the chances of a neural tube defect by at least 50%.

spinal cord injury (paraplegia, quadriplegia)

An insult to the spinal cord that results in alteration of autonomic, motor, and sensory function below the level of injury. Paraplegia involves the lower extremities; quadriplegia involves all extremities. Injury to the cord may result in incomplete or total transection.

Etiology and incidence: Spinal cord injury (SCI) may be caused by external trauma or internal disease or degeneration. Common traumatic causes of spinal cord injury include vehicle accidents (48%), falls (21%), acts of violence (15%), and sports injuries (14%). Metastatic carcinoma, spinal cord tumors, spondylosis, and vertebral disk degeneration are common nontraumatic causes of spinal cord injury. The worldwide incidence of SCI is about 55 per million per year with about 35 individuals per million of those surviving the acute insult. The prevalence of SCI survivors worldwide is estimated to be between 700 to 900 individuals per million. About 10,000 cases occur in the United States annually, and 150,000 to 200,000 individuals are living with SCI in the United States today. About 55% of individuals are quadriplegic, and the remaining 45% are paraplegic. Traumatic injury occurs most often in young adult men 18 to 25 years of age, whereas nontraumatic injury is more common in individuals of both genders who are over age 50.

Pathophysiology: Injury may be direct or indirect. Direct injuries involve compression or transection of the cord by the causal agent (e.g., bone fragments, bullets, or other external debris in the cord; external severing of the cord; tumor growth on the cord, or bony overgrowth of the spine that squeezes the cord). Tissue necroses around the site of injury. Indirect injury involves compression, overstretching, rotation, wedging, or misalignment of the cord, which results in edema, swelling, and localized hemorrhage. This in turn reduces vascular perfusion, decreases oxygen tension, and increases the norepinephrine concentration, producing ischemia and tissue necrosis. Necrosed tissue is removed by bodily functions within a month of injury and is gradually replaced by connective scar tissue and glial fibers.

Clinical Manifestations

Manifestations differ by level and completeness of injury.

Initial phase (spinal shock)	Partial or complete flaccid paralysis below injury level; partial or complete loss of proprioception, pain, touch, pressure, temperature, spinal reflexes, vasomotor tone, and visceral and somatic sensation below injury level; loss of ability to perspire below injury level; dysfunction of bowel and bladder; impaired or absent respiration if injury is above C5; bradycardia; hypotension
Autonomic hyperreflexia	Onset occurs after resolution of spinal shock and return of reflex activity; affects mostly those with an injury at T6 or above; paroxysmal hypertension, bradycardia, pounding headache, profuse sweating and flushing above injury level, nausea, nasal stuffiness
Long term	Muscle spasms, exaggerated deep tendon reflexes, contractures, hyperesthesia immediately above injury level, paresthesias, neuropathic pain; impotence, trophic ulcers, dry skin, nail changes, skin breakdown

Complications

The immediate complications are generally life threatening and include respiratory failure, hemorrhage, and cardiac failure. Long-term complications include pneumonia and atelectasis, cardiovascular disease, orthostatic hypotension, severe bradycardia, hyperkalemia, deep vein thrombosis, pulmonary embolism, gastric atony, ileus, bladder and kidney infections, decubiti, pathological fractures, heterotrophic ossification, degeneration of upper extremity joints, emotional debility, and suicide.

Diagnostic Tests

Clinical evaluation	Absence of reflexes, flaccidity, loss of sensation below injury level; examination of dermatomes and muscles to determine level of injury

Spinal x-rays	Vertebral fractures, bony overgrowth
CT/MRI scans	Evidence of cord compression and edema or tumor formation
Lumbar puncture/ myelography	Spinal blockage

Therapeutic Management

Surgery	*Initial:* Laminectomy or fusion for decompression and stabilization, wound débridement, placement of cervical tongs or halo traction for stabilization, tracheotomy for mechanical ventilation if needed
	Long term: Myotomies, tenotomies, rhizotomies, and muscle transplantation to treat spasticity; contracture release; débridement of decubiti; spinal instrumentation to halt scoliosis; penile implant for impotence; colostomy for atonic colon; urinary diversion for incontinence or retention; implant of an intrathecal Baclofen pump to control spasticity
Drugs	*Initial:* Massive corticosteroid therapy to improve outcome, prophylactic antiinfective drugs for open wounds, analgesics for pain, anticoagulants to prevent emboli and thrombus formation, antihypertensives for hyperreflexia, antianxiety agents to reduce emotional stress
	Long term: Muscle relaxants for spasms, stool softeners and laxatives for constipation, anticholinergics for bladder spasticity
General	*Initial:* Spinal stabilization with backboard or cervical collar on initial transport; mechanical ventilation if necessary; cardiac monitoring; blood gases; monitoring of intake and output; vital signs and neurological vital signs; maintenance of skeletal traction and body alignment; repositioning, turning every 2 hours; passive range-of-motion exercises; footboard; all activities of daily living (ADLs) performed for person; monitoring of bowel and bladder function; monitoring of skin integrity

Long term: Bowel training using digital stimulation, gravity, high-fiber diet, regularity, adequate hydration; bladder training using intermittent catheterization; physical therapy to diminish orthostatic hypotension, increase strength and endurance, decrease muscle spasticity, prevent contractures, teach functional mobility skills (e.g., transfer techniques, wheelchair manipulation); occupational therapy to aid adaptation of ADLs (e.g., feeding, bathing, hygiene, grooming, dressing) and to teach use of adaptive equipment; respiratory therapy to increase vital capacity and tidal volume; recreational therapy to enhance quality of life; speech therapy if injury is high enough to affect swallowing or when permanent ventilation requires alternative communication systems; long-term medical follow-up by physical medicine, urology, gastroenterology, and respiratory specialists to reduce complications; vocational training; counseling of individual and family for support and adaptation; instruction in bowel and bladder programs, skin inspection, pressure relief, decubitus ulcer prevention, prevention or early treatment of urinary tract and upper respiratory infections, and recognition of hyperreflexia

stomach cancer (gastric cancer)

Most malignant lesions of the stomach are adenocarcinomas (95%). The rest are lymphomas and leiomyosarcomas.

Etiology and incidence: The cause of stomach cancer is unknown but is thought to be related to dietary factors connected to food preservation and preparation. Gastritis, gastric atrophy, and genetic factors are believed to be interactive factors. The incidence varies worldwide. Stomach cancer is the most common malignancy in Japan, and the incidence is extremely high in Iceland and Chile. The number of cases has declined significantly in western Europe and the United States. About 23,000 new cases are seen in the United States each year, with more than 14,500 deaths reported per year. The incidence is higher in men than in women (2:1 ratio) and higher in black men than in white men (1.5:1 ratio). It occurs most often in individuals ages 50 to 70. The peak decade is for men in their 70s and women in their 80s.

Pathophysiology: Cancer cells usually begin to grow in the distal end of the stomach in the lesser curvature. The cells form a tumor that spreads along the mucosa, eventually invading and moving through the stomach wall. The tumor then spreads directly to surrounding structures such as the spleen, esophagus, pancreas, colon, duodenum, and peritoneum. The cancer is also spread via the lymphatics to regional nodes and via the bloodstream to the liver.

Risk Factors

Diet (low fat or low protein consumption, low intake of vitamins A and C)

Ingestion of food preservatives used in salting, pickling, smoking

Lack of refrigeration or poor food preparation techniques

Use of well water with high nitrate concentrations or *Helicobacter pylori* bacteria colonies

Smoking

History of gastric atrophy, chronic gastritis, gastric surgery or *H. pylori* infection, celiac sprue pernicious anemia or late onset immunoglobulin deficiency

Occupations such a coal miner or rubber worker

Clinical Manifestations

No specific symptoms appear in the early stages. Most people have generalized gastrointestinal (GI) complaints such as indigestion, burping, and fullness after eating. Later signs may include vomiting, dysphagia, anorexia, weight loss, and back pain.

Complications

The prognosis for long-term survival is poor (16%), primarily because most cases are diagnosed after metastasis has occurred. Complications include malnutrition and GI obstruction.

Diagnostic Tests

Double-contrast x-ray studies of the stomach can delineate suspicious lesions. The definitive diagnosis is made by endoscopy with brush biopsy.

Therapeutic Management

Surgery	Excision of the tumor and regional lymph nodes; subtotal or total gastric resection or gastrectomy for resection for cure, depending on tumor location; gastroenterostomy for palliation
Drugs	Systemic chemotherapy to treat advanced metastatic disease
General	Radiation for palliation of GI obstruction

S

stomatitis

An inflammation or ulceration of the mouth that may be locally or systemically induced

Etiology and incidence: Causes of stomatitis include viral or bacterial infection; drugs or toxic agents (barbiturates, antibiotics, chemotherapy, radiation, lead, mercury, acids, heavy metals); trauma from cheek biting, mouth breathing, or ill-fitting orthodontia; overuse of tobacco or alcohol; sensitivity to toothpaste, mouthwash, food dyes, or preservatives and spices; poor nutrition; and poor oral hygiene. Thrush, a common form of stomatitis, is seen in more than 80% of individuals with HIV or AIDS. Canker sores are also common and are commonly seen in adolescence or young adulthood. Herpetic stomatitis, the most common virally induced stomatitis, is seen in infants and small children. Mechanically induced stomatitis is often seen in older individuals with dentures that are difficult to fit because of continuing deterioration of gum and bone. Necrotizing ulceration is often seen in individuals using certain antibiotics and in people who have depressed immune systems.

Pathophysiology: The pathophysiology depends on the cause, but it involves a process that creates tissue inflammation in the oral mucosa or gums. These inflammatory changes lead to redness, ulceration, and fissures in the mouth.

Risk Factors

Side effects from use of prescribed drugs (e.g., antibiotics, barbiturates, inhaled steroids, immunosuppressants, chemotherapeutics)

Tobacco use (cigarettes, chewing tobacco)

Alcohol abuse

Exposure to radiation, lead, mercury, acids, heavy metals

Trauma from cheek biting, mouth breathing, or ill-fitting orthodontia

Sensitivity to toothpaste, mouthwash, food dyes, preservatives and spices

Poor nutrition

Poor oral hygiene

History of cancer, HIV, AIDS, iron-deficiency anemia, gastrointestinal disease, diabetes mellitus

Clinical Manifestations

Manifestations vary by type of stomatitis.

Allergic	Shiny erythema with slight edema, itching, drying, burning
Thrush	White, raised, milk-curd patches; bleeding; dryness of the mouth; diminished taste; pain; fever; lymphadenopathy
Gingivitis	Redness, swelling, bleeding of gums; gum retraction from teeth
Herpetic	Ulcers 3 to 4 cm in diameter scattered over mucous membranes; swollen, inflamed gums; enlarged lymph nodes
Canker sores	Small, yellowish, hardened, painful sores with red, raised margins that often appear singly or in groups on the lips or in the corner of mouth
Necrotizing	Necrotic ulceration of mucous membranes with severe pain, increased salivation, and inability to eat; fetid breath; bleeding gums; difficulty talking and swallowing; pseudomembrane on ulcers

Complications

Tissue sloughing from necrosis may create craters and other altered tissue topography.

Diagnostic Tests

The diagnosis is made on the clinical history and a physical examination. Cultures or smears may aid in identification of the causative organism in cases arising from infection.

Therapeutic Management

Surgery	None
Drugs	Topical anesthetics for pain; antiinfective drugs (topical, systemic) for bacterial or fungally induced stomatitis

General   Meticulous oral hygiene; mild mouthwashes for comfort; treatment of underlying causes (stopping drugs, avoiding toxins, refitting orthodontics, eliminating allergens); bland, soft, pureed, or liquid diet if eating is a problem; avoidance of alcohol and tobacco products

streptococcal disease

See Rheumatic Fever and Scarlet Fever.

stroke

See Cerebrovascular Accident.

substance abuse and/or dependence

Substance abuse: The maladaptive pattern of using tobacco, alcohol or drugs to induce a sense of well-being or pleasure that has actual or potential undesirable effects on the body

Substance dependence or addiction: Continued substance use despite related difficulties, resulting in more serious physical and emotional problems

Etiology and incidence: Trend data in the United States indicate that the use of tobacco, alcohol, and illicit drug use is on the rise and is a major public health problem. Data from the 1996 and 1997 National Household Survey on Drug Abuse (NHSDA) stated that 111 million Americans age 12 and older had used alcohol during the 30 days before the interview, 64 million reported smoking, and 13.9 million individuals used illicit drugs. Of these, 2.5 million used marijuana, including 1 in 10 youths, ages 12 to 17; 1.1 million had used hallucinogens; and 1.5 million individuals use cocaine. A direct and increased correlation exists between smoking, alcohol use, and illicit drug use. For example, the NHSDA reports that of 11.2 million persons who reported that they were heavy drinkers (five or more drinks on the same occasion or at least on 5 different days during the past month), 30% or 3.3 million of these individuals were also current illicit drug users.

Pathophysiology: Many theories exist about why an individual becomes dependent and abuses elicit substances, alcohol, and tobacco. Among the most prevalent theorized social causes are feelings of low self-worth, inadequacy, and social inadequacy; stress; family- and work-related problems; and economic difficulties. Genetic factors and chemical imbalances may also contribute to substance use, dependence, and abuse.

Risk Factors

Familial history of substance abuse or past personal history of problem
Mental or physical disorder or disability
Poor self-esteem, negative sense of self-worth
Instability in relationships or divorce, death of spouse, retirement, household income, unemployment
Lack of support network

Clinical Manifestations

Erratic performance or failure to perform normal roles and functions at home, school, or work. In addition, each type of substance may present with different clinical manifestations

Alcohol	Alcohol odor on the breath or clothing, decreased alertness, impaired judgment, nausea, vomiting, staggering, slurred speech, emotional impulsivity, uncharacteristic behavior, delayed reaction times, dizziness, confusion, agitation, stupor, hangover
Amphetamines/ stimulants	Euphoria, agitation, irritability, hyperactivity, chest pain, insomnia, sweating, elevated blood pressure, headache, chills, fever, confusion, impaired judgment, paranoid behavior, seizures, possible death
Cocaine/crack	Impulsivity, compulsivity, hyperactivity, disinhibition, hypervigilance, anxiety, irritability, dilated pupils, sweating, slow pulse, increased blood pressure, slowed shallow breathing, rhinitis, nose bleeds
Hallucinogens	Bizarre behavior, mood swings, agitation, aggression, paranoia, feelings of depersonalization, dilated pupils, sweating, hypertension, tachycardia, flushing, tremors, nystagmus, violent outbursts, convulsions, possible death
Heroin/opiates	Euphoria with tranquillity, slowed reaction, drowsiness, impaired function with psychomotor retardation, watery eyes, constricted pupils, shallow slow breathing, decreased muscle tone, increased pulse and blood pressure
Inhalants	Giddiness, silliness, drowsiness, disorientation, slurred speech, headache, nausea, vomiting, increased vital signs, stupor, delirium, coma

Marijuana	Giddiness, laughter, lightheadedness, slow movements, drowsiness, increased appetite, red eyes, increased vital signs
Sedatives	Slurred speech; motor impairment; disorientation; drowsiness; clammy skin; depression; unconsciousness; slow, shallow respirations; weak, rapid pulse

Complications

Personal instability and inability to function and contribute to society, family, and self. Secondary medical problems specific to the type of abused substance may occur.

Diagnostic Tests

Toxicology and blood levels for suspected abused substances

Therapeutic Management

Surgery	Surgery may be required for treatment of conditions that may occur as a result of addiction
Drugs	Medications may be required to treat toxification and specific secondary problems related to the substance abuse Methadone for treatment of heroin addiction Antabuse for treatment of alcohol addiction
General	Detoxification and treatment of physiological complications is the first level of treatment. Counseling, self-esteem building, and support groups to enhance individual's self-worth and provide avoidance support

S

sudden infant death syndrome

The sudden, unexplained death of an infant under age 1 that remains unexplained after a complete postmortem examination

Etiology and incidence: The cause of sudden infant death syndrome (SIDS) is unknown. One widely accepted hypothesis is that it is related to a brainstem abnormality in the neurological regulation of cardiorespiratory control. SIDS is the most common cause of death in infants age 2 weeks to 1 year. Distribution is worldwide, and the incidence in the United States is 1.5 in 1000 live births. More than 7000 infants die each year in the United States alone. Males are affected more often than females, as are Native Americans and blacks. The incidence is higher in the winter, with January the peak month of occurrence.

Pathophysiology: The pathophysiology is unknown, but pathology results on autopsy are consistent and include findings of pulmonary edema and intrathoracic hemorrhages.

Risk Factors

Prematurity
Low Apgar scores
Familial history
Multiple births
Central nervous system or respiratory disturbances
Prone sleeping position, use of soft bedding, pillows, excess
    blankets
Overheating from too many layers of clothing and blankets
Maternal smoking, and/or drug use

Clinical Manifestations

The infant is usually found dead in the bed or crib. The bedclothes tend to be disheveled, and the infant is often huddled in a corner face down with the covers over the head. The infant's hands are often clutching the sheets. Frothy, blood-tinged fluid is in the mouth and nose, and stool and urine fill the diaper.

Complications

The syndrome is fatal.

Diagnostic Tests

The diagnosis is confirmed by postmortem examination, including examination of the site of death.

Therapeutic Management

Management focuses on helping the family to cope and on preventing the disorder in infants seen as high risk.

Surgery	None
Drugs	Respiratory stimulant medications for high-risk infants to prevent SIDS
General	Intensive psychological and emotional support of the family from the time of health care contact for at least 1 year, including time to say good-bye to the infant at the emergency center, arranging transportation home, an immediate home visit to allow family to talk and to discuss SIDS (written supplemental material is desirable), support group and counseling referrals, follow-up home visits
Prevention	Identification of infants with high-risk profiles (one or more previous apparently life-threatening events, preterm, SIDS history of two siblings in family, episode of apnea, excessive periodic breathing, central hypoventilation); use of home monitoring devices; supine or sidelying sleeping position for all infants using a firm mattress and no pillows or soft bedding materials

S

suicide

Suicidal ideation: Presence of thoughts or contemplation about suicide; no self-destructive action occurs related to these thoughts

Suicide threats: Direct or indirect statements that hint, suggest, or declare the intent to end one's life; usually occur before overt suicide actions

Suicide gestures: Acts of self-injury

Suicide: Self-directed act that results in death

Etiology and incidence: It is estimated that one in four persons experiences some type of mood disorder during his or her lifetime. Major depression is the most common of the mood disorders, and an estimated 15% of the general population experiences a major depression sometime throughout the lifetime. Women between the ages of 18 and 44 are two times more likely then men to experience major depression. Suicide, suicide ideation, and suicide threats are adverse responses to individuals who are unable to cope with their life situation and/or depression. The National Institute of Mental Health estimated the lifetime prevalence of suicide attempts. Findings indicate that in individuals with no lifetime history of any psychiatric disorder, the suicide rate is 1% of the general population and among persons with a lifetime history of major depression, the suicide rate is 18%.

Pathophysiology: Major depression generally precedes a suicide attempt. Careful screening and determination of risk factors and/or suicidal ideation may prevent a suicide event.

Risk Factors

Individual or family history of depression or bipolar disorder
Prior suicide attempts
Mood changes including depression
Psychosis including hallucinations and/or delusions
Cognitive changes including suicidal ideation
Behavioral or social changes resulting in depression or feelings of sadness or hopelessness; isolation; anxiety; stress
Loss of significant other
Loss of social and economic resources

General medical illnesses; organic brain disorders including
   delirium and/or dementia
Impulse control disorders

Clinical Manifestations

The individual talks of suicide prior to actual event and
discusses a method of suicide with specific plans. He or she has
the tools in hand to carry out the event (e.g., gun, medication,
etc.), discusses the plan with others, puts his or her affairs in
order, and says good-bye to others.

Complications

Death results.

Diagnostic Tests

Clinical suicide risk assessment	Standardized risk assessment using one of the standardized evaluation tools (*Hopelessness Scale, Suicide Assessment Scale, and others*)
Laboratory tests	Clinical tests for depression: TRH, DST, sleep and waking electroencephalogram, thyroid function test

Therapeutic Management

Surgery	None
Drugs	Antidepressants and other medications that treat underlying cause
	Caution: Provide medications only as prescribed. Do not leave excess medications with individual. Keep all medications in a safe environment away from depressed individual.
General	Ensure that the individual is in a safe and protected environment. Provide frequent checks to ensure that the individual is safe. Do not leave excess medications or other items with individual that may be used to harm self. Provide counseling to determine underlying cause of depression and feelings of suicide.

S

syphilis

A contagious, sexually transmitted systemic disease characterized by sequential clinical stages with intervening years of symptomless latency

Etiology and incidence: Syphilis is caused by the *Treponema pallidum* spirochete. The primary mode of transmission is sexual contact, although the disease may be transmitted transplacentally from an infected mother to her fetus. Syphilis is transmissible by blood in the incubation period and through intimate sexual contact in the primary and secondary stages. It occurs worldwide and is on the increase, particularly in women and neonates. The incidence in the United States is decreasing steadily. The peak incidence occurs among males age 15 to 30 with multiple sex partners. About 68,000 cases are reported each year in the United States. A striking relationship exists between syphilis and HIV-positive individuals; one fourth of the syphilitic population in some urban clinics also have HIV.

Pathophysiology: Syphilis occurs in five distinct stages: incubation, primary, secondary, latency, and late. Incubation lasts 10 days to 10 weeks and begins with penetration of a mucous membrane by *T. pallidum*. Some spirochetes remain at the site, whereas others migrate to regional lymph nodes and then across all organ systems. The inflammatory response in the endothelial tissue produces perivascular infiltration of lymphocytes and plasma cells, causing edema of the endothelium and endarteritis in the capillaries and terminal arterioles. Vessels thicken as fibroblasts proliferate and cause fibrosis and necrosis. The primary stage is marked by the appearance of a single lesion (chancre) at the site of infection. Serum infiltration and accumulation in the associated connective tissue produce a firm, hard lesion. The lesion heals spontaneously in 1 to 5 weeks. Satellite lesions may form in adjacent tissue or in regional lymph nodes. Nodes are swollen and nontender. The secondary stage begins as the primary stage disappears and generally lasts 2 to 6 weeks. Parenchymal, systemic, and mucocutaneous processes occur throughout the body. After the second stage a 1- to 40-year latency period ensues, followed by the late stage, in which the cardiovascular and nervous systems degenerate.

Risk Factors

Unprotected sexual contact (vaginal, anal, oral) with an infected partner

Sharing needles with an infected individual when using IV drugs

Multiple sex partners

Infants of infected mothers

History of sexually transmitted disease, HIV, AIDS

Clinical Manifestations

The disease can appear at any stage without manifestations from the previous stages.

Incubation	Asymptomatic; report of sexual contact with infected partner
Primary	Single lesion starting as a red papule and eroding into a painless ulcer that exudes a clear fluid; red areola around lesion; common sites include penis, anus, rectum, vulva, cervix, perineum, lips, tongue, buccal mucosa, and tonsils; swollen regional lymph nodes
Secondary	Symmetric, pale red (in whites) or pigmented (in blacks) macules, papules, or pustules that predominate on flexor and volar body surfaces, particularly the palms and the soles of the feet; grayish-white erosive patches on mucous membranes; patchy hair loss; generalized swelling of lymph nodes
Latency	May see early mucocutaneous relapse signs but seldom after first year; asymptomatic period that may last rest of individual's lifetime or may move at any time to late stage
Late	Lesions (gummas) of skin, bone, viscera, heart, and nervous system; lesions are indolent, increase slowly in size, and resolve slowly to painless ulcerations that scar on healing; deep, boring pain in bones with lump over involved site; dilation of ascending aorta with aortic insufficiency; meningovascular signs (e.g., headache, dizziness, confusion, lassitude, insomnia, stiff neck, blurred vision, aphasia, hemiplegia); mental deterioration,

dementia, delusions; locomotor ataxia; body
tremors; urinary retention; impotence;
joint degeneration

Complications

Complications occur as a result of untreated disease; they
include periostitis, Charcot's arthropathy, aortic regurgitation or
aneurysm, meningitis, and widespread damage to the central
nervous system, resulting in paresis or dementia paralytica.

Diagnostic Tests

Serology	Positive Venereal Disease Research Laboratory, rapid plasma reagin, automated reagin, or reagin screen tests useful for screening in primary and secondary stages (many false positive results with these tests); tests for fluorescent treponemal antibody (absorbed) and *T. pallidum* agglutination and microhemagglutination done to confirm positive screening tests (they become reactive in the early primary stage and remain reactive in late-stage disease)
Darkfield microscopy	Examination of exudate from lesion is positive for *T. pallidum* in primary and secondary stages

Therapeutic Management

Surgery	None
Drugs	Antiinfective drugs to kill spirochete are effective at all stages
General	Mandatory report to local health authority, tracking of all sexual contacts, refraining from sexual activity until examination of exudates is negative, instruction about sexually transmitted diseases and the importance of completing the full antibiotic course and of returning for all follow-up examinations

temporomandibular joint syndrome

A disorder of the temporomandibular joint structure characterized by pain, muscle spasm, and changes in jaw movement

Etiology and incidence: Predisposing factors for temporomandibular joint (TMJ) disorders include congenital and developmental anomalies (agenesis); joint diseases (arthritis, ankylosis, neoplasms, or lupus); internal derangements of the intraarticular disk; fractures and dislocations from trauma; teeth grinding or clenching; and prolonged stress.

Pathophysiology: The precise pathophysiological process is dictated by the predisposing factor. Congenital and developmental anomalies and fractures and dislocations produce a shift in the mandible and a severe malocclusion, which leads to asymmetric jaw movements, muscle spasms, and pain. Underlying disease processes lead to inflammation and infection in the joint, which limits jaw movement and causes pain. Teeth grinding and jaw clenching habits set up increased muscle tonus, which induces muscle fatigue and spasm.

Clinical Manifestations

Common signs and symptoms include muscle spasm and pain at the joint, temples, mandible, or masticatory muscles that worsens with jaw movement or finger pressure on the joint. Cracking, clicking, and popping sounds may occur with jaw movement. Pain may be referred to the neck and shoulders and may be accompanied by headache, tinnitus, and earache.

Complications

Freezing of the joint may be a complication.

Diagnostic Tests

Radiology	To evaluate joint and determine predisposing factor
Occlusion analysis	To evaluate bite
CT/MRI	To detect soft tissue abnormalities and degenerative changes
Mandibular kinesiography	To assess degree of jaw dysfunction

Therapeutic Management

Surgery	Arthroscopy to débride joint, lyse adhesions, or reposition or remove disk if condition is unresponsive to more conservative management; jaw reconstruction to correct facial deformities and realign jaw; condylectomy to remove condyle; osteotomy to excise bony overgrowth
Drugs	Analgesics for pain; nonsteroidal antiinflammatory drugs; muscle relaxants for spasm; antianxiety agents if disorder is stress related
General	Nightguard, bite plate to prevent grinding and clenching; splint to realign malocclusion; moist heat and ultrasound to induce muscle relaxation and enhance analgesia; cold to reduce muscle spasm and inflammation; jaw exercises to stretch muscles; biofeedback or relaxation exercises to relieve stress

tendinitis, tenosynovitis

An inflammation of the tendon (tendinitis) and lining of the tendon sheath (tenosynovitis) characterized by pain on movement of the associated joint

Etiology and incidence: The etiology is often unknown, but individuals are thought to be more susceptible as degenerative changes occur in the vascularity of the tendons, causing a slower response to repetitive microtrauma. Repetitive movements, strain, or excessive, unaccustomed exercise may be causes. Underlying systemic disease (e.g., rheumatoid arthritis, gout, sclerosis, and disseminated gonococcal infections) may also be a cause. Middle-age and older adults, athletes, or individuals with occupations requiring repetitive motion are at greatest risk.

Pathophysiology: Repetitive microtrauma damages the fibers in the common extensor tendon of the involved joint, causing extravasation of tissue fluid and setting up an inflammatory process. Over time, healing builds fibrous, inelastic tissue and scarring, which often bind the tendon and sheath together, limiting joint motion.

Clinical Manifestations

The involved tendons usually show visible swelling; the joint may be tender and hot to the touch; motion of the joint causes pain. Joint motion may be restricted because of pain and edema.

Complications

Rupture of the tendon is a possible complication.

Diagnostic Tests

The diagnosis is based on a history of repetitive motion or underlying disease and physical examination of the joint. Radiology may show calcium deposits in the tendon or tendon sheath.

Therapeutic Management

Surgery	Removal of calcium deposits in cases unresponsive to other treatment; release of fibro-osseous tunnels associated with de Quervain's disease; tenosynovectomy for chronic inflammation associated with rheumatoid arthritis
Drugs	Oral or locally injected corticosteroids to relieve inflammation; analgesics/antiinflammatory drugs to relieve pain
General	Moist heat compresses to joint; rest of joint with controlled progressive exercise program

testicular cancer

Most carcinomas of the testes are germ cell in origin and are either seminomas or nonseminomas

Etiology and incidence: The etiology of testicular cancer is unknown, although it occurs 40 times more often in men with undescended or atrophic testicles and is believed to be tied to genetic factors. There is a wide geographic difference in reported incidence, with Scandinavia, Switzerland, and Germany reporting the highest per capita rates. Rates are lowest in Africa and Asia. Testicular cancer accounts for only 1% of all cancer in men in the United States, with about 6000 cases and 350 deaths reported per year. However, it is the most common solid malignancy in males under age 30. It is also seen in infants and men over age 60. White males are much more susceptible than black males (5:1 ratio). Male offspring of mothers who received diethylstilbestrol during pregnancy are at greater risk.

Pathophysiology: The cells arise from the primordial germ cell and grow within the testis itself. The cancer forms a solid mass and then metastasizes via regional lymph nodes to the retroperitoneum and distantly to the lungs.

Risk Factors

Caucasian
Ages 25 to 40
Undescended testis (not surgically corrected)
Diethylstilbestrol exposure of mother during pregnancy
History of testicular atrophy (Klinefelter's syndrome, viral
    orchitis), HIV, or AIDS

Clinical Manifestations

The most common presenting sign is a scrotal mass with or without local tenderness and pain.

Complications

The prognosis is excellent if the condition is treated before metastasis occurs in the lymph nodes. Ureteral and bowel obstructions are complications.

Diagnostic Tests

Palpation and ultrasound and CT scans are used to locate suspicious lesions. Alpha-fetoprotein and human chorionic gonadotropin serum markers are elevated. A biopsy through orchiectomy is used for definitive diagnosis.

Therapeutic Management

Surgery	Inguinal orchiectomy with or without transabdominal retroperitoneal lymph node dissection is the primary treatment; testicular implants
Drugs	Chemotherapy (cisplatin alone or in combination) to promote regression of tumors, making them more amenable to surgery
General	Radiation to treat seminomas; counseling for altered sexual functioning, infertility; referral for sperm banking for future children; instruction in testicular self-examination

tetanus (lockjaw)

An acute infectious disease of the central nervous system characterized by intermittent tonic spasms of the voluntary muscles

Etiology and incidence: Tetanus is caused by the tetanospasmin exotoxin produced by the spore-forming *Clostridium tetani* bacillus. The organism enters the body through a wound contaminated with soil and feces containing viable spores. The incidence is sporadic, and the disease occurs worldwide. It is rare in developed countries, where immunization is common. In developing countries, newborns are at particular risk as the unhealed umbilical cord serves as a convenient port of entry.

Pathophysiology: The bacillus spores enter and multiply in a skin wound to produce the tetanospasmin toxin. The toxin travels to the central nervous system via the bloodstream and peripheral motor nerves and binds to ganglioside membranes, blocking release of an inhibitory transmitter. This induces a hyperexcitability in the motor neurons that results in tonic rigidity and spasms of the voluntary muscles. Once bound, the toxin cannot be neutralized by an antitoxin.

Clinical Manifestations

The incubation period ranges from 2 to 50 days, with an average of 5 to 10 days before symptoms occur. The most common symptom is stiffness of the jaw. Others include irritability, restlessness, headache, fever, sore throat, stiff neck, and difficulty swallowing. As the disease progresses, the person has difficulty opening the mouth, facial spasms, and rigidity with a fixed grin; opisthotonos; painful, generalized tonic spasms; profuse sweating; cyanosis; and exaggerated reflexes.

Complications

The worldwide mortality rate is 50%, and prognosis is poor when the incubation period is short and the symptoms progress rapidly. Complications include cardiac and pulmonary failure and muscle rupture.

Diagnostic Tests

The diagnosis is made by history and physical examination. Blood and wound cultures and tetanus antibody tests are commonly negative.

Therapeutic Management

Surgery	Débridement of deep penetrating wounds; tracheotomy if needed for prolonged respiratory management
Drugs	Tetanus toxoid with subsequent booster shots for primary immunity; tetanus antitoxin or tetanus immune globulin may be given at time of penetrating injury with no history of recent vaccination; muscle relaxants to treat rigidity and spasm; antiinfective drugs for infection; analgesics for pain
General	Prompt, thorough débridement of wound; intubation and mechanical ventilation if needed; tube feedings or hyperalimentation to manage nutrition; catheterization to manage urinary retention; coughing, turning, and deep breathing to prevent pneumonia; cardiac and hemodynamic monitoring; adequate fluids and electrolytes; instruction in the importance of maintaining immunization with routine booster every 10 years

thrombocytopenia

A platelet disorder in which the platelet count falls below $200,000/mm^3$, leading to bleeding into the skin, mucous membranes, internal cavities, and organs

Etiology and incidence: Thrombocytopenia may be idiopathic, or it may occur secondary to another process that reduces the number of platelets or produces defective platelets. These processes include use of drugs that can cause platelet destruction (heparin, quinidine, sulfa, oral hypoglycemics, gold salts, rifampin); underlying disease (leukemia, aplastic anemia, cirrhosis, disseminated intravascular coagulation); severe infection; hypothermia; hypersplenism; and alcohol ingestion. Idiopathic thrombocytopenia purpura (ITP) may be either acute or chronic. The acute form usually follows a viral infection such as rubella or chickenpox and affects mostly children between ages 2 and 6. The chronic form is linked to immunological disorders such as lupus and HIV and usually affects adults of all ages, particularly women.

Pathophysiology

ITP is thought to be associated with an autoimmune process in which the platelets are prematurely destroyed by circulating antibodies. The pathophysiology in secondary forms of the disease is related to the causative agent.

Clinical Manifestations

Common manifestations include petechiae and ecchymoses on the skin, particularly the lower extremities; easy bruising; bleeding from the nose and gums; melena in stools; hematemesis; heavy menses and breakthrough bleeding; and hematuria.

Complications

Complications include hemorrhage into organs such as the brain, gastrointestinal tract, or heart, which can be fatal without treatment.

Diagnostic Tests

Other platelet disorders must be ruled out.

Platelets	Count decreased; size and morphological appearance may be abnormal in ITP
Platelet survival	To help distinguish between ineffective and inappropriate platelet production
Bone marrow	Abundance of megakaryocytes
Bleeding time	Prolonged
Coagulation time	Normal
Capillary fragility	Increased

Therapeutic Management

Surgery	Splenectomy for severe thrombocytopenia related to hypersplenism or splenomegaly
Drugs	Corticosteroids to enhance platelet production and promote capillary integrity; immunosuppressants when disease does not respond to steroids; immune globulin to prepare severely thrombocytic individuals for surgery; discontinuing any drug that may be causing the disorder
General	Platelet transfusions for severe bleeding; safety precautions to prevent bruising; balance of rest and activity; monitoring for bleeding episodes; instruction in infection precautions for those taking immunosuppressants

thrombosis, venous (phlebothrombosis, thrombophlebitis)

An abnormal vascular condition in which a thrombus develops in a vein. *Thrombophlebitis* refers to a thrombus accompanied by inflammation of the vein (phlebitis). *Phlebothrombosis* refers to a thrombus with minimal inflammation. Dislodgment and migration of a thrombus are known as *thromboembolism*. (See also pulmonary embolism.)

Etiology and incidence: A number of factors acting in concert contribute to thrombus formation, including intimal damage to the vein from indwelling catheters, injection of irritating substances or septic phlebitis; hypercoagulability related to underlying disorders (idiopathic thrombocytopenia purpura, malignancies, blood dyscrasias) and use of oral contraceptives; and stasis from prolonged immobilization or postpartum or postoperative states. Venous thrombosis is the most commonly seen venous disorder except for varicose veins. Individuals at greatest risk are postoperative patients and those receiving IV therapy.

Pathophysiology: Most thrombi begin forming in the valve cusps of deep calf veins. Tissue thromboplastin is released and forms thrombin and fibrin that trap RBCs to form a clot. The clot continues to enlarge until it eventually occludes the lumen of the vessel. It may break off and migrate to the systemic circulation.

Clinical Manifestations

Deep veins	Calf pain and tenderness; positive Homans' sign (calf pain on foot dorsiflexion); dilated superficial veins; edema, increased size of involved extremity; redness and warmth over vein site
Superficial veins	Redness, warmth, and tenderness over affected vein, which is visible and palpable

Complications

Chronic venous insufficiency and pulmonary embolus are the most common complications of thrombosis.

Diagnostic Tests

A physical examination is the primary diagnostic tool in detecting venous thrombosis and in distinguishing arterial from venous obstructions. Noninvasive tests include ultrasonography and plethysmography, which show reduced blood flow. Contrast venography is the most accurate and the confirming diagnostic tool.

Therapeutic Management

Surgery	Ligation, clipping, plication, and thrombectomy when thrombosis fails to respond to conservative therapy; extravascular vena cava interruption with possible placement of intracaval filter when emboli are probable
Drugs	*Superficial:* Nonsteroidal antiinflammatory drugs for pain and inflammation
	Deep vein: Fibrinolytics to lyse clots; anticoagulants (heparin for acute treatment, warfarin for maintenance) to augment thrombolysis; antiplatelets to prevent thrombus formation; analgesics *(aspirin is contraindicated because it interferes with platelet function)*
General	*Superficial:* Moist compresses to treat discomfort
	Deep vein: Bed rest with elevation of affected extremity above the level of the heart; warm, moist packs; antiembolism hose when ambulatory; monitoring of prothrombin time and partial thromboplastin time during anticoagulant therapy; monitoring for signs of pulmonary embolus; instruction about bleeding precautions while undergoing anticoagulants

thrush

See Stomatitis.

thyroid cancer

Papillary carcinomas are the most common type of thyroid cancer (60% to 70%). Follicular carcinomas account for 15% to 20% of diagnosed cases, anaplastic carcinomas for 10%, and medullary carcinomas for less than 5%.

Etiology and incidence: There is a strong link between radiation therapy to the neck region (a popular childhood treatment to shrink tonsils, adenoids, and thymus glands in the 1950s) and papillary cancer of the thyroid. Other suspected precursors of thyroid cancer include prolonged secretion of thyroid-stimulating hormone (TSH), iodine deficiencies, and chronic goiter. Familial predisposition (autosomal dominant trait) is strongly suspected in medullary cancer. About 14,000 cases of thyroid cancer are diagnosed and about 1100 deaths are reported in the United States each year. It can occur at any age, although anaplastic carcinoma is seen almost exclusively in the elderly. Thyroid cancer is two to three times more common in women than in men.

Pathophysiology: Papillary and follicular carcinomas begin in the epithelial cells of the thyroid, growing slowly and forming nodules in the gland. Papillary tumors are usually nonencapsulated, extend to adjacent tissue beyond the thyroid, and metastasize to local cervical lymph nodes. Distant metastasis is rare. Follicular tumors are encapsulated, invade local tissue and cervical nodes, and metastasize to distant sites (e.g., lungs, bone) through the bloodstream.

Anaplastic carcinomas arise from the epithelium of the thyroid and are characterized by rapid, painful invasive growth to the trachea and major blood vessels, with metastasis to the bones and liver. Medullary carcinoma arises from the parafollicular cells of the thyroid and causes excessive secretion of calcitonin, lowering serum calcium and phosphate levels. Amyloid and calcium deposits are common. The tumor grows rapidly and metastasizes through lymphatics to cervical and mediastinal nodes and to the liver, lungs, and bone, leaving dense calcifications in its wake.

Risk Factors

History of radiation to thyroid gland (papillary cancer)
History of prolonged secretion of thyroid-stimulating hormone, or chronic goiter

Use of steroids
Diet deficient in iodine or very high in iodine
Female gender (2 to 3 times as common in females)
Familial predisposition (medullary cancer).
Advanced age (anaplastic cancer)

Clinical Manifestations

The most common presenting sign is a palpable, symptomless lump in the neck.

Complications

The prognosis is excellent for papillary and follicular cancers if they are treated before distant metastasis occurs. Medullary and anaplastic cancers have a much higher death rate. Medullary tumors are treated successfully only if detected very early, before any tissue invasion is evident; anaplastic tumors are resistant to treatment and spread so rapidly they often cause death within 6 months of diagnosis. Complications include dysphagia, stridor, and tracheal obstruction.

Diagnostic Tests

X-ray examination, thyroid scans, ultrasound and CT scans, and magnetic resonance imaging are used to visualize the size and extent of the tumor and calcifications. A calcitonin assay for elevated levels of calcitonin is a reliable indicator for medullary carcinoma. The definitive diagnosis is made through fine needle aspiration biopsy.

Therapeutic Management

Surgery	Thyroidectomy with or without lymph node dissection as primary treatment; modified radical neck resection for recurrence or metastasis
Drugs	Palliative treatment in widespread disease; thyroid hormone as replacement therapy and to suppress TSH production
General	Radioactive iodine ablation as adjuvant to surgery or alone for palliation; instruction about lifelong use of thyroid replacement hormones

tinnitus

The perception of sound in the absence of an acoustic stimulus, which may be intermittent, continuous, or pulsatile

Etiology and incidence: The etiology is unknown, but tinnitus occurs as a symptom in nearly every disorder of the ear. Contributory factors include obstruction of the external ear canal; infection and inflammation; use of certain drugs (salicylates, quinine, aminoglycoside antibiotics, thiazide diuretics); exposure to certain toxins (carbon monoxide, heavy metals, alcohol); damage to cranial nerve VIII; underlying cardiovascular disease, anemia, or hypothyroidism; and acoustic or head trauma. An estimated 30 million individuals in the United States are thought to suffer from tinnitus.

Pathophysiology: The pathophysiological mechanisms of tinnitus remain obscure.

Clinical Manifestations

The primary manifestation is a sound variously described as ringing, roaring, sizzling, whistling, humming, buzzing, hissing, or clicking. It may be intermittent, continuous, or pulsatile and may be accompanied by a hearing loss.

Complications

Tinnitus that is loud, high pitched, and continuous has been known to drive some individuals to attempt suicide if treatment fails.

Diagnostic Tests

An audiological examination is done to rule out underlying systemic disease or disease of the ear known to produce tinnitus. The examination will also reveal any hearing loss. Measurements of tone masking also are done. Pulsatile tinnitus calls for a workup of the vascular system for aneurysm, obstruction, and neoplasm.

Therapeutic Management

Surgery	None
Drugs	Antianxiety agents and anticonvulsants (e.g., carbamazepine [Tegretol]) combined with primidone (Mysoline) or phenytoin (Dilantin) at night for sedative effect
General	Correction of any associated hearing loss, treatment of underlying disease, use of background noise to mask tinnitus, use of a tinnitus masker worn in the ear to produce a more pleasant sound, avoidance of causative drugs or toxins

tonsillitis

An inflammation of the palatine tonsils

Etiology and incidence: Tonsils normally filter out bacteria and other microorganisms to prevent infections to the body. If they become overwhelmed by bacteria or viral infection, they may become enlarged, causing tonsillitis. *Streptococcus* (*B*-hemolytic streptococci group A) is the most common cause of tonsillitis. Tonsillitis may be acute or chronic and occurs most often in children.

Pathophysiology: The classic symptoms of tonsillitis are a sore throat, swollen tonsils, and enlarged and tender anterior cervical lymph nodes. The tonsils are swollen, reddened, and inflamed with pus or exudate (often yellow pustules). Some cases may have referred pain to the ears. If the exudate is scraped from the tonsils, bleeding may result.

Risk Factors

Children with frequent colds
Winter season

Clinical Manifestations

Symptoms include moderate to severe sore throat lasting longer than 2 days; difficulty swallowing; pain referred to the ears; enlarged anterior cervical nodes; fever and chills; headache; muscle and joint pain; anorexia; increased secretions from the throat; enlarged, reddened, inflamed tonsils; pus or exudate on the tonsils; halitosis; or edematous or inflamed uvula. Symptoms often last 2 to 3 days after treatment is initiated.

Complications

If not treated, the following can occur: peritonsillar abscess, airway occlusion, rheumatic fever and subsequent cardiovascular disorders, kidney failure, or poststreptococcal glomerulonephritis.

Diagnostic Tests

Direct inspection
Throat culture

Therapeutic Management

Surgery	Tonsillectomy may be recommended if tonsillitis is severe, recurs often, or does not respond to antibiotics.
Drugs	Antiinfective agents if cause is bacterial
General	Rest; warm, bland fluids or very cold fluids may alleviate discomfort; saltwater gargles, adequate fluids

toxic shock syndrome

An acute bacterial infection that may progress rapidly to severe shock

Etiology and incidence: The exact etiologic mechanism of toxic shock is unknown, but all cases have reported infection with exotoxin-producing strains of *Staphylococcus aureus*. The syndrome was first reported in children and adolescents in 1978. In 1980 a large number of cases occurred in young menstruating women who used tampons. Changes in the composition of tampons and their use have drastically reduced the incidence in this group. Cases have subsequently been detected in postoperative patients, after nasal reconstruction cases with packing, in those with infected insect bites, and in those with burns. Reported mortality rates range from 8% to 15%.

Pathophysiology: It is presumed that those at risk harbor a preexisting colonization of *S. aureus* in their bodies. The mechanisms that turn the bacteria into a toxin are unclear but seem to be associated with possible mechanical or chemical factors at work on the harbored bacteria. Once the toxin is produced, it is thought to enter the bloodstream through a break in the skin or mucosa and spread systematically.

Clinical Manifestations

The onset is sudden and marked by high fever, headache, sore throat, nonpurulent conjunctivitis, lethargy, confusion, vomiting, diarrhea, and a sunburnlike skin rash. Within 48 hours the syndrome progresses to syncope, orthostatic hypotension, diminished urine output, and shock. Peripheral and pulmonary edema, hepatitis, and myolysis then occur. After 3 to 7 days, the skin sloughs off on the palms and soles.

Complications

Toxic shock syndrome can lead to residual neurological or psychological deficit, renal failure, respiratory failure, and death.

Diagnostic Tests

The Centers for Disease Control and Prevention has set up diagnostic criteria. At least three of the following conditions must be present on a clinical examination or laboratory test: (1) gastrointestinal effects, including vomiting and profuse, watery diarrhea; (2) muscular effects, with severe myalgia and a fivefold increase in serum creatinine phosphokinase; (3) mucous membrane effects; (4) renal involvement, with blood urea nitrogen or serum creatinine at least double normal levels; (5) hepatocellular damage, with serum bilirubin, alanine aminotransferase, and aspartate aminotransferase double the normal levels; (6) blood involvement, with thrombocytopenia and a platelet count under $100,000/\text{mm}^3$; and (7) central nervous system effects, such as confusion without focal signs.

Therapeutic Management

Surgery	Tracheostomy if needed for ventilation
Drugs	Antiinfective drugs specific to *S. aureus* to prevent recurrence; antidiarrheal drugs and antiemetics to reduce diarrhea and vomiting; analgesics for pain
General	Immediate treatment for septic shock if indicated: fluid and electrolyte replacement, packed RBCs, monitoring of intake and output and central venous pressure; universal precautions for secretions and discharges; vital signs, neural vital signs, and reorientation for confusion; safety measures to prevent falls from orthostatic hypotension; mechanical ventilation if necessary; instruction about susceptibility to recurrence and the safe use of tampons

transient ischemic attacks

Recurrent, focal neurological disturbances of sudden onset and brief duration characterized by loss of sensory, motor, or visual function

Etiology and incidence: Most transient ischemic attacks (TIAs) are caused by cerebral emboli that break off from atherosclerotic plaques in the carotid or vertebral arteries in the neck. Hypertension, atherosclerosis, heart disease, diabetes mellitus, and polycythemia serve as predisposing factors. The attacks are most common in adults past middle age and often presage a stroke. Occasionally TIAs are seen in children with severe cardiovascular disease and an elevated hematocrit.

Pathophysiology: An atherosclerotic plaque breaks off from an artery in the neck and travels to the brain, where it temporarily impedes the blood flow in the carotid-middle or vertebral basilar artery in the circle of Willis.

Clinical Manifestations

TIAs appear suddenly, usually last 2 to 30 minutes, and then subside with no neurological sequelae. They may occur daily or two or three times a year. The manifestations are specific to the artery occluded.

Carotid	Ipsilateral blindness described as a shade being pulled down over the eye; contralateral hemiparesis; paresthesias; slurred speech
Vertebrobasilar	Confusion, vertigo, diplopia or binocular blindness, unilateral or bilateral muscular weakness and paresthesias, drop attacks with buckling of the legs, slurred speech

Complications

TIAs may precede a stroke.

Diagnostic Tests

The diagnosis is made on the clinical history with an ultrasound scan or arteriography, which confirms the presence of stenosis and atherosclerosis of the carotid or vertebral arteries.

Therapeutic Management

Surgery	Endarterectomy to remove atherosclerotic plaque from the artery is considered if the artery is at least 70% occluded; intracranial anastomosis to revascularize the brain
Drugs	Antiplatelet agents and anticoagulants for 2 to 3 weeks to interfere with clot formation; aspirin therapy long term to interfere with platelet aggregation
General	Monitor for bleeding; long-term follow-up

traumatic brain injury (head injury)

Physical injury to the brain or other structures in the cranium, which may be open with skull fracture or penetration or may be closed with impact and rapid jarring. Concussion is the least serious injury and is characterized by a transient loss of consciousness with no gross damage to the brain and no neurological sequelae. Contusions and lacerations indicate a more serious injury, and there is bruising of brain tissue with bleeding and tearing of the cortical surface.

Etiology and incidence: Leading causes of head trauma include falls, industrial accidents, vehicular accidents (particularly involving motorcycles, or automobile accidents with passengers who were not wearing seat belts), assaults, sports injuries (boxing, diving, football), and intrauterine and birth injury. Alcohol use is a common related factor. Traumatic brain injury (TBI) causes more death and disability than any other neurological disorder in individuals under age 50. It is the leading cause of death in men under age 35. More than 77,000 individuals die of TBI each year in the United States, and 55,000 more are left with permanent neurological damage.

Pathophysiology: Damage occurs from skull penetration or rapid brain acceleration and deceleration, which injure brain tissue at the point of impact, at its opposite pole (contrecoup), and diffusely in the frontal and temporal lobes. Blood vessels, meninges, and nerves can be ruptured, sheared, and torn. This results in neural disturbances, ischemia, hemorrhage, and cerebral edema. Laceration of meningeal arteries or sinuses can cause subdural or epidural hematomas and leakage of cerebrospinal fluid (CSF).

Clinical Manifestations

Clinical manifestations vary by the structures and brain tissue involved, whether the injury was open or closed, and the severity of the injury. The manifestations listed below are all possible.

Level of consciousness	Ranges from anxiety and irritability to restlessness, confusion, delirium, stupor, and coma; posttraumatic and retrograde amnesia

Pain	Mild to severe headache
Cranial nerve injuries	Anosmia; diplopia, strabismus, nystagmus, or blindness; deafness; vertigo; trigeminal paresthesias
Motor function	Weakness, paresis, paralysis; decorticate and decerebrate posturing; areflexia
Meningeal effects	Nuchal rigidity, positive Kernig's sign, positive Brudzinski's sign
Fractures	*Linear:* No bone displacement, possible epidural hematoma
	Depressed: Focal deficits and cranial nerve injuries
	Basilar: CSF otorrhea or rhinorrhea, periorbital ecchymosis, conjunctival bleeding
Cerebral edema	Increased intracranial pressure (ICP) with slow respirations, bradycardia, nausea, vomiting, altered or loss of consciousness, seizures, weakness
Hematoma	*Epidural:* Ipsilateral pupil dilation, rapidly increasing ICP
	Subdural: Lethargy, headache, seizures, minimal dilation of pupil on affected side; widening pulse pressure; fixed, dilated pupils; hemiplegia; decorticate rigidity
Vital signs	Decreased blood pressure; pulse slow (intracranial hypertension) or rapid and feeble (hemorrhage); shallow respirations with possible Cheyne-Stokes; hyperthermia with hypothalamic injury

Complications

Complications include infection, seizure disorders, hydrocephaly, organic brain syndrome, permanent residual neurological deficits (memory loss, loss of impulse control, loss of initiation skills, decrease in cognition and abstract reasoning, decrease in judgment and problem solving); physical deficits (paralysis, weakness, spasticity, loss of fine motor abilities); and death.

Diagnostic Tests

Skull x-rays	To detect fractures and bone fragments
CT/MRI scans or angiography	To detect subdural or intracranial hematoma, shift, or cerebral ventricle distortion
Echoencephalography	To detect midline shifts
Cisternography	To detect dural tear
CSF sampling	*May be contraindicated with signs of ICP, since it may lead to cerebral herniation;* normal findings with cerebral edema and concussion, increased pressure and blood in CSF with laceration and contusion

Therapeutic Management

Surgery	Débridement of open injuries; ventriculostomy or shunting procedures for ICP or hydrocephalus; craniotomy to elevate severe skull depressions, to stop hemorrhage from vessel lacerations or to evacuate hematoma; trephine to relieve pressure from hematoma; bolt placement to monitor ICP pressure; tracheostomy if needed for ventilation
Drugs	Antiinfective drugs to prevent infection with open injury and leaking CSF; osmotic diuretics to control cerebral edema; corticosteroids to reduce cerebral edema; polar beta-blockers to control transient hypertension; anticonvulsants for seizures; analgesics for pain *(medullary depressants such as morphine are contraindicated, since they may interfere with level of consciousness);* muscle relaxants or paralyzing agents for decorticate and decerebrate posturing and restlessness in coma; stool softeners and suppositories

T

to prevent constipation; artificial tears to prevent corneal damage with coma; histamine antagonists and antacids to control gastric reflux with tube feedings and reduce the chance of ulcers developing

General   *Initially:* Secure airway, control bleeding, stabilize body on backboard and transport; mechanical ventilation if needed with hyperventilation to control intracranial hypertension; central venous and arterial lines; ICP and cardiac monitoring; blood gases; vital signs and neural vital signs; monitoring of intake and output; enteral feedings or hyperalimentation; indwelling Foley catheter; seizure precautions; passive range-of-motion exercises, turning if comatose; cooling blankets for hyperthermia

Long term: Comprehensive rehabilitation program, including cognitive therapy to address cognitive, memory, and abstract reasoning deficits; speech therapy for communication deficits; physical therapy for residual weakness, paralysis, gait retraining, ataxia; occupational therapy for relearning activities of daily living; respiratory therapy to retain vital capacity; vocational therapy for learning vocational skills; counseling of individual and family to aid in adaptation to residual disabilities and amelioration of behavioral sequelae; transitional living placement to return individual to independent or supervised community living; long-term medical follow-up to reduce complications; instruction of family about the importance of structure and consistency of environment, safety issues arising from impaired judgment and lack of impulse control; instruction in the use of memory books and other memory aids

trichinosis

A roundworm (*Trichinella spiralis)* infection, usually transmitted by eating raw or undercooked pork

Etiology and incidence: The *Trichinella spiralis* is a parasite. Infection occurs when the individual eats contaminated undercooked pork or wild game meat. Because of meat processing and United States Department of Agriculture guidelines in the United States, the disease is uncommon. Approximately 50 to 60 cases are reported each year in the United States. Trichinosis is more prevalent throughout the rest of the world, especially where meats such as undercooked pork, ham, or sausage is eaten. The disease may also be seen in individuals who hunt and prepare their own meat, especially bear, cougar, fox, dog, wolf, horse, seal, walrus, or other wild animals who may be a reservoir for roundworm infection. The infection may be prevented if all meat, especially pork and meat from wild animals, is cooked until well done. Freezing specially prepared meats at subzero temperatures for several weeks kills encysted organisms.

Pathophysiology: The muscles of infected animals contain cysts that are ingested. The acid in the human digestive system breaks down the cyst and the larva hatch within the host (human) intestinal tract to produce a roundworm. It takes only one or two days for the young worm to become an adult roundworm. The adult roundworm then produces numerous larvae that migrate throughout the gastrointesinal system and bloodstream to muscle tissue. There, they produce cysts, and the life cycle repeats.

Risk Factors

Eating raw or undercooked pork, ham, or sausage, especially in
  areas outside of the United States
Eating game meat that has not been properly and fully cooked

Clinical Manifestations

Early: 1 to 2 days after infection	Nausea, vomiting, fatigue, fever, and abdominal discomfort
Late: About 2 to 8 weeks later	Headache, fevers, chills, cough, eye swelling, aching joints and muscle

T

	pains, itchy skin, diarrhea, or constipation
Serious late signs	Difficulty coordinating movements, fatigue, cardiac arrhythmias, respiratory distress

Complications

If not identified and treated, serious cases may cause overwhelming infection and sometimes death.

Diagnostic Tests

CBC may indicate increased eosinophils; creatine phosphokinase to identify elevated level of creatine kinase; serology studies to test for trichinella; and muscle biopsy to locate evidence of the *Trichinella spiralis* roundworm

Therapeutic Management

Surgery	None
Drugs	Antiinfective agents specific to causative organism
General/Prevention	Prevention is the best intervention. Cook all meat products until the juices run clear or to an internal temperature of 170° F. Cook wild game meat thoroughly. Clean meat grinders thoroughly if you prepare your own ground meats. Curing (salting), drying, smoking, or microwaving meat does not consistently kill infective worms.

tuberculosis

A recurrent, chronic, infectious pulmonary and extrapulmonary disease characterized by formation of granulomas with caseation, fibrosis, and cavitation

Etiology and incidence: Tuberculosis (TB) is caused by spore-forming mycobacteria *(Mycobacterium tuberculosis, M. bovis,* or *M. africanum)*. In developed countries the infection is airborne and is spread by inhalation of infected droplets. In underdeveloped countries (Africa, Asia, South America), transmission also occurs by ingestion or by skin invasion, particularly when bovine TB is poorly controlled. The incidence varies widely by country, age, race, gender, and socioeconomic status. The incidence of TB has risen precipitously in the United States with the advent of HIV infection and among certain immigrant populations. Nearly 23,000 new cases are reported annually in the United States.

Pathophysiology

TB has three stages: (1) primary (initial) infection; (2) latent (dormant) infection; and (3) recrudescent (postprimary) disease. During the first stage, the mycobacteria invade the tissues at the port of entry (usually the lungs) and multiply over a period of approximately 3 weeks. They form a small inflammatory lesion in the lung before traveling to the regional lymph nodes and throughout the body, forming additional lesions. The number of lesions formed depends on the number of invading bacteria and the general resistance of the host. This stage is generally asymptomatic.

Lymphocytes and antibodies mount a fibroblastic response to the invasion that encases the lesions, forming noncaseating granulomas. This marks the latent stage, and the individual may remain in this stage for weeks to years, depending on the body's ability to maintain specific and nonspecific resistance. Stage three occurs when the body is unable to contain the infection, and a necrotic and cavitation process begins in the lesion at the entry port or in other body lesions. Caseation occurs and the lesions may rupture, spreading necrotic residue and bacilli throughout the surrounding tissue. Disseminated bacteria form new lesions, which in turn become inflamed and form noncaseating granulomas and then caseating necrotic cavities. The lungs are the most common site for recrudescent disease, but it may occur anywhere in the body. Untreated disease has many remissions and exacerbations.

Risk Factors

Age extremes (under age 3 or over age 65)
Smoking
Drug and alcohol abuse
Occupational history as a silicone and asbestos workers (particularly those who smoke)
Malnourished state
Unsanitary, crowded living conditions
Residence in institutional settings
History of chronic illness, general debilitation, immunosuppression, HIV, AIDS

Clinical Manifestations

Manifestations vary with the systems involved. Symptoms are rarely seen until the recrudescent stage. Individuals are communicable whenever bacilli are present in the sputum.

Pulmonary	Weight loss, fatigue, generalized weakness, anorexia; slight fever with chills and night sweats; nonproductive cough that eventually becomes productive with mucopurulent sputum; tachycardia; dyspnea on exertion; hemoptysis
Cardiovascular	Pericarditis with precordial chest pain, fever, ascites, edema, and distention of neck veins
Gastrointestinal	Peritonitis with acute abdominal pain, abdominal distention, vomiting, anorexia, weight loss, night sweats, gastrointestinal bleeding, bowel obstruction
Neurological	Meningitis with headache, vomiting, fever, declining consciousness, and neurological deficit
Musculoskeletal	Joint pain, swelling, tenderness, deformities; limitation of motion

| Genitourinary | Urgency, frequency, dysuria, hematuria, pyuria; infertility, amenorrhea, vaginal bleeding and discharge; salpingitis with lower abdominal pain |
| Lymphatics | Enlarged lymph nodes |

Complications

Complications include massive destruction of lung tissue, leading to pneumothorax, pleural effusion, pneumonia, and respiratory failure; brain abscess; cardiac tamponade; vertebral collapse and paralysis; liver failure; renal failure; and generalized, massive dissemination of disease that usually is fatal. New drug-resistant strains of tuberculosis are emerging, leading to more frequent progression to complications.

Diagnostic Tests

Skin tests (purified protein derivative/ Mantoux)	Positive reaction indicates past infection and presence of antibodies; it is not indicative of active disease
Sputum culture	Positive for causative agent within 2 to 3 weeks of onset of active disease; it is not positive during latency
Acid-fast sputum smear	Positive for acid-fast bacillus
Tissue biopsy/culture	Positive for causative agent
Pleural needle biopsy	Positive for causative agent
Chest x-ray	May reveal cavitation, calcification, parenchymal infiltrate; not diagnostically definitive

Therapeutic Management

| Surgery | Drainage of pulmonary abscesses; correction of complications such as intestinal obstruction or urethral stricture |
| Drugs | Antiinfective drugs in combinations of primary drugs or primary and secondary drugs to combat causative agent (new strains of bacillus are occurring that are resistant to traditional primary drugs); antiinfective drugs (isoniazid) as che- |

T

moprophylaxis in individuals who have converted from a negative to a positive skin test, particularly those with HIV or other immune-suppressed conditions, insulin-dependent diabetics, those on prolonged corticosteroid therapy, small children, and health care workers who are regularly exposed

General   Sputum precautions until no sputum is evident (10 to 14 days after start of drug therapy); management usually on an outpatient basis unless the disease is in an advanced state with complications; instruction about the importance of uninterrupted drug therapy and the need for periodic recultures of sputum throughout drug therapy, which may last a year or longer; skin testing and examination of close contacts at the time of initial diagnosis and again in 2 to 3 months; long-term medical follow-up to prevent recurrence

ulcerative colitis

A chronic inflammatory mucosal disease of the colon and rectum characterized by bloody diarrhea

Etiology and incidence: The cause of ulcerative colitis is unknown. Immunological factors, infectious agents, toxins, and dietary factors have been studied extensively but with no promising result. The annual incidence of ulcerative colitis in the United States is seven cases per 100,000 persons. The incidence distribution is bimodal, with peak frequencies between ages 15 and 25 and 50 and 70. It is most prominent in whites, especially American and European Jewish individuals.

Pathophysiology: The disease process usually begins in the rectosigmoid area and spreads proximally. Pathological change starts with degeneration of the reticulin fibers beneath the epithelial mucosa. This causes occlusion of the subepithelial capillaries and infiltration of the lamina propria with lymphocytes, leukocytes, eosinophils, mast cells, and plasma. The result eventually is abscess formation, necrosis, and ulceration of the epithelial mucosa. This in turn reduces the colon's ability to absorb sodium and water.

Clinical Manifestations

The primary sign is the presence of frequent spells of bloody, mucoid diarrhea, accompanied by abdominal cramping. As the ulceration extends proximally, the stools become looser and increase in frequency to as many as 20 times daily. Malaise, fever, anorexia, and weight loss may also be present by this time.

Complications

Complications include perforation, toxic megacolon, massive hemorrhage, and a tenfold increased risk of adenocarcinoma of the colon.

Diagnostic Tests

A tentative diagnosis can be made on the history and examination of a stool specimen. Confirmation is made by sigmoidoscopy, which reveals a granular, friable mucous membrane with crypt abscesses, loss of normal vascular pattern, and scattered areas of hemorrhage. Double contrast barium enemas are used to visualize and evaluate disease above the reach of a sigmoidoscope. Plain x-rays of the abdomen may assist in gauging the extent and severity of disease. Stool cultures must be obtained to rule out all possible infectious bowel disorders. They should be negative in ulcerative colitis.

Therapeutic Management

Surgery	Colectomy or proctocolectomy with permanent ileostomy for fulminant disease, hemorrhage, perforation, or toxic megacolon
Drugs	Corticosteroids in retention enema or systemic form, depending on severity of disease; antidiarrheal drugs to control diarrhea; folate supplements; sulfasalazine drugs to help reduce inflammation and maintain remission; analgesics for pain *(avoid aspirin and nonsteroidal anti-inflammatory drugs because they may be irritating; avoid opiates and anticholinergics if disease is severe and the individual is at risk of toxic megacolon);* immunosuppressives used to treat severe, nonresponsive disease in individuals who are not surgical candidates
General	Avoidance of irritating foods (e.g., high-fiber foods, raw fruits and vegetables); adequate fluids; acute attacks treated with bed rest, IV fluids, total parenteral nutrition for severe malnutrition, and blood replacement; referral to support groups for long-term coping with disease; dietary education; ostomy care and instructions if needed; counseling to aid adaptation to altered body image with ostomy

ulcers, peptic (gastric or duodenal ulcers)

A circumscribed excavation of the gastric or duodenal mucosal wall that penetrates the muscularis mucosae and exposes it to acid and pepsin

Etiology and incidence: Infection by *Helicobacter pylori* bacteria is the major etiologic factor in ulcer formation. Other factors that have been implicated include use of certain drugs (e.g., aspirin and other nonsteroidal antiinflammatory agents [NSAIDs]); use of alcohol, cigarettes, and caffeine; and a familial history of ulcers. About 80% of all peptic ulcers are duodenal in origin, and the remaining 20% are gastric. Gastric ulcers strike men and women equally, with the peak incidence occurring between ages 55 and 65. Forty thousand to 80,000 cases are reported annually in the United States. Duodenal ulcers occur in men two to three times as often as in women, and the incidence increases with age. The annual incidence is 200,000 to 300,000, but it has been steadily decreasing since the 1950s.

Pathophysiology: The pathology is unclear, but it is hypothesized that *H. pylori* or other factors may upset the balance between ulcer-promoting factors, such as secretion of acid and pepsin and factors that serve as protectors of the mucosal lining, such as mucus production and replacement of damaged mucosal cells. This sets up an inflammatory process with resultant ulceration, thrombosis, fibrosis, and scarring of the muscularis mucosa layer of the stomach or duodenum.

Risk Factors

Duodenal ulcer

Increased acid production
Blood type O
Male gender (2:1 ratio)
Familial history

Gastric ulcer

Blood type A
Underlying disease processes such as pancreatitis, gastritis, and hepatic disorders

General factors

Use of NSAIDs, acetaminophen, other antiinflammatory drugs
Alcohol abuse
Smoking
Excessive caffeine consumption
Stress, repression of feelings

Clinical Manifestations

Manifestations vary with location, and ulcers are often asymptomatic or associated with vague symptoms. Only about 50% of individuals have a characteristic pattern of symptoms. The characteristic pain is described as burning, gnawing, or aching and is located in a well-circumscribed epigastric area. In duodenal ulcers the pain usually appears midmorning, is relieved by food, and then reappears 2 to 3 hours after eating. It also wakens the individual 2 to 3 hours after falling asleep. It occurs daily for 1 week or longer and may then disappear without treatment. With a gastric ulcer the pain usually occurs after eating food, is located in the left midgastric area, and often radiates to the back. Epigastric pain occurs with an empty stomach. Pain in both instances is typically relieved by antacids or milk.

Complications

Complications include hemorrhage and perforation of the stomach or duodenum, with resulting peritonitis and obstruction of the pylorus or gastric outlet.

Diagnostic Tests

Endoscopy/biopsy	To establish presence of ulcer and determine whether malignancy is present
Upper gastrointestinal series	May reveal ulcers overlooked on endoscopy
Gastric analysis	Increased output with duodenal ulcer; decreased or normal output with gastric ulcer
Carbon 13 urea breath test	Low levels of 13C in exhaled breath indicative of *H. pylori* infection

Therapeutic Management

Surgery	Gastrectomy, gastroduodenostomy, gastrojejunostomy to remove gastrin-producing portion of stomach in intractable cases with complications; fundic vagotomy with chronic duodenal ulcer disease
Drugs	Bismuth preparations in combination with antiinfective drugs (triple combination of amoxicillin, tetracycline and metronidazole) for eradication of *H. pylori* bacteria
	Histamine receptor antagonists to block gastric acid output; antacids to reduce pain; cytoprotectives (Sucralfate) to form a protective coating in the base of the ulcer; omeprazole (Prilosec) to inhibit gastric secretion; prostaglandins are in clinical trials for treatment associated with NSAID use
General	Avoidance of alcohol and tobacco products; avoidance of coffee (caffeinated and decaffeinated), and foods that cause epigastric distress; avoidance of NSAIDs; stress reduction therapy

U

urinary incontinence

Involuntary leakage of urine classified as instability incontinence (sudden urgent desire or detrusor contraction with immediate loss of control), stress incontinence (loss of control on sneezing, coughing, laughing, or straining), overflow incontinence (chronic overdistention of the bladder that results in dribbling), and constant incontinence (continual dribbling)

Etiology and incidence: Causes vary by classification. Instability incontinence is often associated with disease or trauma of the central nervous system (e.g., cerebrovascular accident, parkinsonism, brain tumors, spinal cord injury); bladder outlet obstructions (e.g., benign prostatic hypertrophy); bladder infection; and bladder irritation (e.g., calculi). Other causes of instability incontinence remain unclear and are labeled idiopathic.

Stress incontinence is caused by pelvic relaxation or sphincter incompetence. Pelvic relaxation leads to cystocele, rectocele, or uterine prolapse. Factors associated with relaxation include multiparity, aging, peripheral neuropathy and diabetes, and extensive pelvic surgery. Sphincter incompetence is associated with any factor that loosens the sphincter, such as prostate or urinary surgery or repeat urinary procedures, infection, or a reduction in mucus production.

The two causes of overflow incontinence are deficient detrusor function and bladder outlet obstruction. Detrusor function deficiency is associated with cauda equina syndrome, multiple sclerosis, tabes dorsalis, polio, herpes zoster, pelvic trauma, diabetes, and chronic overdistention. Obstruction is associated with inflammation, benign prostatic hypertrophy, adenocarcinoma of the bladder, urethral stricture in men, and urethral distortion in women.

Constant incontinence results from bypassing of normal sphincter function and failure of the bladder to store urine. Associated factors include urinary fistula, epispadias, urethral ectopia, and surgical conduit.

It is estimated that at least 10 million individuals are incontinent in the United States. It occurs in both men and women and increases with age. As many as 50% of institutionalized elderly individuals experience chronic incontinence, and 20% more experience intermittent incontinence.

Pathophysiology: Stress incontinence occurs when the bladder pressure exceeds the urethral closure pressure. This happens when the urethra is no longer maintained in a normal anatomical position, resulting in inefficient transmission of abdominal pressures along the length of the urethra. Thus sudden increases in abdominal pressure from coughing, sneezing, or straining are not transmitted to the sphincter, and it does not tighten.

Instability incontinence is a result of inappropriate contraction of the detrusor muscle, with loss of coordination between bladder contraction and sphincter release. Overflow incontinence results when the detrusor muscle fails to contract, allowing the bladder to overfill, or when the bladder outlet is blocked and urine backs up and overfills the bladder. Constant incontinence occurs when the sphincter is bypassed and the urine has a new channel or outlet, such as a fistula between the bladder or urethra and the vagina or rectum.

Clinical Manifestations

Involuntary loss of urine is the chief manifestation, and the pattern varies by classification of the incontinence. Abdominal distention and associated urinary tract infection (UTI) are also seen in overflow incontinence.

Complications

Complications include UTI, kidney infection, and skin breakdown.

Diagnostic Tests

Voiding cystourethrography	*Stress incontinence:* Pelvic descent below the pubis, urethral excursion, and leakage of contrast material with straining
	Instability: Detrusor-sphincter dyssynergia
	Overflow: Large bladder capacity, possible blockage
	Constant: Leakage of contrast material through fistula or ectopic structure

U

Urodynamic testing

Stress: Normal capacity, sensations, and compliance; stable detrusor; normal electromyographic (EMG) explosive flow with low-pressure detrusor contraction

Instability: Decreased functional capacity, early sensation, normal compliance, unstable detrusor, normal EMG findings

Overflow with detrusor dysfunction: Enlarged capacity, delayed sensations, abnormal compliance, poor stream, residuals

Overflow with obstruction: Normal or enlarged capacity, normal or delayed sensation, normal or impaired compliance, high detrusor contraction with poor flow

Constant: Impaired urine storage with fistulous tract

Therapeutic Management

Surgery

Stress: Vesicourethral suspension to elevate anatomical structures; artificial urinary sphincter, pubovaginal sling to replace or reinforce damaged sphincter

Instability: Urinary diversions (e.g., suprapubic catheter or ileoconduit)

Overflow: Transurethral resection of enlarged prostate; urethrotomy to correct urethral stricture; reconstruction of bladder or urethra

Constant: Repair or removal of ectopic structures or fistulas

Drugs

Autonomic drugs, spasmolytics to increase detrusor contractility and tone; autonomic drugs to increase or decrease bladder neck tone; muscle relaxants to diminish external muscle tone; antispasmodics to decrease detrusor spasms

General	*Stress:* Kegel exercises to strengthen periurethral muscles; electrostimulation therapy to strengthen pelvic muscles; use of pessary to alter anatomic structure
	Instability: Use of a timed voiding schedule; manipulation of fluid intake, avoiding large-volume intake periods; intermittent catheterization
	Overflow: Double voiding techniques; intermittent catheterization; voiding schedules with manual Credé's maneuvers
Prevention	Good skin care with use of barrier cream to protect irritated skin from moisture and urine; use of incontinence aids (e.g., pads, adult diapers, odor elimination substances, external catheters); referral to continence support group; instruction in intermittent catheterization techniques if needed

U

urinary tract infection, lower (cystitis, urethritis)

An inflammation of the bladder or urethra

Etiology and incidence: Most urinary tract infections (UTIs) are caused by gram-negative bacteria, with *Escherichia coli* accounting for approximately 80% of cases. *Staphylococcus, Klebsiella, Proteus, Enterobacter,* and mixed infections account for most of the remainder. The infecting bacteria are commonly normal intestinal and fecal flora. Interference in urine flow dynamics puts an individual at greater risk; such individuals include those with underlying obstructions (strictures, calculi, tumors, prostatic hypertrophy), neurogenic bladder, vesicoure-thral reflux, and diabetes or renal disease; those who are sexually active or pregnant; and those undergoing medical or surgical procedures, such as catheterization or cystoscopy. Women are 10 times more likely than men to have a UTI because of anatomical construction of the female urinary system. Approximately 20% of women have at least one UTI in their lifetime.

Pathophysiology: Bacteria invade the urethra and bladder when the body defense mechanisms (regular emptying and cleansing of the lower urinary tract by urine flow) are diminished or absent. When urine flow is impeded or interrupted, or when the bladder is retaining residual and static urine, bacteria can ascend the urethra, move into the bladder mucosa, colonize, and multiply; this sets up the inflammatory process.

Clinical Manifestations

Common signs and symptoms include pain; burning on urination; frequency; urgency; nocturia; cloudy, foul-smelling urine; and hematuria.

Complications

The major complications include damage and scarring to the lining of the urinary tract with recurrent infection and ascension of the infection to the kidneys, causing pyelonephritis.

Diagnostic Tests

The diagnosis is based on the history and on urine culture and sensitivity to identify the causative agent and its response to a given antiinfective drug. A complete urodynamic workup may be done in those with recurrent infection or to identify factors contributing to infection, such as obstruction, stricture, and detrusor abnormality.

Therapeutic Management

Surgery	Revision of abnormalities in urinary tract
Drugs	Antiinfective drugs (3- to 5-day course) to kill pathogen and render urine sterile
General	Repeat of culture about 14 days after start of drug therapy; increased fluid intake; evaluation of voiding patterns, sexual practices, and hygiene practices for possible preventive measures

U

urticaria (hives, angioedema)

An allergic reaction that produces wheals and erythema in the dermis (urticaria) or the dermis and subcutaneous structures (angioedema)

Etiology and incidence: Urticaria and angioedema are caused by an allergen that provokes a histamine-mediated response. Common allergens include drugs, insect bites or stings, miscellaneous environmental factors, desensitization injections, and foods (eggs, shellfish, nuts, fruits). About 20% of the general population have an episode of urticaria or angioedema at some time. The peak incidence occurs in adults in their 30s.

Pathophysiology: A histamine response to the allergen induces vascular changes that result in vasodilation and itching. The histamine-mediated response also causes endothelial cells to contract, which allows vascular cells to leak between the cells via the vessel wall to form a wheal on the skin. A more diffuse swelling of subcutaneous tissue accompanies angioedema and is typically seen in the hands, feet, face, and upper airways.

Clinical Manifestations

Pruritus is followed by the appearance of wheals 1 to 5 cm in diameter. These may enlarge and develop a clear center and erythematous border. The wheals may occur singly or in crops. They may appear in one site, remain for several hours, disappear, and then appear in a new site. Angioedema involves edema of subcutaneous tissues, and the wheals are typically larger. Respiratory distress and stridor may be seen if the upper airways are affected.

Complications

Skin abrasion and secondary infection may occur as a result of scratching, and laryngeal edema may occur in angioedema.

Diagnostic Tests

The diagnosis is made by history and clinical examination. Other tests are unnecessary unless the urticaria is chronic and has no apparent allergic cause. In such cases underlying disease (e.g., lymphoma, polycythemia, systemic lupus erythematosus) should be ruled out.

Therapeutic Management

Surgery	None
Drugs	Antihistamines to control histamine response; epinephrine subcutaneously for wheals and by mist for pharyngeal or laryngeal edema
General	Identification and elimination of allergens; avoidance of scratching

uterine bleeding, dysfunctional

Abnormal uterine bleeding not associated with recognizable organic lesion, inflammation, ovulation, or pregnancy

Etiology and incidence: Dysfunctional uterine bleeding (DUB) usually results from an imbalance in the hormone-endometrium relationship when unopposed estrogen stimulates the endometrium. Variation in uterine bleeding is the most frequently encountered health problem in women, and DUB is the most common cause of abnormal bleeding. It is typically seen at the extremes of reproductive life, with 50% of cases occurring after 45 years of age and another 20% in adolescence.

Pathophysiology: Unopposed estrogen stimulation often causes an endometrial hyperplasia. The endometrium becomes thickened by the estrogen, and when it can no longer be maintained, the endometrial lining sloughs in an incomplete and irregular pattern, leading to irregular, prolonged bleeding.

Risk Factors

History of anovulation from factors such as polycystic ovaries, follicle depletion
Obesity
Nulliparity
Use of exogenous estrogen

Clinical Manifestations

The main sign is painless, irregular, heavy vaginal bleeding. Midcycle spotting, oligomenorrhea, or amenorrhea may also be present.

Complications

Anemia is the chief complication.

Diagnostic Tests

The diagnosis is made on the basis of the history, a pelvic examination, and laparoscopy to rule out other bleeding disorders or underlying disorders. Endometrial biopsy can rule out cancer.

Therapeutic Management

Surgery	Laser ablation or fulguration of endometriosis; presacral neurectomy when bleeding is severe and does not respond to other treatment
Drugs	Combination contraceptives to control bleeding
General	Iron replacement or packed cells for associated anemia; adequate nutritional intake; cessation of extreme exercise schedules

U

uterine cancer (endometrial cancer)

Adenocarcinomas account for most endometrial cancer; other tumor types include adenoacanthoma and clear cell and squamous cell tumors.

Etiology and incidence: The cause of endometrial cancer has not yet been firmly established although a long-established link exists to hormone-related disorders. However, approximately 40% of endometrial tumors appear to be autonomous with no known etiology.

Endometrial cancer is the most common of the gynecological malignancies, with more than 35,000 new cases a year in the United States. This cancer is found primarily in postmenopausal women between ages 55 and 60. The women tend to be from highly industrialized countries, and the prevalence has increased sharply.

Pathophysiology: Cells begin as endometrial hyperplasia and change to cancer cells, beginning in the fundus of the uterus and spreading to the entire endometrium. The tumor may then extend down the endocervical canal and involve the cervix and vagina. It also spreads through the uterine wall to the abdominal cavity and adjacent structures and metastasizes to the pelvic and paraaortic lymph nodes, lungs, bone, and brain.

Risk Factors

Infertility

Early onset of menarche (before age 12), late onset of menopause (after age 52)

Nulliparity

Use of unopposed estrogen

Extended periods of anovulation

Morbid obesity

History of hyperplasia of the endometrium, diabetes, hypertension or gallbladder disease

History of breast or ovarian cancer

History of pelvic radiation

Familial history of the disease

Clinical Manifestations

The only significant clinical sign of endometrial cancer is inappropriate uterine bleeding. Approximately one third of postmenopausal women who experience such bleeding have endometrial cancer.

Complications

Advanced disease leads to complications such as bowel obstruction, ascites, and respiratory distress, and the prognosis is poor. Prognosis with early detection is excellent, with a greater than 85% 5-year survival rate.

Diagnostic Tests

A Pap smear is helpful but undependable, because 30% to 40% of smears yield false-negative results. Malignant cells on endometrial biopsy and fractional curettage yield a definitive diagnosis.

Therapeutic Management

Surgery	Hysterectomy
Drugs	Chemotherapy for recurrent lesions and metastasis; hormones (e.g., progestin) to treat metastasis or precancerous lesions
General	Radiation as adjunct to surgery and palliation; counseling for body image and sexual functioning alterations

U

uterine fibroids (leiomyomas, myomas)

Well-circumscribed, nonencapsulated, benign tumors of the uterus

Etiology and incidence: The etiology is unclear, but the tumors tend to grow in response to excess estrogen levels and shrink after menopause. Steroid hormones including estrogen and progestin, and several growth factors have been implicated as causal factors. Fibroids are the most common pelvic neoplasm and occur in about 30% of women over age 35. In the United States, the incidence is higher in black women.

Pathophysiology: Fibroids arise from the smooth muscle within the myometrium of the uterus. They may be seen on the intramural, submucosal, or subserous surface of the uterus or in the musculature of the cervix or broad ligaments. Tumor growth often outstrips blood supply, causing the tumor to hyalinize. The hyaline tissue may then liquefy and calcify.

Clinical Manifestations

Most fibroids are asymptomatic. Symptoms, when present, include prolonged or excessive menstrual bleeding with no change in the cycle interval. Pain, heaviness, or tenderness in the lower abdomen may also be present.

Complications

Complications include hemorrhage, torsion and infection, adhesions, and infertility.

Diagnostic Tests

The diagnosis is made on abdominal and bimanual palpation of the uterus. Ultrasound scanning may be used to distinguish endometriosis from leiomyomas. Cytological tests and cervical biopsy may be done to rule out cancer.

Therapeutic Management

Surgery	Hysteroscopic or laparoscopic myomectomy to preserve uterus for childbearing; hysterectomy to control heavy bleeding
Drugs	None
General	Ongoing gynecological examinations to monitor fibroids

U

vaginitis

Infection and inflammation of the vaginal mucosa, often extending secondarily to the vulva

Etiology and incidence: Most vaginitis is caused by bacteria *(Gardnerella vaginalis)*, protozoa *(Trichomonas vaginalis)*, fungi *(Candida sp.)*, and viruses (human papilloma virus). Other causes include mechanical forces (foreign objects, vigorous wiping or cleansing); irritating chemicals found in douches, deodorant sprays, laundry soaps, and bathwater additives; and sensitivity to spermicides, latex condoms, or latex diaphragms. Tight, nonporous, nonabsorbent underclothing or poor hygiene may foster growth of pathogens. Women exposed to diethylstilbestrol have vaginal adenosis, which can produce a vaginal discharge. Older, postmenopausal women have vaginal and mucosal atrophy, which predisposes them to infection. Vaginitis is a common disorder, and most women can expect to have at least one vaginal infection in their lifetime. All age groups are at risk. In the reproductive years, vaginitis is usually caused by infection. Premenopausal and postmenopausal causes are more often mechanical or chemical.

Pathophysiology: The causative agent sets up an infective or inflammatory process. Infective agents invade and grow in the warm, moist environment of the vagina, often aided by a decrease in acidity and an increase in the sugar level in the vaginal environment. Infective agents are often introduced by sexual activity *(Trichomonas* and *Gardnerella spp.*, papilloma virus) or are part of the normal vaginal flora *(Candida albicans)* that overgrow when vaginal conditions are ripe, such as before menstruation and during pregnancy. Inflammation occurs with mechanical, chemical, or other sensitivity, often with an inadequately lubricated or a thinning vaginal mucosa.

Clinical Manifestations

The most common presenting sign is vaginal discharge with or without itching, odor, or pain.

Mechanical/chemical	Increase in clear, viscous discharge; burning; redness; itching

Bacterial *(Gardnerella)*	Malodorous (fishy) white or grayish yellow discharge; itching, burning
Protozoan *(Trichomonas)*	Copious frothy, bubbly, greenish gray, malodorous discharge; itching, dyspareunia, vulvar edema, hyperemia
Viral (papilloma virus)	Vaginal or vulvar warts, discharge, odor, spotty bleeding
Fungal *(C. albicans)*	Thick, cheesy white or yellow discharge; intense itching, redness
Atrophic	Itching, dryness, redness, irritation, burning, spotty bleeding

Complications

Chronic vulvitis and vulvar dystrophies can occur and are most often seen after menopause.

Diagnostic Tests

The diagnosis is made by the history, a pelvic examination, and a wet smear or culture to identify the causative organisms. Pap smears and biopsies may be done to rule out cancer.

Therapeutic Management

Surgery	Laser therapy, cautery, or cryotherapy to remove warts
Drugs	Topical or systemic antiinfective drugs to treat specific causative pathogen; treatment of sex partner for pathogens; estrogen supplements with atrophic vaginitis
General	Removal of chemical, mechanical, or other sources of irritation; instruction about vaginal hygiene; use of loose underwear that breathes (e.g., cotton)

V

varicose veins

Elongated, dilated, and tortuous superficial veins usually seen in the lower extremities

Etiology and incidence: Varicose veins occur because of incompetency in the valves of the vein, which permits a backflow of blood in the dependent position. The cause of valvular incompetence is unclear, but predisposing factors include familial tendency, inherent weakness in the vein walls, congenital arteriovenous fistulas, pregnancy, ascites, occupations requiring prolonged standing, and vein trauma or occlusion. Varicosities increase with age and are more common in women than in men.

Pathophysiology: The pathophysiology is unclear. The prevailing hypothesis for pathogenesis is that valve failure occurs at the perforator veins in the lower leg, resulting in high-pressure flow and increased volume in the superficial veins during muscular contraction. Over time the superficial veins become dilated, separating the valve cusps and reversing blood flow in the affected veins.

Clinical Manifestations

Initially the vein may be palpated but invisible, and the individual may have a feeling of heaviness in the legs that gets worse at night and in hot weather. Aching also occurs after prolonged standing or walking, during menses, or when fatigued. Over time, the veins can be seen as dilated, purplish, and ropelike.

Complications

Venous insufficiency and venous stasis ulcers are the two most common complications.

Diagnostic Tests

The initial diagnosis is made on inspection and palpation and is checked by a manual compression test that reveals a palpable impulse. A Trendelenburg test can help pinpoint the location of incompetent valves. Plethysmography and ultrasound scans can be used to detect venous backflow.

Therapeutic Management

Surgery	Stripping and ligation of severely affected veins
Drugs	Sclerotherapy (injection of chemicals designed to sclerose the affected veins is sometimes used instead of surgery)
General	Lightweight compression hosiery and avoidance of prolonged standing for mild varicosities; custom-fitted, surgical weight antiembolism stockings with graduated pressure (high at ankle, lower at top) with prescribed exercise program to promote circulation and prevent stasis with moderate varicosities

V

Zollinger-Ellison syndrome

A syndrome marked by hypergastrinemia, gastric acid hypersecretion, and recurrent peptic ulcerations

Etiology and incidence: The cause of Zollinger-Ellison syndrome (ZES) is excessive gastrin secretion produced by a non-beta islet cell tumor in the pancreas. Most individuals have several tumors, and about 50% of the tumors are malignant. ZES often occurs in conjunction with other endocrine abnormalities, particularly of the parathyroids. About 60% of cases are seen in men. The peak incidence occurs between 30 and 50 years of age.

Pathophysiology: The high serum gastrin levels continuously stimulate HCl hypersecretion from parietal cells. This constant production of HCl overcomes the duodenum's ability to neutralize the acid, and peptic ulcers result. The gastrin stimulates intestinal motility and increases secretion of water and electrolytes, and the HCl increases peristalsis. Intestinal pH and fat breakdown are diminished, which inactivates pancreatic lipase and interferes with absorption of a variety of substances in the intestine. Gastrin also stimulates intrinsic factor secretion and interferes with vitamin B_{12} absorption.

Clinical Manifestations

The major manifestations stem from peptic ulcer formation and include burning epigastric pain (relieved by food) and coffee grounds or bloody emesis. Diarrhea, steatorrhea, foul-smelling stools, anorexia, and weight loss may also be present.

Complications

The mortality rate is high because of malignant metastasis to the liver, spleen, bone, skin, and peritoneum and perforation and hemorrhage of the peptic ulcers.

Diagnostic Tests

Serum gastrin	Elevated to 500 pg/ml or higher
Endoscopy/x-ray	To detect ulcers
Provocative tests	Serum gastrin rises within 30 minutes of injection of secretin and calcium
Arteriography	To locate pancreatic tumors

Therapeutic Management

Surgery	Resection of tumor possible in 20% of cases; total gastrectomy when ulcers are not responding to medication
Drugs	Histamine-receptor antagonists to reduce gastric acid output; antacids to relieve pain; anticholinergics in refractory cases; omeprazole or octreotide to reduce gastric acid when resistance to histamine-receptor antagonists develops; chemotherapy to treat malignant tumors; vitamin B_{12} injections, iron and calcium supplements
General	Fluid replacement with diarrhea; monitoring for dehydration and electrolyte imbalance; support to aid in adaptation

Z

bibliography

Acute prostatitis, *Healthway Online,* 1999 (www.healthanswers.com).

American Cancer Society: *Cancer facts and figures,* Atlanta, 1998, The Society.

American Psychological Association: *Diagnostic and statistical manual of mental disorders,* ed 4, Washington, DC, 1994, The Association.

American Psychological Association: *Diagnostic and statistical manual of mental disorders,* ed 5, Washington, DC, 1998, The Association.

American Society of Internal Medicine, Guidelines for thyroid disease screening, *Ann Int Med,* 1998.

Ayers M, Bruno A, Langford R: *Community-based nursing care: making the transition,* St Louis, 1999, Mosby.

Beare PG, Myers JL: *Adult health nursing,* ed 3, St Louis, 1998, Mosby.

Beck AT, Weissman A, Lester D, Trexler L: The measurement of pessimism: the hopelessness scale. *J Consult Clin Psych,* 42:861-865, 1974.

Belcher A: *Blood disorders,* St Louis, 1993, Mosby.

Berkow R, Fletcher A: *The Merck manual,* ed 16, Rahway, NJ, 1992, Merck.

Bourdon KH, Rae DS, Locke BZ, Narrow WE, Regier DA: Estimating the prevalence of mental disorders in U.S. adults from the epidemiological catchment area survey, Public Health Report, 107(6):663-668, November, 1992.

Centers for Disease Control and Prevention: *Trichinosis,* Division of Parasitic Diseases, National Center for Infectious Diseases, September 15, 1998. (www.cdc.gov/ncidod/dpd/trichino.htm).

Centers for Disease Control and Prevention: Disease Information, Ebola Virus: *Fact sheet,* 1999, Public Domain.

Centers for Disease Control and Prevention: Ebola Virus Hemorrhagic Fever: *General information,* 1999, Public Domain.

Centers of Disease Control and Prevention: Hantavirus: General information, 1999, Public Domain.

Dains, JE, Baumann LC, Scheibel P: *Advanced health assessment and clinical diagnosis in primary care,* ed 1, 1998, St Louis, Mosby.

DeLisa JA, Gans BM: *Rehabilitation medicine: principles and practice,* ed 2, Philadelphia, 1993, JB Lippincott.

DeVita VT, Hellman S, Rosenberg SA: *Cancer: principles and practice of oncology,* ed 5, Philadelphia, 1997, Lippincott-Raven.

Ferri F: Practical guide to the care of the medical patient, ed 4, St Louis, 1998, Mosby.

Fraunfelder FT, Roy FN, editors: Current occular therapy, Philadelphia, 1995, WB Saunders.

Gillenwater J et al: *Adult and pediatric urology,* ed 3, St Louis, 1996, Mosby.

Griffith H: *Complete guide to symptoms, illness and surgery,* New York, 1995, Putnam Berkley Group.

Haber J, Krainovich-Miller B, Leach McMahon A, Price-Hoskins P: *Comprehensive psychiatric nursing,* ed 5, St Louis, 1997, Mosby.

Histoplasmosis: Protecting workers at risk. US Department of Health and Human Services, NIOSH Publication No 97-146, September, 1997.

Hoff LA: *People in crisis: understanding and helping,* ed 3, Menlo Park, Calif, 1989, Addison-Wesley.

Houston Chronicle: *Researchers identify third Alzheimer's gene,* July 23, 1998, section A, p 6.

Houston Chronicle: *Most Parkinson's cases caused by chemicals, not genes,* January 27, 1999, section A, p 8.

Houston Chronicle: *Transplant-patient drug may boost cancer growth,* February 11, 1999, section A, p 20.

Houston Chronicle: *Laser device expected to be OK'd by FDA,* February 19, 1999, section A, p 1, 8.

Houston Chronicle: *You can do something about the flu,* February 20, 1999, section D, p 7.

Houston Chronicle: *Advances treat cancer of the cervix,* February 23, 1999, section A, p 1, 6.

Johnson RT, Griffin JH: *Current therapy in neurologic disease,* ed 4, St Louis, 1993, Mosby.

Kelley KJ, Walsh-Kelly CM: Latex allergy: A patient and health care system emergency. *J Emer Nursing,* Vol 24, No 6, December 1998, pp 539-545.

Knowledge and use of folic acid by women of childbearing age - U.S., 1995, *MMWR* 44(38):716-718, 1995.

Kolb LC: The psychobiology of PTSD: perspectives and reflections on the past, present, and future, *J Traum Stress,* 6(3), 293-307, 1993.

Latex allergy: a prevention guide, US Department of Health and Human Services, NIOSH Publication No. 98-113, February 25, 1999.

Lewis S, Collier I, and Heitkemper M: Medical-surgical nursing, ed 4, St Louis, 1996, Mosby.

National Cancer Institute, PDQ, Treatment, *Oropharyngeal Cancer,* 1999.

National Center on Elder Abuse, US Department of Health and Human Services, Administration on Aging, Washington, DC, 1999.

National Center for Health Statistics: Expectation of life by age, race and sex: United States, final 1995 and preliminary 1996, *Monthly Vital Stat Rep,* 46(1) supp 2, 1997.

National Center for Health Statistics: Report of final mortality statistics 1995, *Monthly Vital Stat Rep,* 45(11) supp 2, 1997.

National Center for Health Statistics: Report of final mortality statistics 1996, *Monthly Vital Stat Rep,* 46(1) supp 1, 2, 1998.

National Center for Health Statistics: Report of final mortality statistics 1996, *National Vital Stat Rep,* 47(9), 1998.

National Center for Health Statistics: Report of morbidity statistics 1994, *Vital and Health Stat Rep,* 10(193), 1996.

National Center for Health Statistics: Report of morbidity statistics 1995, *Vital and Health Stat Rep,* 10(199), 1997.

National Center for Health Statistics, Faststats, February 1999, (www.cdc.gov/nchswww/fastats.htm), (www.cdc.gov/nchswww/fastats.htm).

National Clearinghouse on Child Abuse and Neglect Information, Washington, DC, 1999.

National Institutes of Health, National Cancer Institute, Cancer Statistics Branch, Bethesda, MD, 1998.

1997 National Household Survey on Drug Abuse, Office of Applied Studies, Substance Abuse and Mental Health Services Administration, US Department of Health and Human Services, Rockville, Md., 1997 (www.samsha.gov).

Quan L: Diagnosis and treatment of croup, *Am Fam Physician,* 46(3):747-755, 1992.

Rosenthal M, Griffith ER, Bond MR, Miller JD: *Rehabilitation of the adult and child with traumatic brain injury,* ed 2, Philadelphia, 1990, FA Davis.

Schaerf T: New understanding and treatment for epilepsy, part II, *Health Week,* February 1, 1999.

Skidmore-Roth L: *Mosby's 1999 nursing drug reference,* St Louis, 1999, Mosby.

Stein JH: *Internal medicine,* ed 4, St Louis, 1994, Mosby.

Technical Information Bulletin: Potential for allergy to natural rubber latex gloves and other latex products. US House Subcommittee on Oversight and Investigation Hearing of the Education and Workforce Committee, US Newswire release, March 25, 1999.

The American Nurse: It's your health, *Am Nurse,* January/February 1999, 10.

Thelan LA, Davie JK, Urden LD, Lough ME: *Critical care nursing: diagnosis and management,* St Louis, 1994, Mosby.

Thomassian BA: Diabetes and cardiovascular disease: getting to the heart of the matter, *Health Week,* February 15, 1999.

Thompson JM, McFarland GK, Hirsch JE, Tucker SM: *Mosby's clinical nursing,* ed 4, St Louis, 1997, Mosby.

Tonsillitis, Healthway Online, 1999 (www.healthanswers.com).

US Department of Health and Human Services/Office of DPHP: *Clinician's handbook of preventive services,* Washington, DC, 1994, US Government Printing Office.

US Department of Health and Human Services: *Child maltreatment, 1996: reports from the states to the National Child Abuse and Neglect Data System,* Washington, DC, 1998, US Government Printing Office.

Wong DL, Perry SE: *Maternal child nursing care,* St Louis, 1998, Mosby.

index

A

HEV	Hepatitis E virus
Hgb	Hemoglobin
HIV	Human immunodeficiency virus
HIV-1	Human immunodeficiency virus type 1
HIV-2	Human immunodeficiency virus type 2
HLA	Human leukocyte antigen
HPA	Hypothalmic-pituitary adrenal axis
HPRC	Hereditary papillary renal carcinoma
HPS	Hantavirus pulmonary syndrome
HPV	Human papilloma virus
HRC	Hereditary renal carcinoma
HSV-1	Herpes simplex virus type 1
HSV-2	Herpes simplex virus type 2
HTN	Hypertension
IBS	Irritable bowel syndrome
ICP	Intracranial pressure
IDDM	Insulin-dependent diabetes mellitus
IF	Intrinsic factor
IgA	Immunoglobin A
IgE	Immunoglobin E
IgG	Immunoglobin G
IgM	Immunoglobin M
I&O	Intake and output
IOP	Intraocular pressure
IPV	Inactivated poliomyelitis vaccine
ITP	Idiopathic thrombocytopenia purpura
IUD	Intrauterine device
IV	Intravenous
IVP	Intravenous pyelogram
KS	Kaposi's sarcoma
LDH	Lactate dehydrogenase
LDMD	Landouzy-Dejerine muscular dystrophy
LMMD	Leyden-Mobius muscular dystrophy
LV	Left ventricular
MG	Myasthenia gravis
MI	Myocardial infarction
MRI	Magnetic resonance imaging
MS	Multiple sclerosis
MVC	Methotrexate, vinblastine, and cisplatin
NCEA	National Center of Elder Abuse
NHSDA	National Household Survey on Drug Abuse
NIDDM	Non–insulin-dependent diabetes mellitus
NIOSH	National Institute for Occupational Safety